KAPLAN

Kaplan National Physical Therapy Exam

Bethany Chapman, MPT
Mary Fratianni, PT

This publication is designed to provide accurate and authoritative information in regard to the subject matter covered. It is sold with the understanding that the publisher is not engaged in rendering legal, accounting, or other professional service. If legal advice or other expert assistance is required, the services of a competent professional should be sought.

Published by Kaplan Publishing, a division of Kaplan, Inc.
1 Liberty Plaza, 24th Floor
New York, NY 10006

Printed in the United States of America

10 9 8 7 6 5 4 3 2 1

ISBN-13: 978-1-4277-9739-1

AVAILABLE ONLINE

kaptest.com/publishing

The material in this book is up-to-date at the time of publication. However, the test maker may have instituted changes in the tests or test registration process after this book was published. Be sure to carefully read the materials you receive when you register for the test.

If there are any important late-breaking developments, or corrections to the Kaplan test preparation materials in this book, we will post that information online at kaptest.com/publishing.

kaplansurveys.com/books

What did you think of this book? We'd love to hear your comments and suggestions. We invite you to fill out our online survey form at kaplansurveys.com/books. Your feedback is extremely helpful as we continue to develop high-quality resources to meet your needs.

Contents

We would like to thank our families: Rob, Tommy and Taylor Chapman, Joe, and Salvatore and Giuseppe Fratianni for all of the support they gave to us in our endeavor. They allowed us to spend hours at a time away from home or at the computer compiling information for this book. We love you and appreciate you!

—Beth and Mary

PART I

The NPTE

1 Introduction to the NPTE

Congratulations! You have made it through your physical therapy education and you are now ready to prepare to take your National Physical Therapy Examination (NPTE). Once you pass, you will be on your way to becoming a licensed physical therapist!

The practice of physical therapy continues to be one of the fastest-growing professions in the nation. As an expanding field, physical therapy continues to change on a yearly basis. What once was a certificate program has now developed into a doctorate-level degree. As the number of applicants and graduates of physical therapy programs continues to increase, the pressure is on to continue to send knowledgeable and qualified professionals into the world of health care.

Several organizations are in place to see that knowledgeable and qualified professionals are those gaining licensure. The American Physical Therapy Association (APTA) sets the standards of practice for physical therapy with their publication, *The Guide to Physical Therapy Practice*. They also give normative information for the establishment and requirements of accredited physical therapy education programs.

The Federation of State Boards of Physical Therapy (FSBPT) uses the information from the guide along with current best-evidence practices to develop an examination that will measure the knowledge and skills required of an entry-level physical therapist. This is the NPTE. According to the FSBPT, "The focus is on the clinical application of knowledge, concepts, and principles necessary for the provision of safe and effective patient care."

HOW TO USE THIS BOOK

You have already done a good part of the preparation for your licensing examination by making the grade in physical therapy school. This book can further benefit you in three ways:

1. **Develop** test-taking strategies specific for taking the NPTE. Kaplan's vast experience and knowledge of test-taking strategies can help perfect your ability to recognize the best answer and choose it correctly. You can create a confidence in your test-taking skills that may even go beyond this examination to further specialty areas.

2. **Review** a professionally prepared, relevant summary of material that will be on the examination. The review portion of this book is based on recommendations listed on www.fsbpt.org that break down the areas of physical therapy and identify how much emphasis the examination places on each area. We have formatted the chapters to follow some of the objectives set out for review for the examination.

3. **Utilize** the two full-length practice tests, so you may test your abilities before you dive into the real thing.

ROLES OF THE PHYSICAL THERAPIST

The Guide to Physical Therapist Practice by the American Physical Therapy Association describes the roles and responsibilities of the physical therapy profession. According to the guide, the role of a physical therapist is to use his or her background knowledge and education to cooperatively work toward "optimal physical function." By doing this, the physical therapist promotes healthy living and strives to improve the patients' quality of life in a variety of care settings. Physical therapists evaluate and develop intervention plans for patients in home care, acute care, and long-term care settings. They do the same in more clinically based outpatient settings and work environments. In some regions, the term *physiotherapist* is interchangeable with *physical therapist.*

Physical therapists work closely with other allied health professionals and are part of an overall health-care team. Referrals can come from such team members as physicians, chiropractors, dentists, orthodontists, physician assistants, and nurse practitioners. Physical therapists will also work closely with nurses, medical assistants, and other therapy services such as speech, occupational, and recreational. Within many physical therapy departments there will also be interaction with and supervision of physical therapy assistants, physical therapy aides, and reception staff. In addition to working with health-care teams, physical therapists interact with legal and insurance representatives.

The Guide to Physical Therapy Practice further defines the preferred practice patterns that will provide the public with the best care and best outcomes possible. The American Physical Therapy Organization has developed a Code of Ethics for physical therapists. It has also described the physical therapist's scope of practice to define exactly what services and roles are unique to the practice. It urges government agencies to ensure that these services are provided only by licensed physical therapists. Knowing all of the roles is the responsibility of any individual who wants to become a licensed physical therapist.

APPLYING FOR THE NPTE

The NPTE is administered at over 300 sites in all 50 states. Once you have completed the required course work, you are ready to begin the application process to take your licensing examination. You will need to fill out the paperwork given to you by your educational facility. Along with that paperwork you will send the examination fee, which is currently $350 to FSBPT and $65 to Prometric (the test-administrating organization).

That information and fees are sent to the following address:

FSBPT
124 West Street South, 3rd Floor
Alexandria, VA 22314
Phone: (703) 299-3100
Fax: (703) 299-3110
www.fsbpt.org

Once they receive it, the FSBPT will process your paperwork and send you a letter authorizing you to sit for the exam. You then have 60 days from the date of your authorization letter to schedule and take the examination. The phone number for your desired testing center should be on the authorization to test (ATT) letter, or can be found by accessing the website www.prometric.com. Be sure to take into consideration any time needed for travel when scheduling your exam time and date. You must arrive at the test site 30 minutes prior to your test-taking time. At that time you will need to show two forms of identification that exactly match the name on the ATT letter. For added security, you will also be thumb-printed and photographed at the Prometric site.

OVERVIEW OF THE TEST

Before learning some key test-taking strategies, it is important for you to be familiar with the test content, structure, and scoring. This test may be different than any other you have taken in your physical therapy schooling, and knowing these differences can put you at ease when you sit down to actually take the examination.

Once you enter the testing area, you will find an optional tutorial on taking computerized exams. Reading it will take approximately five to ten minutes, and this does not count against your total exam time. It may be beneficial if you are not familiar with computerized exams. An erasable note board is provided as scratch paper during the exam.

Once each section is completed, you *cannot* backtrack to change or review any answers. Within each section, you are able to flag questions to which you would like to return, whether you have answered them or not. You may also still move back through your questions even if you have not flagged them.

Four hours is the allotted time for completing the examination. There is a 15-minute scheduled break after completion of the second section. The physical therapy examination also has three unscheduled breaks that you may take between any of the five sections of the test. During these unscheduled breaks, the exam clock continues to run.

There is no penalty for incorrect answers, so it is most beneficial to answer all of the questions.

Test Content

The FSBPT gives a blueprint of information that will be covered on the multiple-choice NPTE. This is the breakdown of the test content outline directly from the website www.fsbpt.org, effective March 2008:

Content Topic	% on Exam	Number of Items on Exam
Clinical Application of Foundational Sciences	14.5%	29
Examination	13%	26
Foundations for Evaluation, Differential Diagnosis, & Prognosis	23.5%	47
Interventions	18.5%	37

Content Topic	% on Exam	Number of Items on Exam
Equipment & Devices; Therapeutic Modalities	11%	• 10 (equipment & devices) • 12 (therapeutic modalities)
Safety & Professional Roles; Teaching/Learning; Research	19.5%	• 15 (safety & professional roles) • 11 (teaching & learning) • 13 (research)

The "meat" of the exam is the first four topics listed on the table above. Each of those four can be further broken down as follows:

Content Topic	% on Exam	Number of Items on Exam
Cardiovascular & Pulmonary Systems	11.5%	23
Musculoskeletal System	18%	36
Neuromuscular & Nervous Systems	17%	34
Integumentary System	7%	14
Other systems (includes metabolic & endocrine, gastrointestinal, genitourinary, multisystem)	16%	32

Test Scoring

There are 250 questions on the examination. Fifty of those questions will not be scored but are considered pretest questions and are used to determine if they may be appropriate to be test questions in the future. The 250 questions are divided into five sections of 50 questions each.

Your final score is based on the number of correct answers. The scoring scale converts the raw score out of 200 questions to a scaled score of up to 800. This is done because the exam offers several variations in level of difficulty. The scaled scores allow for more difficult exams to require fewer correct answers than easier exams. The nationally adopted scaled score that you need in order to pass the NPTE is 600. Once the exam is scored by the FSBPT, the results are forwarded to the appropriate licensing authority in your state. The final letter awarding licensure will come from that source. If the test taker's score on the first attempt is below passing level, the FSBPT allows up to three retakes within a 12-month period of time from the initial test date. Some licensing jurisdictions have more restrictive allowances.

Take Control of the Test

2

In 2006, the first-time passing rate for physical therapists taking the NPTE was 86 percent. The fact that the passing rate is not 100 percent means it's not an easy test that just anyone can pass. Suddenly you are about to sit for what you are anticipating may be one of the harder tests you have ever taken.

TEST-TAKING STRATEGIES

Along with preparation for your examination, this Kaplan review book provides some key test-taking strategies that will help you on your way to physical therapy licensure.

1. Relax!

Having the right mind-set plays a large part in how well people do on a test. Those who are nervous about the exam and are hesitant to make guesses often fare much worse than students who have an aggressive, confident attitude.

2. Pace yourself

One of the most nerve-wracking aspects of the NPTE is the fact that it is timed, so learning to pace yourself throughout the exam will help ease your worries about not finishing in time. The better you pace yourself in each section, the more time you will have to go back at the end of that section and review your answers, if you choose to. Poor pacing causes students to spend too much time on some questions—to the point where they run out of time before getting a chance at every question.

3. Use the two-pass system

Using the two-pass system is one way to help your pacing on a test. The key idea is that you don't simply start with question 1 and trudge onward from there. Instead, you start at the beginning but make a first pass through the test to answer immediately all the questions that are easy for you. If you encounter a tough question, you spend only a small amount of time on it and then move on in search of the questions that are easier for you. On the computerized NPTE, you are able to flag questions so you can go back to recheck or answer them before completing each section. This way you don't get bogged down on a tough question when you could be earning points answering later questions that you *do* know. Your second pass takes you back through the section to answer all the tougher questions that you passed over the first time. In the second pass you should be able to spend a little more time on them, and this extra time might help you with the answers. Even if you don't reach an answer, you might be able to use techniques (such as the process of elimination) to cross out some answer choices and then take a guess.

4. Use the process of elimination

On every multiple-choice test you ever take, the answer is given to you. The only difficulty resides in the fact that the correct answer is hidden among incorrect choices. Even so, the multiple-choice format means you don't have to pluck the answer out of the air. Instead, you can eliminate the answer choices you know are incorrect; and when only one choice remains, that must be the correct answer.

5. Identify patterns and trends

The key word here is the *standardized* in standardized testing. Being standardized means that tests do not change greatly from year to year. Sure, the questions will not be identical, and different topics will be covered from one year's test to the next, but there will also be a lot of overlap from year to year. That's the nature of standardized testing: if the test changed wildly each time it came out, it would be useless as a tool for comparison. Because of this, certain patterns can be uncovered about any standardized test. Learning about these trends and patterns can help students who are taking the test for the first time. These standards are given to us by the FSBPT.

6. Don't go into the test "cold"

People who take a test "cold" or have not thought about the test itself or the information it contains have more problems than those who take the time to learn about the test beforehand. In the end, factors like these mark the difference between people who are good test takers and those who struggle even when they know the material.

7. Beware of the "not" or "except"

Read each question carefully and look for the negative words to indicate you are looking for the one answer that does not fit with the others. In this case, you don't want to quickly identify the one correct answer; instead, you're looking for the one incorrect answer. Often the negative words are in capital letters or bolded.

8. An educated guess is better than not answering

The FSBPT scores only the questions that you have answered correctly. There are no deductions for answering incorrectly—plain and simple, you just don't get the score for those. It is in your best interest to make sure you have answered every question and left none blank.

9. Take a break!

The fact that you are taking a four-hour exam on a computer necessitates some break time. Take advantage of the scheduled break after section 2, and step away from the computer if you are comfortable. If you feel you don't want to lose your rhythm, at least take the opportunity to look away from the computer screen at times to give your eyes (and your brain) a rest!

Kaplan's Strategies for Multiple-Choice Questions

The NPTE is made up of 250 multiple-choice questions, so that means you need to prepare to answer only one type of question. You don't have to worry about searching your memory for answers to essay or fill-in questions. But there are some things to keep in mind that will help you move efficiently through the array of questions. These ideas, as part of the two-pass system, can keep you from getting frustrated with working though each question in numerical order and will keep you on pace!

Short question stem

In test-speak, the portion of a problem that comes before the answer choices is typically called the question stem. Stem length varies on the NPTE from short, memory recall–type questions to longer descriptions of hypothetical situations. Either way, while you're reading the question stem, time is ticking away. The longer the stem, the more time it takes you to read it. If you're a fast reader, this might not be very much time. If you read at a more methodical rate, you might try saving the wordier problems for your second pass.

Choose topics you like

On your first pass through the section, answer all the questions that deal with concepts you like and about which you are knowledgeable. When you come to a question that is on a subject that's not one of your strong points, skip it and return to it later. The overarching goal is to use your available time to answer correctly as many questions as possible. This also prevents you from being frustrated with more difficult questions or spending too much time on any one question initially.

You don't have much time to ponder every tough question, so trusting your instincts can help keep you from getting bogged down and wasting time on a problem. You might not get every educated guess correct; but again, getting a perfect score is not the goal. The goal is to get a good score to pass the exam and to survive hard questions by going with your gut feelings.

Strategies That Don't Work

The following are strategies that will NOT work favorably when taking the NPTE:

1. Cramming

Trying to memorize and cram into your brain hundreds of facts about anatomy, physiology, and physical therapy patient care, all in the week before the examination, will not pay off. The examination evaluates your ability to apply concepts that you have already learned.

2. Selecting the response that is a different length compared to the other choices

One answer choice being longer or shorter than the others does not necessarily mean it is the right one! Think of your answer carefully and then look for it in the response choices.

3. When in doubt, choosing C

There is no correlation between choice C and the correct answer!

CRITICAL APPLICATION AND CRITICAL THINKING

On some of the examination questions you may have no inkling of what the correct answer should be. In that case, turn to the following key idea: critical thinking. By using critical thinking skills, you can distinguish which answers are NOT correct to better guide you toward the correct choice. The NPTE is given to reward good physical therapists with a license to practice physical therapy. It covers the fundamental science behind physical therapy and clinical application skills. Since this is a multiple-choice test, there have to be three incorrect answer choices around every single right answer. So if you don't know how to answer a question, look at the answer choices and think about what a good physical therapist would do or know. This may lead you to identify some poor answer choices that can be eliminated.

Many times examination questions are going to be in clinical application format. In that case, what could be a more simplified recall or recognition question has been hidden in a more complicated wording. For example, let's look at this sample question:

> A 63-year-old woman underwent a total knee replacement seven days ago. She enters your outpatient clinic for evaluation and treatment. Upon inspection, you notice that she has extreme redness and edema in her knee, and the knee feels very warm to the touch. What question should you ask next to confirm or deny your suspicion?
>
> (A) No questions; this is a normal presentation.
>
> (B) "Have you experienced any fever?"
>
> (C) "Do you have any allergies?"
>
> (D) "Do you have any cold sensitivity?"

We know that the reason for the redness, edema, and warmth of the knee is infection, but that is not one of the answer choices. We can then look further into the answer choices and find that a fever is another indication of a systemic problem such as infection. Instead of simple recall or recognition, the answer requires clinical application and more critical thinking skills. How do we further interview the patient to get to the final answer? Choice B is the best answer to confirm that the patient is presenting with signs and symptoms of infection.

LEARNING METHODS

As you prepare to enter the review portion of this book, it is important that you take a moment to figure out what kind of learner you are. Do you think predominantly in images or in words? By knowing which type you are, you will be better able to study in a way that fits your learning style, and you will answer questions with less frustration. Read the following sentence:

A physical therapist walks into a room and finds the patient with her arm in a sling.

As you read the sentence, were you hearing yourself read the words? Or did you visualize a physical therapist walking into a room and seeing a patient wearing a sling? If you heard the words, you more likely think in words. If you visualized the scenario, you more likely think in images or pictures.

If you are more of a visual person, you might find yourself thinking that you have more difficulty remembering what you've read in a book than what you see firsthand. You may also feel that you have to read things repeatedly to get the concept down. For some people, imagery is necessary to understand ideas and concepts. If this is true for you, you need to visualize the information that you are learning. As you prepare for the NPTE, try to form mental images of anatomy, patient care, and clinical principles. For example, if you're reviewing information about manual muscle testing but you have difficulty remembering positions and grades, it would be helpful for you to have done manual muscle testing on a subject.

If that isn't possible, find a picture of the application in question. As you read each topic in the review, think of a photo of patient care to visualize. If you can visualize the theory that you are trying to learn, it will make recall and understanding of concepts much easier for you. It is also important that you visualize test questions. As you read the question and possible answer choices, picture yourself going through each suggested action. This will increase the likelihood of your selecting correct answer choices.

As with any test, make sure you have given yourself plenty of sleep both the night before and two nights before your exam date. Make sure you are not hungry at test time—eat well that morning or noon, depending on the time of day of your exam. Wear comfortable clothing in layers so you can adjust your temperature based on the temperature of the room. On the day of your exam, be sure you bring your reading glasses or contact lenses, if needed.

Finally, *use all the strategies discussed in this chapter* when you are taking the practice exams. Trying out the strategies there will help you become comfortable with them, and you should then be able to put them to good use on the real exam. These test-specific strategies—combined with the factual and clinical information covered in your educational preparation and in this book's review—are the one-two punch to help you succeed on this specific test.

Of course, all the strategies in the world can't save you if you don't know anything about the art and science of physical therapy. The next section of the book will help you review the primary concepts and facts that you can expect to encounter on the NPTE.

PART II

Diagnostic Test

Diagnostic Test

HOW TO USE THIS DIAGNOSTIC TEST

The purpose of this test is to help identify possible weak areas that are in need of some extra attention before attempting the full 250-point practice examinations. Our recommendation is that this test be taken before any review is done. As the exam is corrected you will see that each question is subdivided into the system or chapter it comes from. There are a total of 5 questions for each chapter in this book. Once you have corrected your exam, you will be able to see which chapters may be strong or weak for you.

For example, if you only score 1 of 5 in the Cardiac, Pulmonary, and Vascular Systems questions, you may need to spend a little more time reviewing that chapter in this book and referring to your own school's cardiopulmonary textbook. If you score 5 of 5 in the Musculoskeletal System Questions, you may be able to just do a quick overview of the chapter before moving onto the full practice examination. There is no need to time yourself for this exam as it is purely to aid in identifying weak areas, but do try to do the exam without any other assistance. Good luck!

Diagnostic Test

1. A physical therapist is reviewing the medication list of a patient recently referred for physical therapy. The patient has an intermittent history of corticosteroid prescription. What potentially harmful side effect can this drug have on this patient?

   (A) Osteoporosis

   (B) Arterial insufficiency

   (C) Diabetes mellitus

   (D) Diabetes insipidus

2. What is one normal age-related change related to the integumentary system?

   (A) Increased inflammatory response

   (B) Increased risk of injury

   (C) Increased subcutaneous fat

   (D) Decreased pain perception

3. What treatment technique focuses on diagonal and spiral movement patterns to simulate and encourage normal movement patterns?

   (A) Neurodevelopmental techniques

   (B) Proprioceptive neuromuscular facilitation

   (C) Brunnstrom's techniques

   (D) Rood's techniques

4. A physical therapist is working with a patient in their home after a 10-day hospital stay. The patient has a history of angina. On the physical therapist's second visit, the patient complains of chest pain. What medicine can the patient take (if prescribed and available to treat this acute angina?

   (A) Albuterol

   (B) Lasix (furosemide)

   (C) Nitroglycerine

   (D) Levaquin (levofloxacin)

5. A physical therapist is reviewing the chart of a patient he is to see in the hospital. He reads in the recent labs that the patient has had bithermal caloric testing. What pathology is this type of test looking for?

   (A) Vascular insufficiency

   (B) Vestibular dysfunction

   (C) Nerve conduction dysfunction

   (D) Muscular wasting

6. A patient has had frostbite to his right foot and a right leg fracture. He is seeing a physical therapist for increased mobility. The patient asks the physical therapist what happened in his right foot due to the cold exposure to cause damage. How should the physical therapist respond?

   (A) Ice crystals formed in your tissues due to the extreme cold.

   (B) The blood vessels in your skin constricted, causing your injury.

   (C) Your injury was caused by increased metabolism due to the extreme cold.

   (D) Your blood froze and that is what caused your injury.

7. A patient is performing pelvic floor muscle strengthening for urinary incontinence. While practicing her long holds the physical therapist notices her abdomen rises and her face turns red. What is the physical therapist observing?

(A) Normal accessory motion
(B) Excessive posterior pelvic tilt
(C) Valsalva maneuver
(D) Excessive rectus abdominis firing

8. A physical therapist is treating a patient who has a diagnosis of cerebrovascular accident. The patient's symptoms include homonymous hemianopsia, thalamic pain syndrome, and memory deficits, and contralateral sensory loss. What vessel does the physical therapist suspect was affected in this stroke?

(A) Anterior Cerebral Artery
(B) Middle Cerebral Artery
(C) Vertebrobasilar Artery
(D) Posterior Cerebral Artery

9. A physical therapy student reads a research article about prenatal factors and the development of cerebral palsy. One prenatal factor is found to have no relationship to the development of cerebral palsy. The correlation coefficient for this factor is closest to what number?

(A) –1.0
(B) 0
(C) +1.0
(D) 10

10. A patient is burned in an explosion. The areas of his skin that are burned are bilateral arms (anterior and posterior), anterior thorax, and his head. What percentage of his skin is burned?

(A) 36%
(B) 45%
(C) 54%
(D) 63%

11. A physical therapist is manual muscle testing the supraspinatus muscle of the shoulder. Which position best isolates this muscle to test strength?

(A) Arm neutral, elbow flexed 90°, resist external rotation
(B) Arm neutral, elbow flexed 90°, resist internal rotation
(C) Arm abducted 90°, horizontally adducted 30°, internally rotated, resist shoulder flexion
(D) Arm abducted 90°, horizontally adducted 30°, externally rotated, resist shoulder flexion

12. A physical therapist is observing a tech performing ultrasound on a patient. As she talks to the patient, she pauses briefly from continuously moving the sound head. What adverse effect can this have on the tissues?

(A) Unstable cavitation
(B) Cyclic vasoconstriction and vasodilation
(C) Refraction
(D) Reflection

13. A physical therapist is treating a patient in a nursing home. The patient has sustained a recent right hip fracture and has Alzheimer's dementia. She complains of pain with all mobility and requires maximum assistance for transfers. She has subsequently developed a pressure ulcer on her left heel. The left heel has a large blister that affects the epidermis and the dermis. What stage of pressure ulcer is this?

(A) Stage I
(B) Stage II
(C) Stage III
(D) Stage IV

14. A physical therapist is treating a patient who has low back pain. The patient is morbidly obese and has a sedentary lifestyle. The physical therapist plans to help the patient to begin a cardiovascular and strengthening exercise program. The physical therapist emphasizes to the patient the danger of a sedentary lifestyle and the patient's susceptibility to chronic medical problems due to her lack of exercise and obesity. The physical therapist helps the patient to eliminate or minimize any barriers to exercise. Finally, the physical therapist encourages the patient that she is able to incorporate exercise in her daily routine. The physical therapist has educated the patient on the threat, the susceptibility to medical problems, the benefits and barriers of exercise, and finally tried to encourage the patient's self efficacy. What health behavior change model has the physical therapist used to assist this patient?

(A) Health Belief Model
(B) Attribution Model
(C) Transtheoretical Model
(D) Social Cognitive Model

15. A patient is being treated by a physical therapist following a right transfemoral amputation. The physical therapist is working with the patient on gait training using a prosthesis. The physical therapist notes that the patient walks with a lateral trunk bend. What is the most likely source of muscular weakness in this patient based on this gait deviation?

(A) Illiopsoas weakness
(B) Gluteus medius weakness
(C) Erector spinae weakness
(D) Quadriceps weakness

16. What is a normal age-related change seen in the respiratory system?

(A) Increased tidal volume (TV)
(B) Decreased tidal volume (TV)
(C) Decreased residual volume (RV)
(D) Decreased vital capacity

17. A physical therapist is documenting her initial evaluation of a patient. Which of the following includes all of the necessary components of a long-term goal?

(A) The patient will have full range of motion in four weeks.
(B) The patient will report 0/10 pain in her left elbow
(C) The patient will be able to use her arm to dress herself without pain in four weeks.
(D) The patient will be able demonstrate active motion from 0-140°.

18. A physical therapist is treating a patient who has a wound with moderate exudate. The wound is deep. There is a sparse amount of necrotic tissue, which the physical therapist plans to debride with tweezers. What dressing would be appropriate for this wound?

(A) Alginate
(B) Hydrogel
(C) Transparent dressing
(D) Non-adherent dressing

19. A patient has been referred for physical therapy for evaluation of leg pain. He describes his symptoms as worse with walking and standing and better if he squats down to the floor. Which of the following differential diagnoses could account for this presentation?

(A) Spinal stenosis
(B) Intermittent claudication
(C) Disc herniation
(D) Sciatica

20. A patient is hospitalized with active tuberculosis and is on airborne precautions. Which of the following is one of the proper guidelines for prevention of disease transmission?

(A) A private room with positive airflow
(B) Limited transport of patient using a surgical mask on the patient
(C) Anyone else in contact with a patient must wear a surgical mask
(D) The patient may be co-horted with others on airborne precautions

21. Which one of the following is not an electrolyte ion?
    (A) Sodium
    (B) Magnesium
    (C) Phosphorus
    (D) Chloride

22. A patient is jogging at a moderate to high intensity on the treadmill when he begins to note some GI distress. Which one of the following is an atypical response of the gastrointestinal system during strenuous or long duration exercise?
    (A) Constipation
    (B) Heartburn
    (C) Abdominal cramping
    (D) Fecal urgency

23. A physical therapist receives a referral for a patient in an acute care setting. From the chart review, the physical therapist knows that the patient has had a traumatic brain injury due to a motor vehicle accident. The physical therapist tests the patient's response of eye opening, motor response and verbal response. What measure is the physical therapist using?
    (A) Modified Ashworth Scale
    (B) Rancho Los Amigos Cognitive Functioning Scale
    (C) Glasgow Coma Scale
    (D) Brunnstrom's Stages of Recoverye

24. A physical therapist is performing a positional release technique to the cervical spine. Her goal in treatment is to open the affected foramen to decrease nerve root irritation. Which position is best for that goal?
    (A) Forward flexion, contralateral sidebending, ipsilateral rotation
    (B) Forward flexion, contralateral sidebending, contralateral rotation
    (C) Forward flexion, ipsilateral sidebending, ipsilateral rotation
    (D) Forward flexion, ipsilateral sidebending, contralateral rotation

25. A physical therapist is documenting a patient's progress toward goals written on the initial assessment. Which portion of the note should this be written under?
    (A) Subjective
    (B) Objective
    (C) Assessment
    (D) Plan

26. A physical therapist is working in a skilled nursing facility with a patient who has had a left hip fracture and subsequent pneumonia. The patient's medical history also includes hypertension, right hip fracture, and transient ischemic attack. During aerobic training on a stationary bike, the physical therapist looks for abnormal responses to exercise. What is one example of an abnormal response to exercise?
    (A) Sweating
    (B) Flushing
    (C) Slight dyspnea
    (D) Decreased heart rate

27. A patient presents to physical therapy with a diagnosis of Guillain – Barré Syndrome. GBS is lower motor neuron disorder. What sign or symptom does the physical therapist expect to find upon evaluation?
    (A) Flaccid paralysis
    (B) Hyperreflexia
    (C) Positive Babinski's reflex
    (D) Clonus

28. A physical therapist is instructing a patient in the use of ice for pain and edema management at home. Her instructions are to use ice for 10-20 minutes once an hour as needed. Which of the following describes the hunting response that may occur after longer than 30 minutes of ice application?
    (A) Frostbite to the superficial structures
    (B) Increased muscle spasm and guarding
    (C) Hypersensitivity to cold
    (D) Cyclic vasodilation

29. A patient in a senior living center has been seen for strengthening exercise and gait training following a prolonged hospitalization. She is taking a diuretic, multi-vitamins and pain medicine as needed. Over the last several days, she has had increased fatigue, leg cramping and palpitations. What other condition may this patient have?

(A) Deep vein thrombosis
(B) Hypokalemia
(C) Delayed onset muscle soreness
(D) Hyperglycemia

30. A physical therapist working in a phase II Cardiac Rehab program provides an educational class entitled "Exercise: What you need to know". The physical therapist includes information on exercising in high heat and humidity. She advises the patients to avoid strenuous exercises in temperatures above 75 degrees or humidity greater than 70%. She also explains why exercise in these conditions may be dangerous. What is one side effect of exercise in high heat and humidity that puts a cardiac patient at risk?

(A) Decreased heart rate
(B) Blood vessels of the skin constrict
(C) Increased heart rate
(D) Delayed onset of angina

31. Which one of the following modalities would be an example of a conversion mechanism of heat exchange?

(A) Hot packs
(B) Ultrasound
(C) Fluidotherapy
(D) Warm whirlpool

32. A physical therapist is evaluating a patient with a known endocrine dysfunction. During muscle testing, which joint would be expected to show a painless weakness?

(A) Hip
(B) Elbow
(C) Ankle
(D) Wrist

33. A physical therapist is recommending aquatic therapy for a patient who does not seem to be progressing well with land-based therapy. What happens to the weight distribution when exercising in the water?

(A) As the level of the water increases, the amount of weightbearing increases
(B) As the temperature of the water increases, the amount of weightbearing increases
(C) As the level of the water increases, the amount of weightbearing decreases
(D) As the temperature of the water increases, the amount of weightbearing decreases

34. A hospitalized patient is referred to physical therapy. His medical diagnosis is cystic fibrosis. The physical therapist assesses the patient and determines that he has increased thickness of mucous and an ineffective cough. The physical therapy treatment plan includes airway clearance techniques. Which of these treatment techniques is considered an airway clearance technique?

(A) Chest wall stretching
(B) Positioning for dyspnea relief
(C) Inspiratory muscle training
(D) Active cycle of breathing

35. A patient is using electrical stimulation as a means of strengthening his VMO following a meniscus repair and 6 weeks of non-weightbearing ambulation. At what amplitude should the stimulation be set to achieve this goal?

(A) Below sensory
(B) Sensory
(C) Motor
(D) Noxious

Diagnostic Test Answers and Explanations

1. A

Prolonged use of corticosteroid medication can lead to bone loss and increased risk of osteoporosis.
(Goodman/Pathology, page 954)
Musculoskeletal System

2. D

As we age, the skin demonstrates impaired pain perception, decreased inflammatory response, decreased risk of injury, decreased subcutaneous fat, and decreased vascularity.
(Goodman/Pathology, page 268)
Integumentary System

3. B

Proprioceptive neuromuscular facilitation focuses on diagonal and spiral movement patterns including D1 and D2. The treatment includes contract-relax, rhythmic initiation, and hold-relax.
(Dobkin, page 221)
Nervous System

4. B

Nitroglycerine is given sublingually to treat acute angina.
(Mosby, page 742)
Cardiac, Vascular, and Pulmonary Systems

5. B

Bithermal caloric testing assesses vestibular function and it's possible contribution to a patient's symptoms of dizziness or loss of balance.
(Goodman/Pathology, page 1133)
Nervous System

6. A

Ice crystals form when tissue is colder than -2°C and extracellular spaces expand. This causes local cold injury. With normal exposure to cold temperature, vasoconstriction occurs. Exposure to extreme cold can cause impaired metabolism.
(Goodman/Pathology, page 300)
Integumentary System

7. C

The Valsalva maneuver is a breath holding technique also known as "bearing down". The abdomen rises, and the patient holds their breath causing the face to turn red. This is an incorrect performance of the desired exercise.
(Stephenson, page 67)
Other Systems

8. D

Posterior Cerebral Artery Syndrome produces visual defects, contralateral sensory loss, memory deficits, and thalamic pain syndrome. It can also cause coma and decerebrate rigidity.
(Goodman/Pathology, pages 1057-1058)
Nervous System

9. B

A correlation coefficient of zero indicates no relationship between variables. A value of –1.0 indicates a strong negative relationship, while a value of 10 indicates a strong positive relationship.
(Hicks page 77).
Research and Evidence Based Practice

10. B

Using the Rule of Nines, this patient has burned 45% of the surface area of his body.
(Hanumadass, page 8).
Integumentary System

11. C

The supraspinatus is best isolated with the arm abducted 90°, horizontally adducted 30°, internally rotated and resisting shoulder flexion in that position.
(Donatelli, page 246)
Musculoskeletal System

12. A

Although not a common problem with proper ultrasound technique, unstable cavitation can occur if the sound head is held in one place too long. This causes the formation and growth of mini gas bubbles under the skin that could rapidly collapse causing tissue damage.
(Behrens, page 63)
Equipment and Devices and Therapeutic Modalities

13. B

A stage II pressure ulcer involves the epidermis, dermis or both. It is superficial and presents as a blister, crater, or abrasion.
(Hanumadass, page 8)
Integumentary System

14. A

The Health Belief Model incorporates threats to health, in particular the severity and susceptibility of the threat, the benefits and barriers to change, and the self-efficacy to change.
(Christiansen, page 422-423)
Teaching and Learning

15. B

Weakness of the gluteus medius can cause lateral trunk bending during ambulation. Also, the prosthesis could be short, misaligned, or positioned in excessive abduction in the socket. Pain along the medial wall can also cause this gait deviation.
(Seymour 230)
Equipment and Devices and Therapeutic Modalities

16. D

The correct answer is decreased vital capacity. Residual volume increases with increased age. Tidal volume remains the same with age. Also, the strength of the diaphragm and other respiratory muscles decreases.
(Lewis, page 34)
Cardiac, Vascular, and Pulmonary Systems

17. C

A long-term goal must indicate a functional improvement that is measurable and observable. It should also be set within a specific time frame, such as 4 weeks or upon discharge.
(Duesterhaus, page 6)
Safety, Protection & Professional Roles

18. A

Alginate is used to absorb exudate in draining wounds. Alginates should not be used in dry wounds. Hydrogels are used for dry wounds. Transparent dressings are used for superficial, non-exudative wounds. Non-adherent dressings are used for superficial wounds.
(Brown, page 61)
Integumentary System

19. A

Pain caused by spinal stenosis is worsened with any extension position, in this case, standing or walking. Pain is lessened by moving into a flexion position of the spine (i.e. Sitting, squatting or bending at the waist).
(Meadows, page 204)
Musculoskeletal System

20. B

Transport out of a private room should be limited. If it is necessary for tests or procedures, the patient must wear a surgical mask. These patients should be in private rooms with negative airflow and closed doors. Any personnel coming into contact with the patient must wear a specialized, filter mask.
(Goodman/Pathology, page 202)
Safety, Protection & Professional Roles

21. C

Sodium(+), magnesium(+) and chloride(-) are all electrolytes. Phosphorus itself is not an electrolyte, but phosphate ($PO4^{3}$) is an electrolyte.
(Goodman/Pathology, page 107)
Other Systems

22. A

Constipation is more typically associated with bed rest or lack of activity.
(Goodman/Pathology, page 629)
Other Systems

23. C

The Glasgow Coma Scale has subscales of eye opening, motor response and verbal response. A score of 7 or less on this scale indicates a coma.
(Rothstein page 426)
Nervous System

24. B

To maximally open the foramen, the neck should be forward flexed, contralaterally sidebent and contralaterally rotated. Option A would be best for opening of the affected facet joint.
(Behrens, page 111)
Musculoskeletal System

25. C

Progress or lack of progress toward goals is written under the assessment portion of the SOAP note.
(Shamus, page 129)
Safety, Protection & Professional Roles

26. D

Sweating, flushing and slight dyspnea are normal responses to exercise. Cold sweat is an abnormal response. Undue dyspnea is an abnormal response. Decreased heart rate with aerobic exercise is abnormal. Normally, heart rate increases with aerobic exercise. Other abnormal responses to exercise are: Exercise hypertension, systolic hypotension, significant angina, confusion, claudication (severe), and excessive fatigue.
(Hillegass, page 695)
Cardiac, Vascular, and Pulmonary Systems

27. A

Lower motor neuron lesions result in flaccid paralysis, hyporeflexia, muscular atrophy and muscular fasciculations. Upper motor neuron lesions result in spastic paralysis, hyperreflexia, positive Babinski's reflex and clonus.
(Kandel page 245)
Nervous System

28. D

According to the theory of the hunting response, after long periods of cold exposure physiologic response cycles from vasoconstriction to vasodilation.
(Behrens, page48)
Equipment and Devices and Therapeutic Modalities

29. B

Loss of potassium or hypokalemia can occur with the use of diuretics. Signs and symptoms of hypokalemia can include fatigue, muscle cramping, dizziness, palpitations and irregular pulse.
(Goodman/Pathology, page 110)
Other Systems

30. C

During exercise in high heat and humidity, the peripheral vasculature dilates and the heart rate must increase to meet this demand. Dehydration can bring about loss of blood volume that also places increased demands on the heart and vasculature. Angina may occur earlier than in the same intensity of exercise at lower temperatures.
(Hillegrass page 704)
Cardiac, Vascular, and Pulmonary Systems

31. B

Conversion is a change in temperature as energy is transferred from one form to another. Ultrasound converts mechanical energy into heat.
(Behrens, page 39)
Equipment and Devices and Therapeutic Modalities

32. A

Endocrine system disease can be manifested with proximal, painless muscle weakness. Of the options listed, the hip is the most reasonable expected weakness.
(Goodman/Pathology, page 323)
Other Systems

33. C

As the level or height of the water on the individual increases, (i.e. Waist deep vs. neck deep), the amount of weightbearing through the joints decreases. Temperature of the water does not affect weightbearing.
(Behrens, page 83)
Musculoskeletal System

34. D

The active cycle of breathing is a method of teaching the patient to clear secretions and expand the thorax. This technique includes breathing control and is done in postural drainage positions. Other Airway clearance techniques are: postural drainage, percussion, vibration, assisted cough, and manual hyperinflation with suctioning.
(Hillegrass, page 653)
Cardiac, Vascular, and Pulmonary Systems

35. C

In order to achieve the goal of strengthening of the quadriceps, a strong motor or muscle contraction must occur with each bout of stimulation. It is not necessary for it to be noxious to achieve results.
(Michlovitz, page 250)
Equipment and Devices and Therapeutic Modalities

PART III

Physical Therapy Review

3

Cardiac, Vascular, and Pulmonary Systems

The cardiac, vascular, and pulmonary systems affect the body as a whole and as a result, a graduating physical therapy student should be familiar with the basic anatomy of these systems. Physical therapists routinely treat patients whose sole diagnosis is dysfunctions of these systems. However, a patient should not just be an "orthopedic patient" or a "neurological patient," as the organ systems are interrelated and the examination and treatment techniques of other systems can directly affect the cardiovascular and pulmonary systems. Your treatment methodologies must consider the patient as a whole and not just the injury or disability for which they are seeking physical therapy. To fully understand the cardiac, vascular, and pulmonary systems, you must first know the anatomy and physiology, including the heart, lungs, and vasculature. Examination of the cardiovascular and pulmonary systems may be included when you are evaluating a patient whose main medical diagnosis does not include these systems. Comorbidities, age, activity level, and psychology of the patient all play into the success of physical therapy as a treatment intervention. In this chapter you will delve a little further, beyond the basics, into the examination and treatment of these important, interrelated systems.

FOUNDATIONAL SCIENCES AND BACKGROUND

A strong understanding of the basic background and fundamental sciences of the cardiac, vascular, and pulmonary systems is necessary before examination, evaluation, interpretation, and intervention can take place. It is necessary to understand how the heart, lungs, and vasculature work, as well as how these organs are interrelated.

Pulmonary Anatomy and Physiology

The **sternum** is located in the center of the thorax and includes the **manubrium** superiorly, the body centrally, and the **xiphoid process** distally. The costal cartilage connects the sternum with the ribs. Thoracic vertebrae provide support and protection posteriorly. Each rib articulates with two thoracic vertebrae.

Characteristics of ribs

- Twelve pairs of ribs
- True ribs: the first seven ribs are joined to the sternum by the costal cartilage anteriorly, and they articulate with the thoracic vertebrae posteriorly
- False ribs: the last five ribs
- Ribs 8–10: attached to the cartilage of rib 7
- Ribs 11–12: floating ribs that do not articulate with other bones or cartilage anteriorly

Muscular Anatomy and Movement Analysis

The **major muscles of inspiration** are the diaphragm, external intercostals, and internal intercostals. A healthy person utilizes the accessory muscles during exercise. A person with cardiopulmonary disease utilizes these secondary muscles at rest.

Accessory muscles of inspiration

- Sternocleidomastoids
- Scalenes
- Serratus anterior
- Pectoralis major
- Pectoralis minor
- Trapezius
- Erector spinae

Movement of the thorax

The upper ribs move in a pump-handle pattern, which increases the anteroposterior diameter. The lower ribs move in a bucket-handle movement pattern. This movement increases the transverse diameter of the thorax.

Inspiration

Inspiration is an active process involving activation of inspiratory muscles. The **phrenic nerve** innervates the **diaphragm**. The diaphragm separates the thoracic cavity from the abdominal cavity. There are three major openings in the diaphragm: for the aorta, vena cava, and esophagus. Other smaller vessels and nerves traverse through these openings as well. The diaphragm's central tendon is the fixed point. When the diaphragm contracts, the central tendon is pulled inferiorly and the lung volume is increased.

Intercostal muscles are located between the ribs. The **intercostal nerve** innervates the **intercostal muscles**. The **external intercostals** rotate the ribs up and out anteriorly, thus increasing the thoracic volume. **Internal intercostals** are used in expiration but are also used to elevate ribs during inspiration.

Expiration

Expiration is passive and occurs with relaxation of the inspiratory muscles. However, the abdominal muscles and the internal intercostals are contracted during forcible expiration. The abdominals are also important in coughing.

Upper Respiratory System Anatomy

The nose is the beginning of the upper respiratory system. The nasal cavity is separated by the nasal septum. The anterior nasal cavity contains skin and hair that trap inhaled particles. The posterior nasal cavity is lined with mucous membranes that produce mucus and serous secretions that trap bacteria and other particles. The pharynx follows the posterior nasal cavity. The inferior segment of the upper respiratory tract is the larynx. The larynx prevents objects such as food and liquids from entering the trachea.

Lower Respiratory System Anatomy

The **trachea** is a cartilaginous tube that sits posterior to the sternum and divides into the right and left main stem bronchi. The trachea contains cilia that beat in a coordinated manner to push secretions out of the lower respiratory tract into the upper respiratory tract to be swallowed or expectorated.

The trachea splits into **bronchi**. The right main stem bronchus is thicker, shorter, and less horizontal than the left main stem bronchus. The right main stem bronchus then branches into right upper, right middle, and right lower lobe bronchi that serve the corresponding lobes of the right lung. The left main stem bronchus is thinner and longer than the right main stem bronchus. The left main stem bronchus splits into the left upper and left lower lobe bronchi. These bronchi continue to divide and get smaller and more numerous until they reach the terminal bronchioles.

The **bronchioles** divide and terminate in alveoli. Cells within the alveoli produce surfactant, a substance that keeps the alveoli expanded.

Right and left lungs are covered with visceral and parietal **pleurae**. Visceral pleurae cover the lungs. Parietal pleurae line the thoracic cavity. Pleural fluid is found in between these linings and prevents friction.

Fissures separate the lungs into lobes. The right lung contains an oblique fissure that separates the lower lobe from the middle lobe. The horizontal fissure of the right lobe separates the middle lobe from the upper lobe. The left lung contains only one fissure. This oblique fissure separates the upper lobe from the lower lobes. Each lung has an **apex** (superior portion) and a **base** (inferior portion). The apex extends on each side above the medial clavicle.

Pulmonary Physiology

Pulmonary physiology includes ventilation, respiration, diffusion, and perfusion.

Ventilation

Ventilation is the movement of air into and out of lungs. Ventilation is under both involuntary and voluntary control. Respiratory centers in the pons and medulla control involuntary respiration. Under normal conditions, the respiratory center of the upper pons controls respiration. Chemoreceptors, found both in the midbrain and in the carotid bodies, are stimulated by changes in the arterial P_{CO2}. When an increase in P_{CO2} occurs, respiration is increased. The chemoreceptors found in the carotid bodies also respond to decreases in P_{O2}. When P_{O2} decreases, respiration increases.

Ventilation (Ve) is the volume of air moved in and out of the lungs in one minute. Ve is the product of the frequency of breathing (f) and the tidal volume (TV), ($Ve = f \times TV$). **Alveolar ventilation** refers to the place where the exchange of gas occurs, the alveoli. Alveolar ventilation (VA) can be calculated by subtracting the dead-space ventilation from the tidal volume.

Respiration

During inspiration, the volume of the thorax is increased and the alveolar pressure is decreased. With this decreased pressure, there is a pressure gradient between the lungs and the external atmosphere. Thus, air flows from the atmosphere (where there is higher pressure) to the lungs (where the pressure is lower). The opposite is true during expiration.

After inspiration the pressure in the alveoli is greater than the atmospheric pressure, and this causes air to flow out of the lungs. Expiration occurs passively with relaxation of the inspiratory musculature and with the return of the lungs to their original position due to elastic recoil. **Compliance** of the lung refers to the distensibility of the lung during inspiration. Compliance is the change in volume compared to the change in pressure of the lungs.

Alveoli need **surfactant** in order to remain open and compliant. Maintenance of the volume of the lungs depends on the pressure of the lungs and the pressure of the chest wall. Normally, these two pressures are in balance. The chest wall exerts a force outward and the lungs exert a force inward, and the volume of the chest cavity remains relatively constant. Airway resistance is found in both the upper and lower respiratory tracts. Edema, changes in tract diameter, mucus, obstructions, and other factors can increase the resistance to the flow of air through the respiratory tract.

Diffusion

Diffusion is the movement of gases between the alveoli and the capillaries. The movement of oxygen and carbon dioxide follows the concentration gradient from areas of high concentration to areas of lower concentration. Oxygen is found in small amounts dissolved in the blood. Most oxygen is bound to hemoglobin molecules in the blood.

Oxyhemoglobin dissociation curve

The **oxyhemoglobin dissociation curve** shows the relationship between the percentages of oxygen saturation of hemoglobin and the partial pressure of oxygen. The partial pressure of oxygen is the amount of pressure that oxygen exerts on the system, and it is directly related to the concentration of oxygen. Small changes in the saturation of hemoglobin can result in large changes in the partial pressure of oxygen. Clinically, this is measured by a pulse oximeter.

Perfusion

Perfusion is the transportation of dissolved gases between the lungs and the cells in the blood, and it is accomplished by the cardiovascular system. Perfusion of the lungs depends on gravity, cardiac output, and peripheral vascular resistance. The **ventilation/perfusion ratio** is the lung ventilation compared to perfusion of blood to the lungs for gas exchange.

Lung Volumes

- **Tidal volume** (**TV**) is the volume of air normally inhaled and exhaled with each breath.
- **Inspiratory reserve volume** (**IRV**) is the additional volume of air available for inspiration, above normal tidal volume.
- **Expiratory reserve volume** (**ERV**) is the additional volume of air available for expiration, beyond tidal volume.
- **Residual volume** (**RV**) is the amount of air left in the lungs after maximal exhalation.
  - **Inspiratory capacity** (**IC**) = TV + IRV
  - **Functional residual capacity** (**FRC**) = RV + ERV
  - **Vital capacity** (**VC**) = IRV + TV + ERV
- **Total lung capacity** (**TLC**) = RV + ERV + TV + IRV

Apnea

Apnea is the absence of ventilation. **Tachypnea** is defined as increased frequency of breathing accompanied by shallow breath depth. **Cheyne-Stokes apnea** is a pattern of varying depths of respirations with periods of apnea. **Biot's apnea** is a pattern of breathing that includes decreased rate, shallow depth, and irregular rhythm accompanied by periods of apnea. **Orthopnea** is difficulty breathing in the recumbent position.

Cardiac System Anatomy and Physiology

The heart is the main organ of the cardiac branch of the cardiopulmonary system.

Characteristics of the heart

- The heart consists of cardiac muscle.
- The pericardium is the sac that encloses the heart.
- The heart is positioned posterior to the lower sternum, with the bulk of the heart lying to the left.
- Fibrous pericardium is the tough outer surface of the pericardium.
- Serous pericardium is the serous membrane on the inner surface of the heart.
- Pericardial fluid is found between these two pericardial surfaces, and it protects against friction from the beating heart.
- Serous pericardium consists of a parietal layer and a visceral layer (also known as the epicardium).

Heart chambers

The heart is split into right and left halves by a longitudinal septum. The heart contains atria (or upper chambers) and ventricles (or lower chambers). Blood leaves the heart via arteries and enters the heart via veins.

Blood flow through the heart

Blood flows through the heart in a specific path. First, the superior and inferior vena cava collect blood from the systemic circulation and return it to the right atrium. The blood then flows through the tricuspid valve into the right ventricle. The blood then exits the heart through the pulmonary valve into the pulmonary arteries and into the lungs. The blood is oxygenated in the lungs and returns via the pulmonary veins to the left atrium. From the left atrium it travels through the mitral valve into the left ventricle. The blood leaves the heart through the aortic valve and the aorta.

Layers of the heart wall

The heart wall has three distinct layers. The **epicardium** is the outer visceral pericardium. The **myocardium** is the middle layer and consists of the cardiac muscle. The **endocardium** is the lining of the inside of the heart chambers.

Characteristics of heart valves

- The heart valves ensure one-way flow of blood through the heart.
- The tricuspid valve has three cusps.
- The mitral valve has two cusps.

- Chordae tendineae and papillary muscles support the cusps.
- Disorders affecting the valves may cause regurgitation of blood in the wrong direction (i.e., back into the atria).

Cardiac blood flow

The cardiac muscle is supplied with blood by the right and left coronary arteries. The left coronary artery is further divided into the anterior descending artery and the left circumflex artery. Cardiac veins enter the coronary sinus, which opens directly into the right atrium.

Electrical conduction of the heart

Electrical conduction of the heart is under both intrinsic and extrinsic control.

Intrinsically, the SA and AV nodes can generate impulses for heart contraction without other nervous input. Normally, the **SA node** sets the pace for the heart. The impulse begins at the SA node and spreads down the heart through the **AV node**, and then through the **bundle of His**. The bundle of His then branches out into the **right bundle branch** and the **left bundle branch**, which terminate in **Purkinje fibers**. The SA node is found in the right atrium, near the opening of the superior vena cava. The AV node is found in the floor of the right atrium. The bundle of His division is found in the ventricular septum. Intrinsically, the SA node fires at 100 beats per minute (bpm) or more. The AV node fires at 40 to 60 bpm.

Extrinsically, the heart rate is under the control of the autonomic nervous system. The vagus nerve lowers the heart rate and is controlled by the parasympathetic branch of the autonomic nervous system. The upper thoracic nerves quicken the heart rate and are under the control of the sympathetic nervous system.

Heart rate

The normal resting heart rate (HR) is 60 to 100 bpm. An HR of less than 60 bpm is termed **bradycardia**, and an HR of greater than 100 bpm is termed **tachycardia**.

A person's **maximal heart rate** can be estimated by the formula "220 minus age in years," but a physical therapist should be sure to consider the effects of medication and other individual differences as well.

Normally, HR is consistent. If drastic changes are measured during exercise or at rest, this could signal a disease process or medication use. An HR of less than 40 bpm is a contraindication to exercise due to cardiovascular impairment. Normally, HR does increase with exercise. Upper-extremity exercises increase HR and blood pressure (BP) more than lower-extremity exercise. After a heart transplant, the heart is denervated and the patient will have an abnormal HR response.

Cardiac output

Cardiac output (CO) is the amount of blood pumped by the heart in one minute. Normal resting cardiac output is four to six liters per minute (L/min).

Blood pressure

Systolic blood pressure is the maximum pressure of the blood on the walls of the arteries, which typically occurs at the end of the left ventricular contraction. **Diastolic blood pressure** is the least amount of pressure of the blood against the walls of the arteries, which occurs during the cardiac cycle. **Mean arterial pressure (MAP)** is the average pressure during the cardiac cycle. MAP is the product of cardiac output and peripheral vascular resistance (MAP = CO × PVR). BP is measured in millimeters of mercury (mm Hg).

Angina

Angina is defined as chest discomfort caused by cardiac muscle ischemia. The **anginal threshold** is individual to the patient and is the product of heart rate and systolic BP (HR × SBP) at the onset of angina. The anginal threshold is also called the **rate-pressure product. Chronic stable angina** is angina that occurs with increased activity or stress when the patient has chest discomfort at the anginal threshold. Chronic stable angina is relieved by rest or nitroglycerin. This anginal threshold is related linearly with myocardial oxygen demand. **Variant angina** (also known as **Prinzmetal angina**) is related to coronary artery vasospasm and is unrelated to occlusive disease. **Unstable angina** occurs when a patient has angina at rest. Unstable angina is often a precursor to myocardial infarction (MI). Often, patients can improve exercise tolerance and pre-anginal workload but cannot change anginal threshold.

Heart murmurs

There are three types of heart murmurs, differentiated by the cause of the murmur. One type of murmur is due to high flow rates through valves. Another type is caused by blood flow through stenotic or abnormal valves. Finally, murmurs can be caused by abnormal backflow through a valve. Murmurs are described on the basis of their timing in the cardiac cycle, intensity, quality, pitch, location, and radiation.

Vascular System Anatomy and Physiology

The vascular system has two divisions: the peripheral circulation and the pulmonary circulation. Both the peripheral and pulmonary circulations start at the heart.

Systemic circulation

Circulation of blood to the body is termed **systemic circulation**. During heart contraction, or systole, blood is ejected from the left ventricle out the aortic valve and into the aorta. The aorta then branches off into arteries. Blood vessels that are closest to the heart are larger and more elastic than those farther from the heart. Arteries branch to form arterioles, which branch to form capillaries. Capillaries then form venules, which pour into veins and then ultimately empty into the vena cava. Veins depend on muscular contraction and pressures to push the flow of blood toward the heart. Veins also contain one-way valves to prevent backflow of blood.

Pulmonary circulation

Circulation of blood from the heart to the lungs is termed **pulmonary circulation**. Pulmonary circulation starts at the right ventricle. With contraction of the heart, the deoxygenated blood in the right ventricle is ejected out the pulmonary valve and into the pulmonary artery. The pulmonary artery is the only artery to carry deoxygenated blood. The pulmonary artery splits into right and left pulmonary arteries, and each of these divides into arteries and arterioles that travel to the lungs. Pulmonary capillaries arise from the arterioles and wrap around the alveoli, where gas exchange occurs. Pulmonary veins then collect the oxygenated blood and return it to the left side of the heart. Pulmonary arteries and capillaries are thinner and wider than systemic arteries. The amount of blood that is contained in the pulmonary circulation is approximately equal to the amount in the systemic circulation, but the resistance and pressure of the pulmonary vessels are much less than in the systemic vessels.

Lymphatic Anatomy and Physiology

The lymphatic system is the body's immune system. The lymphatic system moves fluids and other large molecules into the blood. This system also moves fat-related nutrients from the digestive system into the blood. Lymph is the fluid formed in tissue spaces and is composed of excess interstitial fluid and protein molecules that cannot reenter the capillaries. Lymphatic vessels are the vessels that return the lymph to the circulatory system. Lymph nodes are the nodes along the lymphatic vessels that filter the lymph before it joins the circulation. Major lymph nodes are located in the cervical, submandibular, axillary, inguinal, and popliteal areas. The lymphatic ducts are larger lymphatic vessels that ultimately empty into the two large ducts. These two large ducts are the thoracic duct and the right lymphatic duct. These ducts then empty into the veins of the cervical region. Seventy-five percent of the lymph drains into the thoracic duct. Twenty-five percent of the lymph drains into the right lymphatic duct.

The **thymus** is a lymphatic organ that is larger in childhood and diminishes in size through adulthood. Maturation of T lymphocytes (or T cells) occurs in the thymus. The thymus secretes thymosin, which triggers the maturation of these immunity cells. T cells produce cell-mediated immunity. T cells attach to invading cells and subsequently kill the invading cells.

The **spleen** filters bacteria and other substances out of the blood, destroys old red blood cells, saves iron from the hemoglobin, and can act as a reservoir for blood.

The **tonsils** are composed of lymphatic tissue and provide protection against bacteria. The three types of tonsils are the palatine, pharyngeal, and lingual tonsils.

Lymphatic system physiology

Lymph is formed via three processes. First, excess interstitial fluid that does not re-enter the blood capillaries enters the lymphatic capillaries. Second, larger molecules that may not be able to enter the blood capillaries also enter the lymphatic capillaries. Finally, lipids enter the lymph via lymphatic vessels found in the small intestine. An **antibody** is a compound that is produced by the body to destroy or inactivate an antigen. An **antigen** is a foreign substance in the body that causes formation of antibodies against it.

Pulmonary Pharmacology

There are a variety of pharmaceuticals that are used to treat conditions of the pulmonary system—from acute conditions to chronic conditions, from infections to allergies—and agents to decrease cough and secretions.

Pulmonary Pharmacology

Drug Group	Conditions Treated	Method of Action	Clinical Considerations
Bronchodilators	• Acute bronchospasm	• Bronchodilation	• Dizziness • Hypotension • Tachycardia • Chest pain • Muscle weakness

Decongestants	• Respiratory infections • Common cold • Allergies	• Decrease mucus in upper airways	• Dizziness • Hypertension • Palpitations
Antihistamines	• Allergies	• Decrease congestion and discharge	• Dizziness • Loss of coordination
Antitussives	• Cough	• Suppress cough	• Sedation
Mucokinetics	• Increased secretions of the respiratory tract	• Mobilize and remove secretions	
Antibiotics	• Respiratory bacterial infections	• Varies	• Penicillin allergy

Cardiovascular Pharmacology

Many pharmacologic agents can be used to treat a wide range of problems in the cardiovascular system. Prescription drugs can be used to treat angina pectoris, hypertension, arrhythmias, heart failure, and ischemia.

Drug Group	Conditions Treated	Method of Action	Clinical Considerations
Nitrates	• Angina pectoris • Ischemia	• Smooth-muscle vasodilation	• Headache • Reflex tachycardia • Hypotension, place patient in seated position
Beta-blockers	• Hypertension • Angina pectoris • Ischemia • Arrhythmias	• Decrease HR • Decrease contractility • Decrease CO • Decrease BP	• Decreased HR response to exercise
Calcium channel blockers	• Ischemia • Arrhythmias • Hypertension • Heart failure	• Decrease coronary artery contractions	• Orthostatic hypotension
Antiplatelet agents	• Prophylaxis to thrombus	• Prevent thrombus formation	
Anticoagulants	• Prophylaxis to blood clots	• Prevent blood clot formation	• Bleeds easily
Diuretics	• Heart failure • Arrhythmias • Hypertension	• Decrease blood volume	
Positive inotropes	• Heart failure	• Increase cardiac contractility or cardiac output	• Digitalis toxicity
Vasodilators	• Heart failure • Hypertension	• Reduce afterload or preload	• Orthostatic hypotension
Angiotensin-converting enzyme inhibitors	• Heart failure • Hypertension	• Decrease preload	
Sodium channel blockers	• Arrhythmias	• Prolong refractory period	

Physiology and Environmental Factors

Environmental factors such as air temperature, humidity, altitude, water temperature and depth, and buoyancy affect the physiology of the cardiovascular and pulmonary systems. Properties of water include temperature, depth, and buoyancy.

Air temperature

During exercise, the working muscles produce heat. To maintain homeostasis of body temperature, heat must be lost via other mechanisms. These mechanisms include evaporation of sweat and loss of water vapor through the respiratory tract. The cardiovascular system's responses to increased ambient temperature include: decreased stroke volume, vasodilation of skin, increased heart rate, and vasoconstriction of the viscera.

Responses to cold ambient environment

- Constriction of peripheral blood vessels in order to shunt warm blood flow to the body's core
- Skin temperature decreases while the core remains warm.
- Shivering produces heat via muscular contraction.
- Increased loss of water and heat through the respiratory tract that can result in irritation of the tract

Responses to hot ambient environment

- Heat loss is via radiation of our electromagnetic heat waves, conduction to air molecules and other surfaces the skin is touching, convection, and evaporation of sweat.
- As the ambient temperature increases, heat loss via radiation, conduction, and convection decreases and evaporation is the only means of heat loss available.
- Heart rate increases.
- Cardiac output increases.
- Superficial veins and arteries dilate to shunt warm blood to the body shell and away from the core.
- Skin becomes flushed or reddened due to the vasodilation.
- Vast increases in sweating allow for larger heat loss through evaporation.

Exercise in a hot ambient environment

- Stroke volume decreases.
- Heart rate increases for submaximal workloads.
- Cardiac output is decreased at maximal workloads.
- Vasodilation to superficial blood vessels with vasoconstriction to the viscera
- Increased total vascular resistance
- As dehydration occurs, blood volume decreases.
- Increase in anaerobic metabolism, and resultant increased lactic acid buildup
- Risk of dehydration from excess fluid loss
- Obesity increases the risk of heat stroke. Fat is an insulator and decreases heat loss to the ambient air.

Humidity

Evaporation of sweat to the air depends on the relative humidity of the environment. Higher humidity limits the amount of sweat that can be evaporated from the skin.

At high humidity sweat cannot evaporate, which results in the danger of dehydration and overheating. Proper intake of fluids is key to maintaining hydration so that plasma volume can remain and evaporative cooling can take place. Changes in body weight can be used to establish loss of water during exercise. Pre-exercise and post-exercise body weights are compared.

Altitude

At higher altitudes, the frequency of breathing is increased. Also, both submaximal heart rate and cardiac output increase at higher altitudes. At extremely high altitudes, there is a risk of both altitude sickness and high-altitude pulmonary edema (HAPE).

The main difficulty with high altitudes is the lowered partial pressure of the ambient oxygen (P_{O2}). This results in arterial hypoxia. A small decrease in P_{O2} (on the oxyhemoglobin dissociation curve) results in a small decrease in hemoglobin saturation. Larger changes are seen at higher altitudes and with exercise. In a person at higher altitudes, small changes in oxygen saturation of the blood result in difficulties with exercise.

Acclimatization

Acclimatization is the term used to describe improvements in tolerance to altitude hypoxia. Acclimatization is altitude-dependent, meaning that becoming tolerant to medium altitudes means only partial tolerance to higher altitudes. Acclimatization to higher altitudes requires periods of weeks or months.

Altitude sickness

Mountain sickness (or altitude sickness) is the term used to describe the discomfort felt without acclimatization during acute exposure to altitudes above 10,000 feet. Symptoms are headache, dizziness, nausea, vomiting, decreased vision, insomnia, anorexia, and weakness. Exercise is intolerable and contraindicated for those with mountain sickness. With acclimatization, these symptoms start to disappear. **High-altitude pulmonary edema (HAPE)** is a severe form of mountain sickness that is life-threatening. With HAPE, fluid collects in the lungs and brain. Treatment of HAPE consists of the affected person immediately moving to a lower altitude.

Immediate responses to high altitude

- Hyperventilation
- Increased submaximal heart rate
- Increased submaximal cardiac output
- Stroke volume, maximal heart rate, and maximal cardiac output remain the same or are slightly lowered.
- Fluid loss and risk of dehydration
- Decreased aerobic capacity
- Decreased aerobic power

Long-term responses to altitude

- Continued hyperventilation
- Increased submaximal heart rate
- Decreased stroke volume, maximal heart rate, and cardiac output
- Acid-base equilibrium adjustment: arterial CO_2 is decreased, causing the blood pH to rise and become more alkaline; this respiratory alkalosis is minimized by excretion of base through the kidneys.

- Increased amount of hemoglobin
- Increased amount of red blood cells
- Actual oxygen-carrying capacity of blood approaches sea-level capacity due to the increase in hemoglobin and red blood cells, despite the reduced saturation of the hemoglobin.
- Lowered body mass
- Decreased aerobic power

Cardiopulmonary Changes and Increasing Age

There are changes that occur to the cardiopulmonary system with increasing age:

- Decreased maximal exercise capacity (decreased VO_2 max)
- Valves thicken and calcify.
- Increased size and thickness of blood vessels
- Increased resting BP
- Heart rate decreases with exertion.
- Increased thoracic kyphosis; therefore, increased work of breathing
- Decreased oxygen saturation

Neonatal Cardiopulmonary Considerations

There are many cardiopulmonary considerations related to the neonate. Major pulmonary problems include irregular breathing rhythm and a resting respiratory rate of 40 breaths per minute. Cardiac problems include increased and variable heart rate. Examination of the neonate should include evaluation of primitive reflexes, muscle tone, sucking and swallowing, and postures.

Responses to Exercise and Inactivity

The cardiovascular and pulmonary systems are perhaps the systems that show the most significant changes due to exercise or inactivity. These systems show acute changes that can be seen over the course of one treatment session of exercise; thus, responses need to be monitored closely. Inactivity for as little as three days can lead to detrimental effects that the physical therapist needs to consider, both for tolerance to increased activity and for treatment goals. The therapist should also connect vital sign changes to use of medications and to clinical signs and symptoms, such as dyspnea, heart sounds, angina, and EKG changes.

Normal responses to exercise

- Increased heart rate (HR)
- Increased cardiac output (CO)
- Increased systolic blood pressure (SBP)
- Decreased peripheral vascular resistance (PVR)
- Increased ventilation: this occurs first as a result of increased tidal volume (TV), then of increased respiratory rate or frequency (f)
- Increased tidal volume (TV)
- Increased respiratory rate (f)

- Diastolic BP can increase, decrease, or remain unchanged.
- Blood flow is shunted to working muscles and away from organs and nonworking muscles.

Effects of bed rest and immobility

- Decreased VO_2 max
- Decreased functional abilities
- Increased resting heart rate
- Orthostatic hypotension
- Increased risk of atelectasis
- Atrophy of the accessory respiratory muscles

EVALUATION

During the evaluation process it is important for the examiner to make decisions about what tests and measures are appropriate in order to establish a good list of differential diagnoses to treat the injury or disability. Again, during the examination process the patient must be viewed as a whole. In some instances the examination will be done in a hospital room, a home setting, an outpatient setting, or a long- or short-term care facility. In all cases each part of the examination process must be considered, although it is known that some portions of the examination are more appropriate for certain settings—for instance, special tests may be more appropriate in an outpatient setting, mobility evaluation may be more appropriate in a home setting, and a chart review of labs and medical tests may be more appropriate for the acute-care setting.

Pulmonary Evaluation

Evaluation of the pulmonary system includes observation, chest wall analysis, diaphragmatic analysis, mediate percussion, and auscultation, among other tests.

Observation

- Color of skin (pallor, cyanosis)
- Respiratory rate
- Difficulty breathing/dyspnea
- Diaphoresis
- Breathing pattern
- Appearance of digits and extremities
- Digital clubbing (indicates chronic tissue hypoxia)
- Nail beds (cyanosis can indicate cardiopulmonary or other disease)

Cough evaluation

A normal cough consists of a deep inspiration with trunk extension. The glottis closes, and then there is a sharp expiration with trunk flexion to complete the cough.

Chest wall excursion analysis

Various methods of analyzing the chest wall excursion are available for the evaluation of a patient with pulmonary considerations. The chest wall can be observed, palpated, and measured. The chest wall can also be measured using a plethysmography unit.

Observation

In the observation of the chest wall, visualize the upper chest movement (superior to the xiphoid process) and the lower chest wall movement (inferior to the xiphoid process).

Palpation

The therapist should also palpate the chest wall by placing his hands on the upper and lower chest of the patient. Alternatively, the therapist can place his hands on the posterior thorax as well as the anterior thorax.

Measurement

Chest wall excursion can be measured with a tape measure. Measurements should be taken of the thorax circumference at the end of normal expiration, normal inspiration, and maximal inspiration.

Diaphragmatic movement analysis

The diaphragm is the key muscle of respiration; therefore, impairments such as flattening of the diaphragm and no neural input due to trauma or disease will affect breathing.

If the diaphragm is flattened from COPD, the muscle has little room to descend, and thus its efficiency is compromised. When this occurs, accessory muscles are used in breathing, resulting in an abdominal paradoxical breathing pattern. The upper chest expands outward and the abdomen is drawn inward.

In a patient with a spinal cord injury below C5, neural input to the diaphragm is preserved; however, if abdominal muscle neural input is not preserved, the result is an upper-chest paradoxical breathing pattern. The abdomen is drawn outward and the upper chest is drawn inward.

In a patient with a spinal cord injury above the level of C3, the diaphragm receives no neural input and the patient will need mechanical ventilation.

Diaphragmatic movement can be palpated by placing two fingers under the lower ribs, 8 cm from the xiphoid process. Upon inspiration, the fingers normally should be moved away from the ribs due to the downward motion of the diaphragm.

Auscultation

Breath sounds are auscultated using a stethoscope against the chest wall. Normal breath sounds are heard at a specific time of respiration over a specific part of the chest. Normal breath sounds that are heard at the wrong time of respiration are considered abnormal (adventitious).

Normal breath sounds

- Vesicular: soft, low-pitched, heard at the periphery
- Bronchial: loud, high-pitched, heard at the sternum
- Bronchovesicular: medium-pitched, near the main-stem bronchi
- Tracheal: loud and harsh, heard over the trachea

Adventitious breath sounds

- Crackles: soft, high-pitched, discontinuous
- Wheezes: high-pitched, continuous, heard in constricted airways

Mediate percussion

Mediate percussion is performed to assess lung density. Place one hand on the patient's chest wall, with the middle finger against the chest wall (other fingers off the chest wall). The therapist's other middle finger taps against the tip of the middle finger that is against the chest wall.

- **Resonance**: a normal sound
- **Dull** sound: over dense tissue, such as liver or tumor
- **Tympanic** sound: loud, hollow sound heard over an empty stomach or hyperinflated lung

Exercise testing

Typically exercise testing is completed on a treadmill, on an ergometer, or by simple walking. Pre-, during-, and post-exercise evaluation are performed and include HR, oxygen saturation, BP, rating of perceived exertion, arterial blood gases, and lactic acid levels. Common exercise tests are the 12-, 6-, and 3-minute walk tests.

The 6-minute walk test is an objective test where the patient is monitored for oxygen saturation and other vital signs while walking as far as she can in 6 minutes. Twelve- and 3-minute walk tests are similar except for the time of walking.

Pulse oximetry

Pulse oximetry uses a handheld unit to measure the oxygen saturation of arterial blood.

Borg's Rating of Perceived Exertion

0 = resting

0.5 = very, very weak exertion

1 = very weak exertion

2 = weak or light exertion

3 = moderate exertion

4 = somewhat strong

5 = strong or heavy

6

7 = very strong

8

9

10 = very, very strong (maximal)

Cardiovascular Evaluation

Observation

- Skin color
- Body type, weight
- Jugular vein distention (indicates cardiac dysfunction such as CHF)
- Skin: presence of hair loss, sores, dry skin

Pulse

Palpation of the radial pulse can provide information not only on the patient's heart rate but also on the regularity and strength of the pulse.

Common arteries to use in palpating pulse

- Brachial artery
- Radial artery
- Carotid artery
- Femoral artery
- Popliteal artery
- Posterior tibial artery
- Dorsalis pedal artery

Blood pressure

BP is usually measured with a sphygmomanometer and a blood-pressure cuff. The examiner listens for the Korotkoff sounds. The pressure at which the first sound is heard is labeled as the systolic pressure, and the pressure at which the sounds cease is the diastolic pressure. BP is measured in millimeters of mercury (mm Hg).

Orthostatic BP measurements are blood pressures taken as the patient is first supine, then seated, then standing. **Orthostatic hypotension** is a decrease in BP (systolic greater than diastolic) as the patient assumes a more upright position. Symptoms are dizziness and light-headedness.

Normally, systolic BP (SBP) rises with exercise. The increase in SBP is proportional to the workload. Diastolic BP exhibits little to no change with exercise (±10 mm Hg).

Auscultation of the heart

To listen to the heart sounds, press the bell of a stethoscope lightly on the skin over the heart. Generally, you want to listen over the four cardiac valves:

- Aortic: right of sternum, second intercostal space
- Pulmonary: left of sternum, second intercostal space
- Tricuspid: left sternum, fourth intercostal space
- Mitral: left midclavicular line, fifth intercostal space

Heart Sounds

Name of Heart Sound	Sound	Indicates
S_1	"lub"	• Closure of mitral and tricuspid valves • Onset of systole
S_2	"dub"	• Closure of aortic and pulmonary valves • Onset of diastole
S_3	Often impossible to hear with a stethoscope	• Ventricular filling • Can be pathological or normal
S_4	Often impossible to hear with a stethoscope	• Ventricular filling and atrial contraction • S_4 is an abnormal heart sound

Homan's sign

Homan's sign is a test for deep vein thrombosis. The therapist dorsiflexes the foot and then squeezes the gastrocnemius. If the patient complains of pain, the test is positive and further medical testing should be done, along with referral to a physician or emergency room.

Trendelenburg test of venous insufficiency

The Trendelenburg test can indicate the presence of venous insufficiency. To perform the test, place the patient in supine position and elevate the affected leg to 90° of hip flexion. Place a tourniquet around the patient's thigh to occlude blood flow, then have the patient assume a standing position. Normal venous flow should occur in 30 seconds. Venous insufficiency is present if filling takes longer than 30 seconds. If filling occurs after removal of the tourniquet, insufficiency of saphenous veins is suspected.

Pitting edema scale

The pitting edema scale places a score on the severity of edema. To determine, place pressure on the pretibial area for 10 to 20 seconds. Then measure the indentation left in the skin.

Pitting Edema Scale

Score	Appearance
1+	Barely perceptible depression
2+	Easily identified depression, skin rebounds in less than 15 seconds
3+	Easily identified depression, skin rebounds in 15 to 30 seconds
4+	Easily identified depression, skin takes longer than 30 seconds to rebound

DIFFERENTIAL DIAGNOSIS AND PATHOLOGY

Based on the findings obtained during the evaluation of the musculoskeletal system, a list of differential diagnoses can be made. Each pathology or condition of the nervous system is unique and will dictate the medical management and treatment intervention choices made by the physical therapist. Differential diagnoses and pathologies of the nervous system can each cause a wide range of problems and impairments, based on the location and severity of the injury. This also helps to drive treatment intervention decisions.

Chronic Obstructive Pulmonary Disease

Chronic obstructive pulmonary disease (COPD) is a group of diseases that includes emphysema, chronic bronchitis, bronchiectasis, asthma, and cystic fibrosis. Patients with COPD demonstrate decreased expiratory flow rate and increased residual volume (RV).

Increased RV is due to hyperinflation of the lungs and often results in the typical barrel-chested appearance. Emphysema and chronic bronchitis are not mutually exclusive, and often patients receive a dual diagnosis.

Risk factors for COPD

- Smoking
- Male gender
- Particulate inhalation
- Increasing age
- Low socioeconomic status
- History of childhood respiratory illness

Emphysema

Emphysema is the destruction of the lung parenchyma which results in large dead airspace and decreased surface area available for gas exchange.

Signs and symptoms of emphysema

- Dyspnea on exertion
- Cough
- Deconditioning
- Barrel chest
- Distant breath sounds
- Increased use and hypertrophy of the accessory respiratory musculature

Chronic bronchitis

A diagnosis of chronic bronchitis is made when a person has a productive cough for three consecutive months per year for at least two years. Chronic bronchitis is a mechanical obstruction of the airway.

Signs and symptoms of chronic bronchitis

- Coughing
- Dyspnea
- Respiratory infections
- Poor exercise tolerance
- Increased time of expiration
- Wheezes and crackles of the lungs
- Cyanosis
- Peripheral edema

Bronchiectasis

Bronchiectasis is an irreversible abnormal bronchial dilation and/or obstruction. It can be caused by infection, tumors, foreign bodies, aspiration, immune disorders, and genetic disorders.

Signs and symptoms of bronchiectasis

- Chronic productive cough
- Bronchial markings
- Hemoptysis
- Clubbing of fingers

Asthma

Asthma is a hypersensitivity of the upper airway to irritants such as pollens, medications, certain foods, and exercise. Asthma causes smooth bronchial muscle to spasm and hypertrophy. This condition also causes increased mucus production and inflammation.

Signs and symptoms of asthma

- Dyspnea
- Wheezes
- Increased respiratory rate
- Nonproductive cough

Cystic fibrosis

Cystic fibrosis (CF) is a genetic disorder that affects the exocrine glands, particularly the bronchial mucous glands, exocrine pancreas tissue, and sweat glands. It occurs due to a recessive gene from both parents. Secretions from these glands are abnormal and tend to block the opening of the glands. In the lung, there is also abnormal ciliary function. Patients with CF are at a greater risk for lung infections. This is a disease of children and young adults.

Signs and symptoms of cystic fibrosis

- Tachypnea
- Dyspnea
- Cough
- Wheezing
- Multiple bouts of pneumonia in infancy
- Drastically increased amounts of thick mucus

Respiratory Infections

Respiratory infections are caused by infectious agents and produce conditions such as the common cold, upper respiratory infections, and pneumonia. Respiratory infections can be caused by bacteria, viruses, fungi, or protozoa.

Interstitial Pulmonary Fibrosis

Interstitial pulmonary fibrosis is a condition of the alveolar epithelium. The epithelium is replaced with interstitial fibrosis and inflammatory cells.

Signs and symptoms of interstitial pulmonary fibrosis

- Dyspnea
- Extreme fatigue with minimal activity
- Nonproductive cough

Pulmonary Embolism

Pulmonary embolism (PE) is an embolism that becomes lodged in the pulmonary circulation. Pulmonary emboli most often migrate from a deep vein thrombosis in the lower extremity.

Cardinal symptoms of pulmonary embolism

- Abrupt, acute chest pain
- Striking dyspnea

Pulmonary Edema

Pulmonary edema is an increase in water in the interstitium of the lungs and alveoli.

Signs and symptoms of pulmonary edema

- Dyspnea
- Orthopnea
- Cough
- Wheezing

Occupational Lung Diseases

Occupational lung diseases are lung diseases that are caused by exposure to particulate matter or toxic fumes. Mineral and organic dusts are examples of particulate matter.

Pleural Effusion

Pleural effusion is an increased amount of fluid in the pleural space.

Pleurisy

Pleurisy is an inflammation of the pleura.

Pneumothorax

Pneumothorax is air in the pleural cavity.

Atelectasis

Atelectasis is the collapse of lung tissue that prevents the exchange of gases.

Signs and symptoms of atelectasis

- Decreased breath sounds
- Shift toward the side of collapse
- Fever
- Dyspnea

Acute Respiratory Failure

Acute respiratory failure is the failure of the cardiac and pulmonary systems to maintain adequate gas exchange. This is life-threatening and a medical emergency. Hypercapnic respiratory failure is caused by inadequate ventilation and reduced minute ventilation. Hypoxemic respiratory failure is caused by inadequate oxygen delivery to the tissues and/or disproportionate oxygen consumption by the tissues. Treatment is supplemental oxygen.

Pulmonary Conditions of Prematurity

Premature and low-birth-weight neonates are more susceptible to pulmonary complications. **Respiratory distress syndrome (RDS)** is a surfactant deficiency that results in collapsed alveoli. Signs and symptoms are tachypnea, cyanosis, nasal flaring, and expiratory grunting. If the signs and symptoms of RDS continue and progress past one month of life, **bronchopulmonary dysplasia** is diagnosed. **Meconium-aspiration syndrome** occurs with aspiration of meconium during delivery that causes fetal distress, hypoxia, and secondary lung infections.

Coronary Artery Disease

Coronary artery disease (CAD) can produce ischemia and myocardial infarction. **Atherosclerosis** affects medium and large arteries of the body and also coronary arteries. Atherosclerosis of the systemic arteries can result in thinning of the smooth muscle, weakening of the vessel wall, aneurysm, and rupture. In coronary arteries, atherosclerosis results in stenosis. This results in inadequate blood flow to meet the oxygen needs of the cardiac muscle.

Ischemia is defined as oxygen demand of tissue that is greater than the oxygen supply. The heart is more prone to ischemia than other tissues of the body. During exercise, dysrhythmias can occur due to ischemia. These ischemic dysrhythmias are due to the increased oxygen demands of the cardiac muscle. Reduction in the risk factors for CAD can slow the progression of CAD. Presentation of the signs and symptoms of CAD varies according to the number of affected coronary vessels and the severity of the blockages.

Risk factors for CAD

- Male gender
- Hypertension (SBP >160 mm Hg, DBP >95 mm Hg)
- Smoking
- Hypercholesteremia
- Diabetes
- Lack of exercise
- Family history
- Increasing age
- Obesity

Signs and symptoms of CAD

- Death
- Infarction
- Angina

Myocardial Infarction

A **myocardial infarction (MI)** results from a complete occlusion of a coronary artery. Necrosis of cardiac tissue and scar formation follow the occlusion. Extended ischemia may produce an MI. MIs are diagnosed by medical personnel on the basis of clinical signs and symptoms, serum blood markers, EKG, and radioisotope studies. Serum enzymes and markers that can indicate cardiac injury are creatine kinase, troponin-I, and myoglobin.

Signs and symptoms of MI

- Severe chest pain; pressure or heaviness with or without radiation to the shoulder, arm, and/or jaw
- Lightheadedness
- Nausea and vomiting
- Hypotension
- Dyspnea
- Diaphoresis
- Weakness
- Some MIs are asymptomatic.

Heart Failure

Heart failure is the resting heart's inability to maintain adequate cardiac output. The most common cause of heart failure is hypertension (HTN). The heart hypertrophies due to the increased blood pressure. Pressure then builds in the pulmonary circulation and pulmonary edema can occur. This pulmonary edema causes the right side of the heart to fail. Because the right side of the heart fails, pressure then builds in the peripheral circulation. This ultimately results in peripheral edema.

Congestive heart failure (CHF) is **left-sided heart failure** that leads to congestion in the chest (pulmonary edema) and increased pressure on alveoli that makes breathing difficult. CHF is diagnosed by EKG, chest X-ray, and echocardiogram.

Signs and symptoms of CHF

- Dry cough
- Difficulty breathing
- Sudden weight gain
- Development of a third heart sound
- Orthopnea
- Dyspnea on exertion

Right-sided heart failure can eventually occur due to left-sided heart failure. **Cor pulmonale** is right-sided heart failure that is caused by a pulmonary disease.

Signs and symptoms of right-sided heart failure

- Peripheral edema
- Decreased exercise tolerance
- Hypotension with exercise
- Dyspnea during exercise

Intermittent Claudication

Intermittent claudication is exercise-induced muscle ischemia that causes pain with ambulation.

Pathologies of the Lymphatic System

Lymphedema

Lymphedema is an abnormal accumulation of lymph that causes edema. Inflammation, congenital abnormality, or worms that block the lymphatic vessels can cause lymphedema. Primary lymphedema is either hereditary or congenital. Secondary lymphedema is caused by injury to the lymphatic system, such as trauma, surgery, infection, tumors, venous insufficiency, and/or radiation.

Classification of lymphedema

- Mild: Less than 3 cm difference between affected and unaffected limb
- Moderate: 3 to 5 cm difference between affected and unaffected limb
- Severe: Greater than 5 cm difference between affected and unaffected limb

Lymphoma

A **lymphoma** is a lymphatic tumor that is most often malignant. There are two main types of lymphomas, Hodgkin's disease and non-Hodgki's lymphoma. Signs and symptoms of lymphoma include anemia, weight loss, weakness, fever, and painless enlargement of lymph nodes.

Lymphangitis

Lymphangitis is an inflammation of the lymph vessels.

Medical and Diagnostic Imaging

There are a multitude of diagnostic tests and imaging that can be used to diagnose dysfunctions, conditions, and diseases of the cardiovascular and pulmonary systems. Included here are highlights of the most common tests and imaging techniques.

Pulmonary imaging and tests

Bronchoscopy

Bronchoscopy utilizes a bronchoscope to examine the bronchial tree.

Pulmonary function tests

Pulmonary function tests measure lung volumes, gas flow rates, and diffusion and distribution of gases. These tests help to determine obstructive, restrictive, or combined lung pathologies. There are different methods of administering pulmonary function tests. A spirogram, the helium dilution method, the nitrogen washout method, and body plethysmography are examples of methods of determining lung volumes and capacities.

Pulmonary function tests are used to measure volumes of airflow in inspiration and expiration. Normal values of lung volumes have been established. Besides the lung volumes listed previously in this chapter, forced vital capacity and forced expiratory volume in one second can also be measured and are considered useful. **Forced vital capacity (FVC)** is the volume of air that is expired forcefully after inspiration. **Forced expiratory volume in one second (FEV_1)** is the volume of air that is expired in the first second of a forceful expiration.

Chest imaging

An **X-ray** produces a radiograph. If an area is radiolucent, a dark image appears. This indicates a low density. Air in the lungs is radiolucent. If an area is radiopaque, a white image appears. This indicates a high density. An example of a radiopaque substance is bone. Tomography is a sectional radiograph.

Magnetic resonance imaging (MRI) is performed by placing the body in a magnetic field. The hydrogen nuclei are then excited, radio waves are emitted, and a computer constructs a sectional picture of the body.

Bronchogram is an imaging technique that uses a contrast medium in the bronchial tree. Radiographs are then produced to view the bronchial tree.

Perfusion scan uses a radioactive dye, which is injected intravenously. The patient is then scanned to examine the perfusion pattern of the lungs.

Ventilation scanning uses xenon gas to scan and examine the ventilation pattern of the lungs.

Cardiovascular imaging and tests

Cardiac catheterization

Cardiac catheterization is an invasive procedure that examines the presence of coronary artery disease, valvular insufficiency, and cardiac disease. This procedure can also establish the patient's ejection fraction, cardiac output, and heart pressures.

Doppler ultrasound

Doppler ultrasound is used to diagnose deep vein thrombosis of the extremities.

Ankle brachial index

Ankle brachial index (ABI) is a medical test that compares blood pressure (obtained by Doppler ultrasound) from the dorsalis pedis with the blood pressure in the higher of the two brachial arteries. Normal ABI is 0.9. An ABI that is lower than 0.5 indicates severe occlusive arterial disease.

Echocardiograph

Echocardiograph is an ultrasonic imaging of the beating heart that can provide information on the size of the heart and its cavities, valves, stroke volume, and ejection fraction. Thickness of the myocardial walls and septa is also determined, along with other information.

Electrocardiogram

Electrocardiogram (ECG) is a technique to image the electrical activity of the heart. This technique captures the atrial depolarization (P), ventricular depolarization (QRS complex), and repolarization (T) of the myocardium. ECG provides information on heart rate, rhythm, hypertrophy, and infarction.

Arterial blood gas values
Arterial blood gas values are used to examine the arterial concentrations of gases dissolved in blood, particularly oxygen and carbon dioxide.

Holter monitoring
Holter monitoring uses a multiple-lead transcutaneous electrocardiogram that can record electrical heart activity for 24 hours.

Swan-Ganz catheter
A Swan-Ganz catheter is a catheter placed in the pulmonary artery to assess intracardiac pressures.

Blood laboratory studies

Complete blood cell count
A complete blood cell count includes measuring hematocrit, white blood cell (WBC) count, and hemoglobin. The normal WBC count is 4,500 to 11,000 μL of whole blood. Normal values for hematocrit and hemoglobin are listed in the table below.

Normal Hematocrit and Hemoglobin Levels

	Normal Hematocrit	**Normal Hemoglobin**
Males	40 to 54%	13.5 to 18 g/dL
Females	38 to 47%	12 to 16 g/dL

Blood Lipids

	Normal Value
Total cholesterol	<200 mg/dL
Low-density lipoproteins (LDLs)	<100 mg/dL
High-density lipoproteins (HDLs)	Males: >33 mg/dL Females: >43 mg/dL

Coagulation Profile

	Normal Value
ProTime	11.6 to 13 seconds
PTT	21.5 to 34.1 seconds

Electrolytes
Two of the electrolytes that are measured are sodium and potassium. Critically low levels of K+ can cause arrhythmias. Critically high levels of K+ can cause contractility issues.

Electrolytes

	Normal Value
Sodium (Na+)	136 to 143 mEq/L
Potassium (K+)	3.8 to 5 mEq/L

Blood Laboratory Study Values

	Normal Value
Glucose	70 to 110 mg/dL
BUN	8 to 18 mg/dL
Creatinine	0.6 to 1.2 mg/dL

Medical Treatment and Management

There are several treatments, techniques, and interventions that can be performed by the medical team in the treatment of patients with pulmonary or cardiovascular system impairments. Discussed here are some of the more common methods of medical management.

Implantable cardiac devices

Cardiac pacemakers and cardioverter defibrillators are two types of implantable cardiac devices. Cardiac pacemakers are superficial electronic pulse generators that control arrhythmias. Implantable cardioverter defibrillators (ICDs) are devices that correct life-threatening arrhythmias such as tachycardia, ventricular fibrillation, and bradycardia.

Vascular interventions

There are interventions that are performed to the lumen of the vascular that are often completed by catheterization. A **percutaneous transluminal coronary angioplasty** is performed by balloon penetration of a stenotic lesion of the coronary artery. The lesion is penetrating until the artery is patent. A **directional coronary arthrectomy** is the removal of a stenotic lesion via catheter placed in the lumen of the coronary artery. To keep a cardiac artery patent, **cardiac artery stenting** can be performed by placing a stent in the lumen of the coronary artery. **Carotid endarterectomy** is the surgical removal of plaque in the carotid artery.

Surgical treatment

There are a variety of cardiovascular surgeries that are used to treat patients with dysfunction of the cardiovascular system. Some of the most common are coronary artery bypass grafting, abdominal aortic aneurysmectomy, and peripheral vascular surgery. **Coronary artery bypass graft** (CABG) is the revascularization with grafts to the myocardium due to occlusion of coronary arteries. One or several arteries may be bypassed. **Abdominal aortic aneurysmectomy** is the surgical repair of an abdominal aortic aneurysm. Pulmonary complications are common after this surgery. **Peripheral vascular surgery** is surgery to repair or bypass peripheral vasculature. Occluded vessels may be bypassed and arteries can be reconstructed. If this treatment fails or is ineffective, limb amputation can be the ultimate result.

Organ transplants

In extreme cases, organs of the cardiac and pulmonary systems can be transplanted. Heart, heart-lung, and lung transplants are all possible. One major consideration following heart transplant is that the heart becomes denervated. This means that there is no autonomic system input to the heart to control rate or rhythm. Patients also demonstrate a reduced exercise capacity after heart or lung transplant.

Airway suctioning

Airway suctioning is the mechanical removal of pulmonary secretions. This technique can be used in conjunction with other techniques, including physical therapy techniques of airway clearance.

TREATMENT INTERVENTIONS

Once patient evaluation is completed and the differential diagnosis is listed, it is necessary to choose the proper interventions to treat the patient's impairments. Primary prevention of cardiovascular and pulmonary dysfunction is important. Typically, functional mobility, exercise, range of motion, mobilization, and modalities are combined to work toward the patient's goals in physical therapy. Specific methods of airway clearance techniques, cardiac rehab, and pulmonary rehab are used to treat dysfunction of these systems. The use of assistive devices, implementation of orthotics and prosthetics, and the application of modalities are covered in chaper 8, Equipment and Devices, and Therapeutic Modalities.

Primary Prevention and Reduction of Risk Factors

- Lifestyle change
- Increased daily activity/exercise
- Promotion of smoking cessation
- Maintenance of healthy weight; weight loss
- Proper nutrition

Airway Clearance Techniques

Airway clearance techniques (ACTs) are used to facilitate clearance of secretions from the airways. These techniques are indicated by an **ineffective cough** or **impaired mucociliary transport**. Specific ACTs include postural drainage, percussion, vibration, assisted cough, manual hyperinflation and airway suctioning, and positive expiratory pressure.

Goals of airway clearance techniques

- Reduce airway obstruction
- Increase ventilation
- Increase gas exchange

Contraindications and precautions for airway clearance techniques

- Trendelenburg position increases intracranial pressure.
- Risk of hemoptysis with postural drainage
- Trendelenburg position in children and infants should be avoided due to increased risk of gastroesophageal reflux disease.
- Percussion can cause decreased PaO_2 and dysrhythmias.
- Rib fracture and infection
- Coagulopathy
- Skin impairments of the thorax
- Monitor lines/tubes/catheters

- Avoid barotraumas with manual hyperinflation.
- Unstable angina
- Chest wall pain
- Unstable dysrhythmias
- Untreated tension pneumothorax in neonate

Complications of airway clearance techniques

- Decreased oxygen saturation with percussion
- Risk of injury to those with osteoporosis or coagulopathy with percussion, vibration

Postural drainage

Postural drainage is the positioning of the patient to allow gravity-assisted drainage of secretions. Specific positions are designated for each lobe of the lungs.

Postural Drainage Positions

Lobe/Segment	Bed Position	Patient Position	Therapist Position and Hand Position for Percussion
Upper lobes, anterior segments	Flat	Supine, knees supported	Claps between clavicle and nipple
Upper lobes, posterior segments	Flat	Sitting, leans forward over pillow at 30°	Stand behind; claps over upper back
Upper lobes, apical segments	Flat	Sitting, leans back against pillow at 30°	Support patient behind pillow; claps between clavicle and superior scapula
Left upper lobe, lingular segment	Foot of bed elevated 16 inches	Head down, right side-lying, then quarter-turn backward, knees flexed	Claps over left nipple area
Right middle lobe	Foot of bed elevated 16 inches	Head down, left side-lying, then quarter-turn backward, knees flexed	Claps over right nipple
Lower lobes, anterior basal segments	Foot of bed elevated 20 inches	Head down, side-lying	Claps over lower ribs
Lower lobes, lateral basal segments	Foot of bed elevated 20 inches	Head down, prone, then rotates quarter-turn upward, upper leg supported by pillow	Claps over uppermost region of lower ribs

Lobe/Segment	Bed Position	Patient Position	Therapist Position and Hand Position for Percussion
Lower lobes, posterior basal segments	Foot of bed elevated 20 inches	Head down, prone, pillow under hips	Claps over lower ribs, medially
Lower lobes, superior segments	Flat	Prone with two pillows under hips	Claps over middle upper back at tip of scapula

Percussion

Percussion refers to the manual or mechanical chest percussion performed upon the chest wall to loosen secretions. Manual percussion is performed with cupped hands over the involved lung segment. The rate of percussion is typically between 100 and 480 bpm. Percussion is generally performed in postural drainage positions.

Vibration

Vibration refers to the manual or mechanical vibration performed after deep inspiration. The physical therapist places the hands on the patient's chest wall and gently oscillates. Vibration is generally performed in postural drainage positions.

Assisted cough

Assisted cough techniques use positioning of the patient to maximize the cough while instruction is provided on proper cough techniques. For thoracic surgical patients, this includes splinting the incision with a pillow.

Manual hyperinflation and airway suctioning

Manual hyperinflation and airway suctioning is used for patients who are ventilated mechanically or have a tracheostomy.

Positive expiratory pressure

Positive expiratory pressure uses a device to maintain and open airways during expiration. The device provides resistance to expiration.

Active Cycle of Breathing

The active cycle of breathing is a technique taught to the patient that includes forced expiration performed by the patient in this specific order:

1. Breathing control: diaphragmatic breathing for five to ten seconds
2. Thoracic expansion: in a postural drainage position, deep inhalation with relaxed exhalation
3. Breathing control
4. Thoracic expansion three to four times
5. Breathing control

6. Forced expiration: abdominal contraction with one to two huffs
7. Breathing control

Mechanical Ventilation

Mechanical ventilation may be medically utilized in the acutely ill patient. Physical therapy goals for patients using mechanical ventilation are improved pulmonary function and airway clearance in order to return to spontaneous breathing. Considerations in the process of weaning the patient from mechanical ventilation are:

- Communication with the patient may include simple gestures or blinking, as mechanical ventilation usually interferes with verbal communication.
- Balance the energy expenditure required for breathing with the energy expenditure required for functional mobility or exercises.
- Amount of dyspnea and pain experienced

Positioning

Bed and chair positioning and the use of specific postures of the acutely ill patient can be used to improve pulmonary function. To improve inspiratory movement, shoulder flexion, abduction, and external rotation, an upward eye gaze should be used. To improve expiratory movement, shoulder extension, adduction, and internal rotation, a downward eye gaze can be performed.

Movement of the trunk can also improve pulmonary function. Posterior pelvic tilting assists in diaphragmatic breathing. Trunk flexion assists expiration; trunk extension assists inspiration.

Positions to improve dyspnea work by maximizing the action of the accessory muscles for inspiration. Leaning forward onto the forearms and left side-lying are positions to improve dyspnea.

Breathing Exercises

Breathing exercises include inspiratory muscle training, sniffing technique, diaphragmatic breathing, and segmental breathing exercises. Also included in this category are resisted inhalation, chest wall stretching, incentive spirometry, and pursed-lip breathing.

Inspiratory muscle training

Inspiratory muscle training is performed to increase ventilation and improve dyspnea. Muscles of inspiration are trained to increase strength and endurance. This technique focuses on diaphragmatic breathing.

Sniffing technique

The sniffing technique is useful to begin diaphragmatic breathing. Proprioceptive feedback is provided to the patient by the therapist placing her hands on the patient's abdomen. The patient is instructed to sniff and follow with a slow, relaxed expiration.

Diaphragmatic breathing exercises

Diaphragmatic breathing exercises are used to increase activation of the diaphragm during breathing. This type of exercise also encourages activation of the abdominal muscles during exhalation.

Segmental breathing exercises

Segmental breathing exercises are used to actively direct air to a specific area of the lung by specific movement of the thorax in that area.

Resisted inhalation

Resisted inhalation is useful to improve the strength of the respiratory muscles. Manual resistance is given to the diaphragm by the therapist placing his hands under the patient's rib cage during inspiration.

Chest wall stretching

Chest wall stretching is performed unilaterally or bilaterally, depending on the patient's status. Unilateral chest wall stretching is completed with the patient in side-lying position with the upper arm abducted. The therapist then gives the chest wall a stretch before and during inspiration. Chest wall stretching is also useful during expiration if the lung is hyperinflated due to disease. Bilateral chest wall stretching is completed with the patient semi-reclined or seated. The therapist applies pressure bilaterally to the chest wall.

Incentive spirometry

Incentive spirometry is effective in diaphragmatic breathing training. Patients may need verbal and tactile feedback to learn to properly use the incentive spirometer.

Pursed-lip breathing

Pursed-lip breathing is taught to the patient who has dyspnea or pulmonary dysfunction. The therapist instructs the patient to expire through pursed, circular lips.

Autogenic Drainage

Autogenic drainage is a treatment intervention in which the patient is educated to determine where in his bronchial tree the secretions exist. The patient then is taught to:

1. Perform low-volume breathing to unstick mucus from the periphery of the lungs.
2. Collect secretions in middle to large airways by low-volume breathing.
3. Evacuate secretions to the large airways by high-volume breathing.

Exercise

Individualized exercise programs should include instruction in mode, frequency, duration, and intensity. The patient should be evaluated regularly for adjustment in mode, frequency, duration, and intensity. Vital signs, Borg's Rating of Perceived Exertion (Borg's RPE), anginal complaints, and dyspnea can all be indicators of how well exercise is being tolerated. Often, acutely ill patients with cardiopulmonary impairments will tolerate only low levels of exercise. Patient education goes hand in hand with exercise training and prescription. In the cardiovascular- and pulmonary-impaired patient, patient education can be key. Training a person on heart-rate monitoring, anginal tolerance, signs of exercise intolerance, and when to stop exercise is of utmost importance.

Functional mobility training is one form of exercise or activity that can be prescribed and assisted by the physical therapist. Bed mobility, sitting tolerance, functional transfers, and static standing are often the first treatment interventions used for the acutely ill patient. Simple exercise such as supine and sitting extremity exercises, isometrics (avoiding the Valsalva maneuver), and active range of motion should be the first step in treating the acutely ill patient.

Indicators of exercise tolerance

- Drastic change in vital signs
- High Borg's RPE
- Maximal dyspnea
- Anginal complaints

Complications of exercise

Oxygen saturation can decrease with exercise. Postsurgical patients may have limitations on range of motion of the upper extremities. Following thoracic surgery, patients may also have lifting restrictions. Postsurgical patients have an increased risk of deep vein thrombosis (DVT). Use Homan's sign to assess for DVTs, and encourage elevation and ankle pumps to avoid DVT formation. Early mobilization is also beneficial for avoiding DVT formation.

Cardiac Rehabilitation

Cardiac rehabilitation is a multidisciplinary program that encompasses exercise, education, and lifestyle change to improve patients' cardiac disease function, health, and activity tolerance. Physician, program coordinator, physical therapist, dietician, counselor, and a nurse are common members of the cardiac rehab team.

Phases of cardiac rehabilitation

Phase I: Acute phase

Cardiac rehabilitation begins in the acute-care setting. Basic education, prevention, and exercise are key components. Vital signs are monitored closely.

Phase II: Subacute phase

Phase II begins up to six weeks after discharge from acute care and continues for up to six months. Patients are monitored for vital signs and ECG. Patient education includes the basics of exercise and self-monitoring of exercise tolerance.

Phase III: Intensive rehab

Phase III begins at 6 months after the cardiac event and extends to 12 months. During phase III, resistance training begins and exercise programs continue to progress.

Phase IV: Maintenance program

Phase IV is for patients whose cardiac event was more than 12 months ago. This phase is a self-directed continuation of the cardiac rehab program. Fitness centers and hospitals often offer groups and facilities for these patients to continue their programs.

Cardiac rehab components

- Exercise testing and training
- Monitoring of vital signs, angina, and workload during exercise
- Patient education on smoking cessation, health behavior change
- Nutrition and weight counseling
- ECG monitoring
- Stress management training

Cardiac rehab diagnoses

- Post-MI
- Heart failure
- Cardiac transplant
- CABG
- Valvular replacement
- Stable angina

Pulmonary Rehabilitation

The pulmonary rehab team is similar to the multidisciplinary cardiac rehab team. Exercises can include use of upper- and lower-extremity ergometer, walking, stair climbing, and stretching. Pulse oximetry, heart rate, and blood pressure are monitored. Pulmonary rehabilitation has both inpatient and outpatient components.

Goals of pulmonary rehab

- Health behavior change, including smoking cessation
- Increased tolerance to activity
- Improved nutrition and healthy weight
- Independence with exercise and monitoring
- Decreased dyspnea with activity
- Improved quality of life

Lymphedema Interventions

Manual lymph drainage with complete decongestive therapy is one therapeutic intervention for the management of lymphedema. It is a systematic, intense program to treat lymphedema, including nail and skin care, exercise, compression garments, and manipulation of lymph vessels and nodes. Treatment begins centrally and progresses distally to clear the involved trunk quadrant first and progress to clearing the involved extremity.

Ultrasound at nonthermal levels can also be used to treat lymphedema.

A FINAL WORD

To adequately evaluate and treat a patient or client, you must have a strong knowledge of the foundational sciences and the background, evaluation, differential diagnoses, and treatment interventions of the cardiovascular and pulmonary systems. This chapter, which highlights each of these areas, along with your experience in lab practicals and clinical affiliations, will help prepare you to identify and treat impairments of these systems.

The following pages offer an end-of-chapter practice quiz to test your knowledge of some of the fundamentals of the cardiovascular and pulmonary systems. It is not necessary to time this, as it is a chapter review quiz.

Cardiac, Vascular, and Pulmonary Systems Chapter Quiz

1. A physical therapist works in a phase III cardiac rehab program. The physical therapist should know that the normal heart rate response to submaximal exercise is which of the following?

   (A) Heart rate increases more quickly with leg work than with arm work.

   (B) Heart rate is unpredictable and not related to workload.

   (C) Heart rate increases linearly with increased submaximal workloads.

   (D) Heart rate decreases linearly with increased submaximal workloads.

2. During blood flow through the heart, where does the blood travel after being pumped out of the right ventricle?

   (A) Systemic circuit

   (B) Right atrium

   (C) Pulmonary circuit

   (D) Left ventricle

3. What is the primary (intrinsic) pacemaker of the heart?

   (A) SA node

   (B) AV node

   (C) Purkinje fibers

   (D) Bundle of His

4. A physical therapist auscultates a patient's lungs. What breath sound is normally heard in a healthy person without pulmonary dysfunction?

   (A) Wheezes

   (B) Rubs

   (C) Crackles

   (D) Tracheal breath sounds

5. Right-sided heart failure is usually a result of what condition?

   (A) Cerebrovascular accident

   (B) Peripheral vascular disease

   (C) Left-sided heart failure

   (D) Electrical conduction dysfunction

6. A five-year-old boy is hospitalized due to pneumonia. He also shows signs and symptoms of digital clubbing, crackles and wheezes upon auscultation of the lungs, chronic cough, frequent respiratory infections, and thick mucus secretions. What systemic pathology is suspected?

   (A) Asthma

   (B) Emphysema

   (C) Cystic fibrosis

   (D) Acute respiratory failure

7. A physical therapist receives a referral for a 60-year-old patient who has had a recent heart transplant. What does the physical therapist know about this patient's heart rate?
   (A) The patient's maximal heart rate is 160 beats per minute.
   (B) The patient's maximal heart rate is 220 beats per minute.
   (C) The patient's heart rate response will be abnormal.
   (D) The patient's heart rate will be lower than 40 beats per minute.

8. A physical therapist is asked to give a lecture to residents of a retirement community about the risks, warning signs, and treatment of heart attacks. What are two signs or symptoms of a myocardial infarction on which the physical therapist can educate this population?
   (A) Foot and leg pain
   (B) Sweating and weakness
   (C) Nosebleed and earache
   (D) Increased energy and activity

9. A physical therapist is incorporating treadmill walking for a 65-year-old patient in a cardiac rehabilitation program. The physical therapist adjusts the intensity, duration, and frequency based on the patient's signs and symptoms. Which of these signs or symptoms does *NOT* indicate exercise intolerance?
   (A) Complaints of severe angina
   (B) A decrease in oxygen saturation to 92 percent
   (C) Rating of perceived exertion of 10 (very, very strong)
   (D) Heart rate of 170 beats per minute

10. A patient with chronic obstructive pulmonary disease is referred to pulmonary rehab. The patient asks his physical therapist what is happening in his lungs that causes his barrel-chested appearance. What should the physical therapist tell the patient?
   (A) "Your lungs are underinflated, causing this barrel-chested appearance."
   (B) "Your lungs are overinflated, causing this barrel-chested appearance."
   (C) "Your lungs are infected, causing this barrel-chested appearance."
   (D) "Your frequent coughing causes this barrel-chested appearance."

11. A physical therapist receives a referral from a hospitalized patient for airway clearance techniques. What is one possible secondary effect or complication of percussion for airway clearance?
   (A) Increased ventilation
   (B) Decreased airway obstruction
   (C) Decreased oxygen saturation
   (D) Increased gas exchange

12. A physical therapist evaluates a hospitalized patient following coronary artery bypass grafting (CABG). The patient has bilateral edema in the lower extremities. The physical therapist places pressure on the pretibial area for 10 seconds. There is an easily identified depression left in the patient's skin that takes less than 15 seconds to rebound. How is this properly rated on the pitting edema scale?
   (A) 1+
   (B) 2+
   (C) 3+
   (D) 4+

13. A physical therapist examines the medical record of a patient with known pulmonary dysfunction to see what volume of air the patient normally inhales and exhales with each breath. What lung volume should the physical therapist look for?

    (A) Vital capacity (VC)
    (B) Total lung capacity (TLC)
    (C) Tidal volume (TV)
    (D) Residual volume (RV)

14. A patient is in the intensive care unit following a massive myocardial infarction of the left coronary artery. The left coronary artery splits into the circumflex artery and what other artery?

    (A) Right coronary artery
    (B) Left anterior descending artery
    (C) Coronary sinus
    (D) Superior vena cava

15. A patient is referred to physical therapy. The patient is hospitalized secondary to vascular pathology. What medical test is *MOST* likely to be ordered by the physician to examine arterial occlusion?

    (A) Ankle brachial index
    (B) Pulse oximetry
    (C) Pulmonary function tests
    (D) X-ray

Answers

1. C.

   Normally, heart rate increases linearly during increasing submaximal workloads. Pathology or medication may alter this relationship. Heart rate also increases more quickly during upper-extremity exercise than during lower-extremity exercise.
   (Irwin, page 83)

2. C.

   Blood is received from the systemic circuit into the right atrium and travels into the right ventricle. From the right ventricle, blood is pumped into the pulmonary circuit.
   (Irwin, page 16)

3. A.

   The SA node is the intrinsic pacemaker of the heart. Impulses start at the SA node, which is located in the right atrium.
   (Irwin, page 178)

4. D.

   Tracheal breath sounds are normal breath sounds when auscultated over the trachea. Wheezes, rubs, and crackles are abnormal breath sounds and indicate pulmonary dysfunction.
   (Irwin, page 291)

5. C.

   Right-sided heart failure usually is caused by left-sided heart failure. Right-sided heart failure can also be caused by chronic hypoxia seen in chronic obstructive pulmonary disease.
   (Irwin, page 20)

6. C.

   Patients with cystic fibrosis often have crackles, rhonchi, wheezes, and increased respiratory rate. Progressive obstruction results in increased chest diameter. Digital clubbing is standard in patients older than four years of age. These patients have recurrent respiratory infections, a chronic cough, and thick secretions.
   (Orenstein, page 10)

7. C.

   After a heart transplant, the heart is denervated. It is not under sympathetic or parasympathetic control. Heart rate response to exercise will be abnormal.
   (Pryor, page 524)

8. B.

   Signs and symptoms of myocardial infarction include sweating (diaphoresis) and weakness, severe chest pain and pressure, lightheadedness, nausea and vomiting, and dyspnea. Some myocardial infarctions are asymptomatic.
   (Irwin, page 136)

9. B.

   Oxygen saturation can decrease with exercise, and this is a normal response. A pulse oxygenation of 92 percent does not indicate exercise intolerance. Severe anginal complaints, a perceived exertion rating of 10, and a heart rate faster than the age-predicted maximum all indicate exercise intolerance.
   (Irwin, page 97)

10. B.

    Increased residual volume and hyperinflation of the lungs results in the characteristic barrel-chested appearance of persons with chronic obstructive pulmonary disease.
    (DeTurk, page 157)

11. C.

    Possible complications of percussion include decreased oxygen saturation and risk of injury for patients with osteoporosis or coagulopathy.
    (Frownfelter, page 345)

12. **B.**

To use the pitting edema scale, place pressure on the pretibial area for 10 to 20 seconds. Assess the indentation present in the skin. A score of 2+ indicates an easily identified depression that rebounds in less than 15 seconds.
(Pillages, page 134)

13. C.

Tidal volume (TV) is the volume of air normally inhaled and exhaled with each breath.
(DeTurk, page 250)

14. **B.**

The left coronary artery bifurcates into the left anterior descending artery and the circumflex artery.
(Irwin, page 21)

15. **A.**

The ankle brachial index (ABI) uses a Doppler ultrasound to compare the highest blood pressure of the dorsalis pedis with the highest blood pressure of the brachial artery. Normal ABI is 0.9. ABI of less than 0.4 to 0.5 indicates occlusive arterial disease.
(De Turk, page 310)

Musculoskeletal System

4

As a graduating physical therapy student, you are expected to be familiar with the basic anatomy of the musculoskeletal system. This includes the muscles and bones that make up each functional joint group. There is most definitely overlap among the different chapters in this book, and both evaluation and intervention techniques from other systems may be necessary in evaluating and treating the musculoskeletal system. It is important that you look at the patient as a whole and not just at the injury or disability for which the patient seeks physical therapy. Comorbidities, age, activity level, and psychology of the patient all play into the success of physical therapy as a treatment intervention. This chapter will take you a little further, beyond the basics of names of bones and muscles, into the functions of the individual joints and the evaluation and treatment of the musculoskeletal system as a whole.

FOUNDATIONAL SCIENCES AND BACKGROUND

A strong understanding of the basic background and fundamental science of the musculoskeletal system is necessary before evaluation, interpretation, and intervention can take place. It is necessary to understand how each joint system works, including the skeletal makeup, muscular action, and innervations, as well as other soft-tissue makeup (ligaments, tendons, joint capsules, fasciae, skin, bursae, etc.).

Anatomy and Physiology

As its name implies, the musculoskeletal system is made up of muscles, bones, connective tissues, and the interactions of all of these in order to produce movement and protect the body. In order to best diagnose and treat disorders of the musculoskeletal system, you must know the makeup of each component of the system.

Muscle tissue

Muscle tissue is unique in the fact that it is contractile tissue. It can be stretched for range of motion and can contract during muscle activation. During immobilization, muscle contractures can develop due to the prolonged shortened position of the muscle. Muscle tissue itself is made up of both contractile and noncontractile tissue. The contractile portion is the muscle fiber itself, further broken down into myofibrils. A myofibril is a collection of sarcomeres that are further made up of the actin-myosin cross-bridges. These use a ratchet motion to allow shortening of the myofibril, which is the basis for the muscle contraction. Muscle tissue can be categorized into the following three types:

1. **Slow, oxidative fibers (type I)** are used during moderate-intensity, long-duration exercise. These fibers produce less total muscle tension but are able to maintain that tension for a long period of time (some say up to one hour).

2. **Fast, oxidative-glycolytic fibers (type IIa)** are used in high-intensity, short-duration exercise or after type I fibers begin to fatigue in long-duration exercise. These fibers produce a much stronger tension than the type I but are quick to fatigue (one to three minutes).
3. **Fast, glycolytic fibers (type IIb)** are also used in high-intensity, short-duration exercise (one to three minutes).

In general, muscles are made up of both slow- and fast-twitch muscle fibers. Some muscles have more of one type, which may make them more tonic (more fast-twitch) or more phasic (more slow-twitch). **Postural muscles** tend to be more phasic, whereas **power muscles** such as the gastrocnemius and quadriceps are more tonic.

Connective or noncontractile tissue

Connective or noncontractile tissue in the musculoskeletal system is made up of ligaments, tendons, bursae, and fibrous fasciae. It does not have the elasticity of muscle but instead is collagen-based and can lengthen only through slow, prolonged stretch or mobilization. Connective tissues are made up of differing percentages of collagen, elastin, and reticulin fibers, based on their function in musculoskeletal support.

Collagen fibers

- **Collagen** provides strength, and collagen fibers lengthen temporarily during a light stretch but tighten under a strong stretch. Tendons have collagen fibers set parallel for strength; skin has collagen fibers set randomly, allowing tissue weakness; and ligaments, joint capsules, and fasciae are somewhere in between. Immobilization, inactivity, age, and certain steroid drug therapies cause weakening of the collagen fibers and overall weakening of the connective tissue.

Elastin fibers

- **Elastin** allows flexibility within the tissues. These fibers will lengthen with light stretch but rupture under a strong stretch.

Reticulin fibers

- **Reticulin** does not by itself provide strength or elasticity to the connective tissue but just adds to the thickness of the particular connective tissue.

Many of the connective tissues function just as their name implies: to connect one tissue to another. Others provide protection from injury or add stability to a joint. Ligaments, tendons, bursae, fasciae, and skin are examples of connective tissues.

Ligaments

Ligaments attach bone to bone, adding stability to the joint; provide proprioceptive input; and also help to control the accessory motion of a joint during mobility. Prolonged immobilization of a ligament can greatly decrease its tensile strength and add to its stiffness, thus increasing the stiffness of a joint. Activity that provides low-load stress to a ligament helps to improve tensile strength slightly.

Tendons

Tendons are continuations of a muscle attaching it to its bony insertion.

Bursae

Bursae are fluid-filled sacs found in areas of the body where friction may occur. Bursae help to protect underlying structures from injury as a result of friction to the soft tissue.

Fascia

Fascia is a fibrous connective tissue that is present between the muscles themselves and the muscle-subcutaneous tissue connection. Tightness in a muscle will also pull on the fascia and subcutaneous tissues surrounding it, and likewise tightness in the fascia and subcutaneous tissue will also pull on the muscle.

Length-tension relationship

Length-tension relationship refers to the length of the muscle fibers themselves and the tendency for the muscle to produce the maximum strength at a particular position of muscle length. This is important to keep in mind when strengthening a muscle and in diagnosing muscle injury dependent on the position the muscle is in at the time of its injury.

Stress-strain curve

The **stress-strain curve** depicts the amount of stress or tension a tissue can withstand before deformation or rupture occurs. It compares the relationship between stress and strain and the effects of that relationship on soft tissues.

Body Types and Body Composition

Each individual's body type and body composition can predispose to certain injuries and pathologies, not only in the musculoskeletal system, but also in any other systems. It is important to be aware of each of these predispositions when evaluating a patient and in determining the plan of care for intervention.

Body types

Body types are named for the embryonic development structures that they most closely resemble.

- **Mesomorph:** muscular body characteristics
- **Ectomorph:** thin body characteristics
- **Endomorph:** fatter body characteristics

Body composition

Body composition is used to calculate the percentage of lean or fat body weight. This can be done in several ways, as follows:

- Skinfold measurement is done using calipers to grasp sections of skin and subcutaneous tissue
- Underwater weighing
- Bioelectrical impedance

Generally, normal fat levels for females should be below 18 percent; and for males, below 14 percent. Body fat below 5 percent is considered dangerously low.

Effects of Activity and Exercise

It is obvious that the musculoskeletal system benefits from exercise. Improvements in strength, range of motion, functional mobility, and muscular endurance can be seen with regular physical activity. Resistance exercise also encourages increased osteoblastic activity for bone strength. Physical inactivity decreases the cross-sectional area of the myofibril of the muscle and the number of collagen fibers within connective tissues, causing overall weakening of the support structures. With immobilization, there is atrophy of muscle, weakening of collagen in connective tissues, and overall increased stiffness of the affected joint. Depending on the position of the immobilization, contractures of the muscle-tendon unit can develop.

Strength

Muscular strength develops as exercise increases the actual number of myofibrils within a muscle. The actual cross-sectional area of the myofibril increases, also increasing the muscle's strength. As exercise intensity increases with training, a greater number of motor units can be recruited, also adding to strength.

Endurance

Muscle endurance improves with exercise as the number of capillaries within the muscle itself increases, allowing a greater amount of oxygen and replacement nutrients to move into the muscle for longer-lasting or repetitive contraction.

Range of motion

Movement of the joints, muscles, and connective tissues is directly affected by exercise. With inactivity, there can be contractures of the muscle tissue and stiffening of connective tissues, both of which contribute to overall decreased range of motion of a joint. Over time, this limited range of motion can cause adhesions around the joint.

Functional mobility

The ability to ambulate with a normal gait pattern, transfer at any level, or perform any activity of daily living requires muscle strength, endurance, and range of motion. Exercise can improve mobility indirectly through the changes to soft tissues and joints mentioned above, allowing greater movement and strength.

Environmental Influences

Changes in environment can influence the effects of exercise or activity on the musculoskeletal system. Aquatics, air temperature, and altitude can each have different effects on the outcomes of physical therapy or a home exercise program.

Water submersion

Simply being submersed in water can increase venous return, increase stroke volume, and decrease heart rate. There is an increase in the work of breathing due to chest-wall compression (repeated exposure can be used to strengthen the chest wall). Tissue perfusion is increased, improving delivery of oxygen and removal of waste. There is also increased blood flow to the kidneys, which results in a diuretic effect. There is a decrease in pain due to pressure and warmth, promoting relaxation.

Exercise in water

Exercise in cold water can cause heat loss that is two to four times greater than heat loss in cold air. During swimming in cool water, heat loss via conduction and convection is greatly increased. Body temperature decreases and oxygen consumption increases. Athletes with an increased amount of subcutaneous fat have an increased amount of insulation against heat loss. Exercise in hot water increases cardiac output.

Temperature

Exercise in hot ambient environments can increase the anaerobic metabolism and the resultant lactic acid buildup. In cold temperatures, shivering produces heat via muscular contraction, which also increases oxygen consumption to sustain the shivering. During exercise in the cold, muscular energy metabolism greatly sustains core temperature. Complications of exercise in hot environments could ultimately result in heat illness. The major forms of heat illness are heat cramps, heat exhaustion, and heat stroke.

Heat cramps

Heat cramps are involuntary muscle spasms during or after physical activity, probably due to electrolyte and fluid imbalance.

Heat exhaustion

During **heat exhaustion**, blood accumulates in the peripheral vasculature and blood volume is drastically decreased so as to lower cardiac output. Symptoms are weak pulse, tachycardia, orthostatic hypotension, headache, dizziness, and weakness. Body temperature is not dangerously increased (remains below 104°F [40°C]). Treatment is exercise termination, moving to a cooler environment, and fluid administration.

Heat stroke

Heat stroke requires emergency medical attention. Body temperature is above 104°F (40°C). During heat stroke, thermoregulation fails, sweating ceases, the skin is dry and hot, and the circulatory system effectively fails. Immediate treatment is to aggressively lower body temperature through ice baths, ice packs, cold-water baths, and alcohol rubs. Heat stroke is life-threatening.

Altitude

The immediate responses to exercise at higher altitudes are decreased aerobic capacity and decreased aerobic power. The long-term responses to exercising at increased altitudes are lowered body mass and decreased aerobic power.

Joint Structure and Classification

Each joint in the body is anatomically different from any other joint in terms of the articulating surfaces and the movement allowed at each type of joint. The shape of the joint and the muscles that cross the joint determine what movements are allowed there. Each joint is stabilized to a certain degree by the ligaments that connect the bones.

Head and face

Bony anatomy of the head and face: frontal, parietal, temporal, occipital, sphenoid, ethmoid, maxilla, mandible, orbit, palatine, lacrimal, zygomatic, nasal

The bones of the skull are considered suture joints; these joints close by the age of 18 months and do not allow movement thereafter. The only movement allowed between any of the bones of the face comes at the temporomandibular joint (discussed below). The nose and the ears themselves are made of cartilage and are not osseus.

Cervical spine

Bony anatomy of the cervical spine: atlas, occipital (also in head and face), seven cervical vertebrae

The atlantooccipital (A-O) joint is a plane joint allowing the glide motions of flexion/extension and side-bending. The anterior longitudinal, posterior longitudinal, and alar ligaments and the ligamentum flavum provide support to the A-O joint. The atlantoaxial joint is a pivot joint allowing upper cervical rotation. Ligamentous support is from the cruciform ligament. The A-O and atlantoaxial joints together are responsible for capital flexion, extension, side-bending, and cervical rotation. The facet joints of the cervical spine are plane joints allowing slight gliding motion in the sagittal plane of flexion/extension. The motions of cervical side-bending and rotation are coupled, meaning they occur together but in opposite directions. Cervical vertebral ligamentous stability comes from the anterior longitudinal, posterior longitudinal, supraspinal, and interspinal ligaments, and the ligamentum flavum continuing down from the A-O joint. Between every two vertebrae of the cervical, thoracic, and lumbar spine is an intervertebral disc. The center of the disc is the "shock absorber" and the outside of the disc maintains the disc's shape.

Thoracic spine and ribs

Bony anatomy of the spine and ribs: 12 thoracic vertebrae and 12 ribs

The thoracic spine has articulations between every two vertebrae (intervertebral) as well as between the facets (zygapophysial) similar to the cervical spine. Ten ribs articulate with the thoracic spine at two joints: the costovertebral and costotransverse. The 11th and 12th ribs are considered "floating" and do not articulate with the sternum. The radiate ligament stabilizes the costovertebral articulation, and the intertransverse ligaments stabilize the costotransverse joint. The structure of the thoracic joint is a tighter capsule and an overlap of the downward-angled spinous processes on the vertebral bodies. This allows less segmental movement than the cervical or lumbar spine. The intervertebral joints allow flexion/extension and side-bending, but the facet joints greatly limit this motion due to their interarticulations. Rotation also occurs in the thoracic spine. Ligamentous support of the intervertebral vertebrae comes from the ligamentum flavum, anterior/posterior longitudinal, interspinous, supraspinous, and intertransverse ligaments.

Lumbar spine

Bony anatomy of the lumbar spine: five lumbar vertebrae

Like the cervical and thoracic spine, the lumbar spine has intervertebral and zygapophysial articulations. The facets are oriented sagittally, allowing a greater amount of flexion and extension than the thoracic spine. Side-bending and rotation are also allowed but not as readily. These two motions are also coupled but occur in the same direction in the lumbar spine. Major ligaments of the lumbar spine are the iliolumbar, anterior/posterior longitudinal, supraspinous, interspinous, intertransverse, and ligamentum flavum.

Sacrum and pelvis

Bony anatomy of the sacrum and pelvis: sacrum of the spine and pelvis

The sacrum and the pelvis articulate at the sacroiliac joint and along the anterior surface of the sacrum down to the inferior lateral angle. The sacroiliac joint is also a plane joint, allowing nutation/counternutation at that joint. The sacrum itself can also be rotated or have a torsion in an abnormal state. The long and short posterior sacroiliac, posterior interosseous, anterior sacroiliac, sacrotuberous, sacrospinous, and iliolumbar ligaments give the sacroiliac joint stability. The right and left sides of the pelvis have an articulation anteriorly at the pubic symphysis, but joint motion does not regularly occur here. It is a cartilaginous joint that allows separation for childbirth and can be asymmetrical in a pelvic rotation. The sacralcoccygeal joint where the spine adjoins with the tailbone is also a fused joint where no movement occurs.

Temporomandibular joint (TMJ)

Bony anatomy of the TMJ: mandible and maxilla (also in the face/skull), 32 permanent teeth

The TMJ is a hinge joint that allows flexion/extension to open and close the mouth. It is also a plane joint that allows lateral deviation and protrusion/retrusion of the jaw. There is an articular disc between the mandible and the maxilla. Stability of the TMJ comes from the temporomandibular, sphenomandibular, and stylomandibular ligaments.

Shoulder

Bony anatomy of the shoulder: humerus, scapula, clavicle, sternum, seven ribs

The glenohumeral joint of the shoulder is a ball-and-socket synovial joint that allows motions in all cardinal planes and between planes. It is further deepened with the glenoid labrum that adds stability to the joint. Ligamentous support of the glenohumeral joint is extensive and includes the following: the superior, inferior, and middle glenohumeral; coracohumeral; coracoacromial; and transverse humeral ligaments. Flexion/extension, abduction/adduction, and horizontal abduction/horizontal adduction are the cardinal motions. The shoulder also allows scaption, internal and external rotation, and circumduction.

The sternoclavicular (SC) joint is a plane synovial joint also considered a saddle joint with an articulating disc. Motion at the SC joint includes elevation/depression and protraction/retraction. The anterior and posterior sternoclavicular, interclavicular, and costoclavicular ligaments are what stabilize this joint.

The acromioclavicular (AC) joint is also a plane synovial joint with an articular disc. Stability of this joint comes from the AC and coracoclavicular ligaments. The AC joint allows upward/downward rotation, elevation/depression, and abduction/adduction of the scapula.

The scapulothoracic joint does not have a joint classification but allows movement of the scapula, which is necessary for movement at the glenohumeral joint. Scapular motions include the following: elevation/depression, abduction/adduction, upward/downward rotation, tilting, and winging.

Elbow

Bony anatomy of the elbow: humerus, radius, ulna

The elbow is actually made up of a group of joints: the humeroulnar, radiohumeral, and superior/inferior radioulnar joints. The articulations with the humerus are considered synovial hinge joints and allow flexion/extension. The radiohumeral joint also participates in pronation/supination. The ulnar collateral and radial collateral ligaments stabilize against varus and valgus stress at the elbow. The superior radioulnar joint is a synovial pivot joint that allows forearm pronation/supination. This joint is supported by the annular ligament and the interosseus membrane, both of which connect the radius and the ulna.

Wrist and hand

Bony anatomy of the wrist and hand: radius, ulna, scaphoid, lunate, triquetrum, trapezium, trapezoid, capitate, hamate, pisiform, metacarpals, phalanges

The radiocarpal joint is classified as a condyloid joint with a disc. It allows flexion/extension and radial/ulnar deviation. The distal radioulnar joint is a pivot joint that moves with the proximal radioulnar joint to allow pronation/supination. Stability for all of the joints of the wrist is from the dorsal and palmar ligaments and the continuation of the interosseus membrane. The midcarpal joints are between the two rows of carpal bones but are not classified as the others. Together the joints work as a saddle joint, allowing slight flexion/extension and deviation. The carpometacarpal (CMC) joints of the fingers are plane joints that allow only glide motions that are important for grip and making a fist. The metacarpal-phalange (MCP) joints are also condyloid joints and allow flexion/extension and abduction/adduction. The proximal and distal interphalangeal (IP) joints are hinge joints and each allows only flexion/extension. The base of the thumb itself (carpometacarpal) is a saddle joint and allows flexion/extension, abduction/adduction, circumduction, and rotation. The MCP and IP joints of the thumb are similar to those of the other fingers in that they are condyloid joints, allowing primarily flexion/extension. The thumb and fingers together allow the motion of opposition as well.

Hip

Bony anatomy of the hip: pelvis, femur

The hip is a ball-and-socket joint that is further deepened by a labrum similar to the shoulder. However, it does not allow as much motion as the shoulder. Motion occurs in flexion/extension, abduction/adduction, and internal/external rotation. The stability of the hip comes from the muscles and joint capsule that hold it in place. Ligamentous support comes from the iliofemoral, the ischiofemoral, and the pubofemoral ligaments.

Knee

Bony anatomy of the knee: femur, patella, tibia, fibula

The tibiofemoral portion of the knee is a condyloid joint allowing flexion/extension, and at the end range of extension there is rotation. The patellofemoral joint is a plane joint and can move superiorly/inferiorly and medially/laterally, rotate, and tilt in the femoral groove. The proximal tibia-fibula joint is also a plane joint but only has motion with ankle mobility versus the knee. Ligamentous stability of the knee comes from the medial and lateral collateral ligaments that prevent excessive varus and valgus motion, and from the anterior and posterior cruciate ligaments that cross to prevent excessive anterior or posterior translation of the tibia on the femur. There are two menisci (medial and lateral) that cushion the weight-bearing pressures between the tibia and the femur. The medial collateral ligament does have fibers that adjoin to the medial meniscus and the medial portion of the joint capsule.

Ankle and foot

Bony anatomy of the ankle and foot: tibia, fibula, talus, calcaneus, navicular, cuboid, cuneiforms, metatarsals, phalanges

The ankle itself is actually comprised of multiple articulating joints that contribute to the multiple planes of motion necessary for mobility. The distal tibiofibular (tib-fib) joint is a syndesmosis joint without movement, and the proximal tib-fib is a plane joint that allows slight superior/inferior glide and rotation during ankle motion. The anterior and posterior tib-fib, the inferior transverse, and the interosseus ligaments stabilize the tib-fib joints. The talocrural joint is a hinge joint that allows dorsiflexion and plantar flexion. Ligamentous support comes from the anterior talofibular, posterior talofibular, calcaneofibular, and deltoid ligaments at the talocrural joint. Below the talocrural joint is the plane subtalar joint that allows inversion/eversion. The lateral and medial talocalcaneal ligaments give connective-tissue support to the subtalar joint. The midtarsal joint is actually two joints: the talonavicular and calcaneocuboid, making up the midfoot. Both joints are concave-convex articulations, and collectively they allow inversion/eversion of the midfoot. The tarsometatarsal (TMT) and metatarsophalangeal (MTP) joints make up the forefoot. The TMTs are plane joints that allow flexion/extension and rotation. The MTPs, similar to the fingers, are condyloid joints allowing flexion/extension and abduction/adduction. The IP joints of the toes are hinge joints allowing just flexion/extension. Significant ligaments of the midfoot, forefoot, and toes include the calcaneonavicular ligament (or spring ligament) medially and the long plantar ligament.

Pharmacology

The effects of medication or drug therapy must always be considered in the evaluation and treatment of musculoskeletal disorders. Different drugs can have adverse or valuable effects on the rehabilitation process, depending on how and when the drugs are used. Below is a list of common drugs prescribed for musculoskeletal system impairments.

Analgesics

As their name indicates, **analgesics** are used for pain control. These drugs are further divided into opioids and non-opioids.

Opioids are used to relieve the more severe, unrelenting pain of chronic syndromes, cancer, and surgeries. Drowsiness and gastrointestinal (GI) upset are the most common adverse side effects of these drugs. Opioids can also be dangerous because of their ability to cause physical dependence. Morphine, fentanyl, methadone, meperidine, propoxyphene, hydrocodone, oxycodone, and tramadol are examples of analgesic opioids.

Non-opioids are more commonly used for pain relief of musculoskeletal injuries and also have anti-inflammatory benefits. Physical dependence is not an issue with non-opioid analgesics. Non-opioids are cyclooxygenase (COX) inhibitors, working to prevent the formation and release of prostaglandin, a hormone that is responsible for the pain and inflammation that often accompany injury. Long-term use of nonsteroidal anti-inflammatory drugs (NSAIDs) can cause GI upset, drowsiness, dizziness, and possible fluid retention. Some commonly used non-opioid analgesics are acetaminophen, aspirin, diclofenac, nabumetone, ibuprofen, naproxen, meloxicam, celecoxib, and valdecoxib.

Glucocorticoids

Glucocorticoids are most commonly used for their anti-inflammatory effects. They can be either systemic or locally topical. The benefits of fighting inflammation are obvious, but there can also be long-term adverse effects. Prolonged use of glucocorticoids can cause bone loss to the point of osteoporosis, muscle loss that causes weakness, connective tissue breakdown, high blood pressure, cataracts, and poor control of blood glucose. Glucocorticoids break down tissues such as muscle, tendon, and bone. Patients who are under long-term glucocorticoid drug therapy may have increased risk for injury to tissue and skin breakdown. Generic names of glucocorticoids include: cortisone, hydrocortisone, betamethasone, methylprednisolone, dexamethasone, prednisolone, prednisone, and cortisol.

Muscle relaxers

Muscle relaxers are commonly used to treat spastic conditions or to allow pain relief through relief of muscle spasms that result from injury or disease. The benefits of muscle relaxers are huge for patients with spasticity that is central in origin because the relaxers allow muscles that are always in a contracted state to relax, to unclench. Clinically, muscle relaxers can be used in conjunction with functional training and range-of-motion activity. Obvious adverse side effects of muscle relaxers include drowsiness, weakness, and CNS depression which may possibly cause motor impairment. Baclofen, diazepam, cyclobenzaprine, metaxalone, and tizanidine are generic names of common muscle relaxers.

Anesthetics

Anesthetics are used for pain management/relief, most typically related to surgical intervention. Epidurals and spinal nerve blocks are also used as anesthetics to block the pain pathway. Additionally, anesthetics may allow the patient functional improvements in mobility and range of motion that are otherwise limited by pain. The adverse effects of anesthetics can include the complete shutdown of the CNS or cardiovascular systems. Procaine, lidocaine, bupivacaine, etidocaine, prilocaine, and ropivacaine are all examples of anesthetic drugs.

Glucosamine and chondroitin sulfate

Glucosamine and chondroitin sulfate are supplements that are thought to help decrease the joint degeneration associated with osteoarthritis. Both are components of naturally made synovial fluid. There is conflicting information on the true benefits of these supplements and on appropriate dosage levels.

EVALUATION

While you are examining a patient, it is important for you to make decisions on what tests and measures are appropriate and will give you a good list of differential diagnoses in order to treat the injury or disability. Again, during the examination process the patient must be viewed as a whole. The examination may take place in a hospital room, a home setting, an outpatient setting, or a long- or short-term care facility. In all cases, each part of the examination process must be considered, although some portions of the examination are more appropriate for certain settings (i.e., special tests may be more appropriate in an outpatient setting, mobility evaluation may be more appropriate in a home setting, etc.).

Patient Interview

These questions are designed to elicit the details about the patient's chief complaint and its possible origin. Some of this information may be found on the patient questionnaire.

- What is the history of the present illness or injury, including surgical history and when the surgery(ies) occurred?
- What is the patient's occupation/social history/support system?
- What is the mechanism of the injury or trauma?
- What is the description of the pain, if there is pain: location (specific location or general area), intensity (visual analog scale, numerical scale), type (dull, sharp, burning, throbbing, etc.), constant or intermittent, duration, improving or worsening symptoms?
- What are aggravating or alleviating activities (time of day, sleep disturbance, activities of daily living, recreational activities, occupational activities)?
- What are the functional limitations (i.e., what activities cannot be done due to the pain/injury/dysfunction)?
- Is there any significant past medical history or related familial history?
- Are there any changes in sensation?
- Are there any joint abnormalities: clicking, popping, locking, grinding, giving out, or instability?
- Has there been any swelling, discoloration, or abnormal skin reaction(s)?
- Has there been any other recent medical testing, radiologic workup, or blood work?
- Is there any contributing pharmacology?
- Are there any "red flag" concerns, including indications of symptoms related to other systems (fever, malaise, change in bowel/bladder habits, weight loss/gain, nausea, etc.)?

Postural Assessment

Correct posture requires the least amount of muscle activity to maintain. Poor posture causes strain on the muscles because of increased and prolonged activation. Poor posture over a prolonged time can also have effects on the skeletal system and connective tissues. For postural assessment, male patients should be wearing only shorts, and female patients should wear shorts and bras; preferably, neither should wear shoes or socks.

In Standing Patient, Anterior View

	Normal	Abnormal
Feet	• Angled slightly outward • Arches present • Malleoli level • Ankles nearly touching	• Pigeon-toed (medial tibial torsion) • Duck-footed (excessive lateral tibial torsion • Pes planus/pes cavus
Knees/ lower leg	• Fibular heads level • Patella facing forward • Inferior patellar poles level • Knees slightly apart (two fingers' width)	• Frog-eyes patella (faces outward) or squinting patella (faces inward) • Genu varum/genu valgum • Bowing of the bone

In Standing Patient, Anterior View

	Normal	Abnormal
Hips/pelvis	• Pubis symphysis level • ASIS level • Iliac crest level	• Pelvic asymmetry (leg-length discrepancy, pelvic rotation, up-slip, torsion, or flare)
Upper extremities	• Arms hang equally from trunk • Carrying angle of the elbow 5–15° • Symmetrical clavicles and shoulders (dominant side may be slightly lower)	• Asymmetry in upper extremities
Trunk	• Rib cage symmetrical	• Protrusion or asymmetry of rib cage or sternum
Head	• Head is at midline • Nose lines up with sternum and umbilicus • Jaw and lips together, teeth slightly apart, tongue at back of top teeth	• Head tilted/rotated (torticollis) • Asymmetry at the jaw line

In Standing Patient, Lateral View

	Normal	Abnormal
Head	• Earlobe aligns with acromion and iliac crest	• Forward head
Trunk/upper extremities	• Cervical lordosis • Thoracic kyphosis • Lumbar lordosis • Shoulders aligned with earlobe and iliac crest • Pelvic cavity tipped slightly anterior (PSIS above ASIS)	• Excessive lordosis or kyphosis at any segment • Flattened spinal curves • Rounded (protruded) shoulders • Prominence or depression of the sternum • Excessive pelvic rotation (anterior or posterior)
Lower extremities	• Knees slightly flexed	• Genu recurvatum • Excessive knee flexion

In Standing Patient, Posterior View

	Normal	Abnormal
Feet	• Heels straight • Achilles straight	• Rear-foot varus/valgus • Angled Achilles (pes planus)
Knees	• Popliteal creases level	• Creases uneven (tibial length difference) • Bowing of the femur
Hips/Pelvis	• Gluteal folds level • PSIS level	• Pelvic asymmetry (leg-length discrepancy, pelvic rotation, up-slip, torsion, or flare)
Trunk	• Spine straight • Ribs symmetrical	• Lateral spinal curve (scoliosis)
Upper extremities	• Arms hang equally from trunk • Shoulders and scapulae symmetrical (dominant may be slightly inferior)	• Scapular winging, positional or size differences
Head	• At midline	• Side-bent or rotated

In sitting

Observation of front-to-back or left-to-right asymmetry is done the same as in a standing patient. Particularly, comparison of the pelvis (iliac crests and PSIS) should be made, as this may rule in or rule out leg-length discrepancy. Note any differences from observations in the standing position.

In supine or prone

Again, observe for asymmetry and compare landmarks of the pelvis, noting any differences compared to other positions.

Movement Analysis of Gait

One of the first things to observe in evaluating a patient is gait. Evaluation of gait can be divided into phases, based on the position of the limb as open-chain or closed-chain. With each portion of each phase, different forces and counterforces act at each of the weight-bearing joints.

Stance phase (closed chain)

The **stance phase** (closed chain) of gait is movement from heel strike, to foot flat, to mid-stance, to heel-off, to toe-off. This makes up 60 percent of the gait cycle in walking and 40 percent in running.

Step length

Step length is the distance from the heel strike of one foot to the heel strike of the opposite foot during midstance. (Normal: 35–41 cm)

Stride length

Stride length is the distance that one foot travels during one gait cycle (measured from the heel strike of one foot to the heel strike of the same foot). (Normal: 70–82 cm)

Base width

Base width is the distance between the heels of the feet in standing or during gait. (Normal: 5–10 cm)

Cadence

Cadence is the number of steps per minute. (Normal: 90–120)

Swing phase (open chain)

The **swing phase** (open chain) is movement from acceleration through midswing through deceleration. This accounts for 40 percent of the cycle in walking and 30 percent in running (the remaining 30 percent in running is divided into two 15 percent "float" phases).

Lateral shift

Lateral shift is the lateral movement of the pelvis during gait to maintain a balance over the center of gravity. (Normal: 2.5–5 cm)

Vertical shift

Vertical shift is the vertical movement of the pelvis during gait, measured from the center of gravity at two inches anterior to S2. (Normal: <5 cm oscillation)

Pelvic rotation

Pelvic rotation is the degree of forward rotation needed at the pelvis to advance the same-side lower extremity during swing phase. (Normal: 40°)

Phases of gait in a normal pattern

In a normal gait pattern, each joint moves through a specific range of motion and calls upon the work of a specific pattern of muscle interaction in order to propel the body ahead. Specific muscle and joint actions occur at each division of the stance and swing phases.

Stance phase (five phases)

- **Heel strike** occurs as the heel of the foot comes into contact with the ground and the involved leg begins weight acceptance.
- **Foot flat** occurs when the entire foot first comes into full contact with the ground.
- **Midstance** occurs when the entire foot is in contact with the ground, full weight is through the loaded leg, and the opposite leg is in swing.
- **Heel-off** occurs when the heel begins to lift off the ground and the weight shifts forward on the foot.
- **Toe-off** occurs when the great toe is in maximum extension and begins to push off to begin swing phase.

Joint and Muscle Activity at Each Stance Phase of Gait

	Joint Position	Muscle Activation	Possible Dysfunctions
Heel strike	• Rear foot everted • Foot supinated • Ankle dorsiflexed • Tibia laterally rotated • Knee extended • Hip flexed	• Tibialis anterior • EDL/EHL • Quadriceps • Gluteus maximus • Hamstrings	• Heel pain with contact • Knee instability if weak or unable to flex (buckling or locked extension) • Patellofemoral pain can inhibit the lateral tibial rotation
Foot flat	• Rear foot inverted • Foot supinated • Ankle plantar flexed • Tibia medially rotated • Knee 20° flexed • Hip extending to neutral	• Tibialis posterior • FHL/FDL • Quadriceps • Gluteus maximus • Hamstrings	• Weak dorsiflexors (foot slap) • Knee instability if weak or unable to flex (buckling or forced extension)
Midstance	• Foot/tibia neutral • Ankle slightly dorsiflexed • Knee 15° flexed • Hip extended	• Gastrocsoleus • Peroneals • Quadriceps (less) • Gluteus medius • Iliopsoas	• Painful joints decrease stance time (arthrogenic gait) • Patellofemoral pain preventing 15° knee flexion • Gluteus medius weak (Trendelenburg) • Gluteus maximus weakness causing extensor lurch • Plantar flexion weakness causing decreased step length contralateral, decreased stance time same leg, and decreased cadence
Heel-off	• Foot supinated • Ankle 15° dorsiflexed • Tibia neutral • Knee 5° flexed • Hip extended	• Gastrocsoleus • Peroneals • Iliopsoas	• Limited ankle dorsiflexion ROM causing compensation proximally • Gastrocsoleus weakness causing decreased push-off

	Joint Position	Muscle Activation	Possible Dysfunctions
Toe-off	• Foot supinated • Ankle plantar flexed • Tibia neutral • Knee 30° flexed • Hip extended	• FHL • Gastrocsoleus • Peroneals • Quadriceps • Hip adductors • Iliopsoas	• Pain/arthritis in the great toe, limiting extension ("turf toe")

Swing phase (three phases)

- **Initial swing** occurs as the foot leaves the ground and accelerates into the swing.
- **Midswing** occurs as the foot clears the ground.
- **Terminal swing** occurs as the foot/leg decelerates the swing and prepares for the heel-strike phase of stance.

Joint and Muscle Activity at Each Stance Phase of Gait

	Joint Position	Muscle Activation	Possible Dysfunctions
Initial swing	• Foot supinated • Ankle dorsiflexed • Knee 65° flexed • Hip moving to flexion • Pelvis dropped	• Tibialis anterior • Hamstrings • Quadriceps (as hip flexors)	• Forced forward pelvic rotation to compensate for quad weakness
Midswing	• Foot supinated • Ankle 20° dorsiflexed • Knee flexion • Hip flexion • Pelvis dropped	• Tibialis anterior • Hamstrings • Quadriceps (as hip flexors)	• Dorsiflexor weakness causing toe drag, requiring excessive hip flexion needed to clear foot (steppage gait) • Inability to flex knee to swing, causing a vaulting gait • Limited hip ROM, requiring compensatory knee or lumbar motion
Terminal swing	• Foot supinated • Ankle dorsiflexed neutral • Tibia laterally rotated • Knee extending • Hip flexion	• Tibialis anterior • Hamstrings	• Hamstring weakness preventing eccentric control of extension to heel strike (callus on heel or forced knee hyperextension)

In a normal gait pattern there should be reciprocal arm swing. The trunk and upper extremity should rotate opposite the pelvis and lower extremity. Step length and stance phase time should be equal bilaterally. There should be normal base of support, unrestricted joint motion, and appropriate muscular concentric and eccentric contraction as discussed above.

Specific abnormalities of gait

There are some specific abnormalities of gait that have characteristic deviations from the normal patterns discussed above.

Peripheral neuropathy

Peripheral neuropathy can cause the need for a wider base of support and for visual assistance to help add stability.

Joint fusions

Joint fusions at any lower-extremity joint cause obvious problems with the affected joint as well as compensatory requirements of surrounding joints.

Pain

Antalgic gait is any gait that is abnormal due to pain. It can affect stance time, step length, and cadence. The arm swing may also be abnormal to help keep the weight off the involved limb.

Trendelenburg gait

Trendelenburg gait occurs when there is an abnormal lateral pelvic shift during gait. It is often due to weakness in the gluteus medius.

Ataxia

Ataxia describes an exaggerated, jerky, and unbalanced gait that is usually due to cerebellar or other CNS dysfunction.

Equinus gait

Equinus gait (toe walking) refers to the tendency to avoid heel strike and to keep the weight more forward on the balls of the feet at all times. This is common in children with clubfoot or cerebral palsy.

Circumduction

Circumduction occurs when the foot/leg is unable to clear the ground during the swing phase of gait. This can be due to muscle weakness or joint restriction, or from a neurogenic cause such as a stroke or paralysis.

Parkinsonian gait

Parkinsonian gait is characterized by short, shuffling steps and a flexed joint posture. Arm swing is nearly absent.

Psoatic limp

Psoatic limp is characterized by external rotation, flexion, and adduction of the hip causing difficulty with advancing the involved leg.

Scissoring

Scissoring occurs when the lower extremities are unable to maintain the normal base width and instead begin to cross over the center line. It can be seen in individuals with cerebral palsy or paraplegia.

Palpation of Structures

Palpation can be used to isolate or pinpoint areas of patient complaint. Palpation can be used to detect tissue continuity/discontinuity, atrophy, tension, inflammatory response, and/or abnormal joint mechanics. Palpation should include soft-tissue, joint, and skin examination. Crepitus or audible clicking in a joint can be attributed to nonpathologic tendon movement, abrasive rubbing on a tendon or articular cartilage, internal derangement, or meniscal tears. Crepitus is more concerning when other symptoms are present and are progressing coincident with it.

Movement Analysis of Joint Range of Motion

Range of motion is assessed both actively and passively to assess differences in quality and amount of motion and the presence of pain. Active range of motion (AROM) evaluates joint mechanics, contractile tissue, and gliding of neural tissue. Special observation should be made during AROM to look for substitution patterns that compensate for lack of available motion. Also note any painful or problematic arc of motion. Depending on the patient's history, the motions may be either sustained or repeated to simulate the pain-provoking action. Passive range of motion (PROM) better evaluates noncontractile tissue as well as joint mechanics and neural tissue. The examiner should note any differences left to right, any pain, any abnormalities, and the end feel. Generally, contractile tissue is not painful during PROM, and noncontractile tissue involvement is not painful during AROM. Painful ROM assessment can indicate acute injury, whereas limited ROM may indicate a more chronic problem. Generally, the dominant arm shows a lesser ROM than the nondominant arm. During ROM assessment of any particular joint, it is always important to do a quick motion assessment of the surrounding joints as well. It is possible that a ROM deficit at one joint can affect the motion of a distal or proximal joint or cause substitution patterns there as well.

Contraindications to examining range of motion on a patient include the following:

- Movement of the joint near a healing fracture
- Recent surgical history to the involved joint with necessary healing restrictions
- Movement of a joint involved in an acute injury with signs of active bleeding or instability

The table below lists normal ROMs; these should be considered averages.

Normal Range of Motion Measures

Upper cervical:	
Head nodding	0 to 15–20°
Head side-bending	0 to 10°
Cervical:	
Flexion	0 to 90°
Extension	0 to 70°
Side-bending (side flexion)	0 to 20–45°
Rotation	0 to 75–90°
Thoracic/lumbar:	
Flexion	0 to 80°
Extension	0 to 25°
Side-bending	0 to 35°
Rotation	0 to 45°

Shoulder:	
Flexion	0 to 170°
Extension	0 to 50°
Abduction	0 to 180°
Scaption	0 to 170°
External rotation	0 to 90°
Internal rotation	0 to 70°
Adduction	0–50°
Elbow:	
Flexion	0 to 150°
Extension	0°
Pronation	0 to 80°
Supination	0 to 80°
Wrist:	
Flexion	0 to 80°
Extension	0 to 70°
Radial deviation	0 to 20°
Ulnar deviation	0 to 30°
Fingers:	
MCP flexion	0 to 90°
MCP extension	0 to 45°
PIP flexion	0 to 100°
DIP flexion	0 to 90°
DIP extension	0 to 10°
Thumb CMC abduction	0 to 70°
Thumb MCP flexion	0 to 50 °
Thumb DIP flexion	0 to 80°
Hip:	
Flexion	0 to 120°
Extension	0 to 30°
Abduction	0 to 40°
Adduction	0 to 30°
Internal rotation	0 to 45°
External rotation	0 to 45°
Knee:	
Flexion	0 to 140°
Hyperextension	0 to 10°
Ankle:	
Dorsiflexion	0 to 20°
Plantar flexion	0 to 50°
Forefoot inversion	0 to 35°
Forefoot eversion	0 to 15°
Rear-foot inversion	0 to 5°
Rear-foot eversion	0 to 5°

Hypomobility, or decreased ROM, can result from soft-tissue tightness, capsular tightness, or joint tightness. This can be further diagnosed with assessment of physiologic versus accessory joint limitations. **Hypermobility**, or excessive ROM, can result from trauma to supportive soft tissue (muscle injury or ligament sprain) or the capsule, "creep" from surrounding joint hypomobility, or poor muscle control. Many times, hypomobility and hypermobility exist together as part of a total joint impairment. **Instability** is a more severe type of hypermobility in which the supporting structures are no longer intact. This includes muscular, ligamentous, and capsular tears or avulsions.

Strength Measures of the Musculoskeletal System

Muscle strength testing can be done either manually or with a dynamometer. Most commonly, manual muscle testing (MMT) is done to evaluate strength and integrity of contractile tissues. It is typically done in mid-range to best evaluate a particular muscle's maximum force. Muscle testing is an isometric hold against resistance that is maintained for three to five seconds. Special consideration is taken to alter MMT positions if further evaluation of a particular muscle is needed, based on the patient's complaints of pain or weakness with a particular movement or activity. During MMT, any weakness in a myotomal pattern should be noted as well (see chapter 5, Nervous System).

Muscle testing is graded as defined in the table below:

Muscle Testing*

Grade 5	Completes full ROM against gravity, holds against maximum resistance
Grade 4	Completes full ROM against gravity, breaks against maximum resistance
Grade 3+	Completes full ROM against gravity, holds against minimal resistance
Grade 3	Completes full ROM against gravity, does not tolerate any resistance
Grade 2	Completes full ROM in a gravity-eliminated position
Grade 2–	Completes partial ROM in a gravity-eliminated position
Grade 1	Muscle contraction elicited but no movement
Grade 0	No muscle contraction

**Strength testing may be modified to alternate positions if the patient cannot move through full ROM against gravity (those below a grade 3). See current muscle-testing manuals or texts.*

Major muscle action and primary movers are:

Muscle Action, Primary Movers, and Primary Nerve Supplies*

Muscle Action	Primary Movers	Primary Nerve Supply
Eyeball elevation	Superior rectus	Cranial nerve III
Eyeball depression	Inferior rectus	Cranial nerve III
Eyeball adduction	Medial rectus	Cranial nerve III
Eyeball abduction	Lateral rectus	Cranial nerve VI
Eyeball lateral rotation	Superior oblique	Cranial nerve IV
Eyeball medial rotation	Inferior oblique	Cranial nerve III

Muscle Action	Primary Movers	Primary Nerve Supply
Eyelid opening	Levator palpebrae	Cranial nerve III
Eyelid closing	Orbicularis oculi	Cranial nerve VII
Wrinkling bridge of nose	Procerus	Cranial nerve VII
Elevates eyebrows	Frontalis	Cranial nerve VII
Furrows/frowns eyebrows	Corrugator	Cranial nerve VII
Closes/puckers mouth	Orbicularis oris	Cranial nerve VII
Smiles mouth	Zygomaticus	Cranial nerve VII
Frowns mouth	Depressor anguli	Cranial nerve VII
Sucks in/blows out cheeks	Buccinator	Cranial nerve VII
Protrudes lower lip	Mentalis	Cranial nerve VII
Jaw opening	Lateral pterygoid, suprahyoid	Cranial nerve V
Jaw closing	Masseter, temporalis, medial pterygoid	Cranial nerve V
Jaw lateral deviation	Medial and lateral pterygoids	Cranial nerve V
Jaw protrusion	Medial and lateral pterygoids	Cranial nerve V
Capital extension	Rectus capitis posterior major/minor, longissimus capitis, obliquus capitis superior/inferior, splenius capitis, semispinalis capitis	C4-C6
Capital flexion	Rectus capitis anterior/lateralis, longus capitis	C1-C3
Capital rotation	Trapezius (opposite side), splenius capitis, longissimus capitis, semispinalis capitis, obliquus capitis inferior, sternocleidomastoid (opposite side)	C3-C4
Cervical extension	Longissimus cervicis, semispinalis cervicis, iliocostalis cervicis, splenius cervicis	C6-C8
Cervical flexion	Anterior, middle, posterior scalenes, sternocleidomastoid	C2-C6

Muscle Action	Primary Movers	Primary Nerve Supply
Cervical side-bending	Levator scapula, splenius cervicis, iliocostalis cervicis, longissimus cervicis, semispinalis cervicis, multifidus, intertransversarii, scalenes, sternocleidomastoid, oblique capitis, rotators	C3-C4
Cervical rotation	Same as cervical side-bending, causing rotation to the same side	C1
Thoracic extension	Iliocostalis thoracis, longissimus thoracis, spinalis thoracis, semispinalis thoracis, multifidus, rotators	T1-T12
Lumbar extension	Iliocostalis lumborum, multifidus, rotators	L1-L5
Lumbar flexion	Rectus abdominis, internal/external obliques, psoas major/minor	T7-T12, L1-L5
Trunk rotation/side-bending (coupled)	Iliocostalis thoracis, longissimus thoracis, intertransverse, internal/external obliques, semispinalis, multifidus, rotators, transverse abdominis	T7-T12, L1-L5
Inspiration	Diaphragm, intercostals	C4
Expiration	External/internal obliques, transverse abdominis, rectus abdominis, intercostals	T7-T12
Shoulder flexion	Deltoid, supraspinatus, pectoralis, coracobrachialis, biceps	C5-C7
Shoulder abduction	Deltoid, supraspinatus, infraspinatus, subscapularis, teres minor, biceps (if externally rotated)	C5-C7
Shoulder adduction	Pectoralis major, latissimus dorsi, teres major, subscapularis	C5-C8
Shoulder extension	Deltoid, teres major and minor, latissimus dorsi, triceps	C5-C8
Shoulder scaption	Deltoid, supraspinatus	C5-C6
Shoulder horizontal adduction	Pectoralis, deltoid (anterior)	C5-C6
Shoulder horizontal abduction	Deltoid (posterior), teres major and minor, infraspinatus	C5-C6

Muscle Action	Primary Movers	Primary Nerve Supply
Shoulder internal rotation	Subscapularis (in neutral), pectoralis major, deltoid (anterior), latissimus dorsi, teres major	C5-C6
Shoulder external rotation	Infraspinatus, teres minor, deltoid (posterior)	C5-C6
Scapular elevation	Trapezius, levator scapula, rhomboids	CN XI, C3-C5
Scapular depression	Serratus anterior, pectoralis major and minor, latissimus dorsi, lower trapezius	CN XI, C5-T1
Scapular protraction	Serratus anterior, pectoralis major, pectoralis major, latissimus dorsi	C5-T1
Scapular retraction	Trapezius, rhomboids	CN XI, C5
Scapular upward rotation	Upper and lower trapezius, serratus anterior	CN XI, C3-C6
Scapular downward rotation	Levator scapula, rhomboids, pectoralis minor	C3-C5
Elbow flexion	Brachialis, biceps brachii, brachioradialis	C5-C8
Elbow extension	Triceps, anconeus	C7
Forearm supination	Supinator, biceps brachii	C5-C6
Forearm pronation	Pronator quadratus, pronator teres, flexor carpi radialis	C6-T1
Wrist flexion	Flexor carpi radialis, flexor carpi ulnaris	C7
Wrist extension	Extensor carpi radialis longus, extensor carpi radialis brevis, extensor carpi ulnaris	C6-C8
Finger MP flexion	Lumbricales, interossei	C8-T1
Finger PIP/DIP flexion	Flexor digitorum superficialis, flexor digitorum profundus	C8-T1
Finger MP extension	Extensor digitorum, extensor indicis, extensor digiti minimi	C6-C8
Finger abduction	Dorsal interossei, abductor digiti minimi	C8-T1
Finger adduction	Palmar interossei	C8-T1
Thumb MP/IP flexion	Flexor pollicis brevis, flexor pollicis longus	C8-T1

Muscle Action	Primary Movers	Primary Nerve Supply
Thumb MP/IP extension	Extensor pollicis brevis, extensor pollicis longus	C6-T1
Thumb abduction	Abductor pollicis longus, abductor pollicis brevis	C6-C7, C8-T1
Thumb adduction	Adductor pollicis	C8-T1
Opposition	Opponens pollicis, opponens digiti minimi	C8-T1
Hip flexion	Psoas major, iliacus, rectus femoris, sartorius, tensor fascia latae, adductors, pectineus	L2-L4
Hip extension	Gluteus maximus, semitendinosus, semimembranosus, biceps femoris	L5-S3
Hip abduction	Gluteus medius, gluteus minimus, tensor fascia latae (in flexion), gluteus maximus	L4-S2
Hip adduction	Adductor magnus, adductor brevis, adductor longus, pectineus, gracilis	L2-L4
Hip external rotation	Obturators, quadratus femoris, piriformis, gemelli	L5-S2
Hip internal rotation	Gluteus minimus/medius, tensor fascia latae	L4-S2
Knee flexion	Biceps femoris, semitendinosus, semitendinosus	L4-S2
Knee extension	Rectus femoris, vastus medialis/lateralis/intermedius	L2-L4
Ankle plantar flexion	Gastrocnemius, soleus (in flexion)	L4-S2
Ankle dorsiflexion	Tibialis anterior	L4-S1
Foot inversion	Tibialis posterior, flexor digitorum longus, flexor hallices longus, gastrocnemius	L4-S2
Foot eversion	Peroneus longus/brevis/tertius, extensor digitorum longus	L4-S1
Toe MP flexion	Lumbricales	L5-S2
Great-toe MP flexion	Flexor hallices longus, interossei, flexor digiti minimi, flexor digitorum longus/brevis	L5-S3

Muscle Action	Primary Movers	Primary Nerve Supply
Toe PIP flexion	Flexor digitorum brevis	L4-S1
Toe DIP flexion	Flexor digitorum longus	L5-S1
Great-toe IP flexion	Flexor hallices longus	L5-S2
Great-toe extension	Extensor digitorum brevis, extensor hallucis longus	L5-S1
Toe extension	Extensor digitorum longus/brevis	L4-S1

**For a complete description of muscle-testing positions at all grades, see your institution's current textbooks or those listed in the references.*

Myotomal patterns

During muscle testing, it is important to also take note of myotomal patterns that could indicate a neurologic impairment rather than pure musculoskeletal system involvement. Myotomes link muscle action to the appropriate dominant nerve root supply. Myotomal muscle testing must be held for at least five seconds to assess for weakness.

Myotomes

Nerve Root	Muscle Action
C1-2	Cervical flexion
C3	Cervical side-bending
C4	Shoulder elevation
C5	Shoulder abduction
C6	Elbow flexion and wrist extension
C7	Elbow extension and wrist flexion
C8	Thumb extension and ulnar deviation
T1	Hand intrinsics
L2	Hip flexion, hip adduction
L3	Knee extension
L4	Ankle dorsiflexion
L5	Ankle plantar flexion
S1	Ankle eversion

End Feels

During ROM evaluation and movement analysis of any movable joint, there is an end feel, or quality of end range of motion of that joint. There are normal and abnormal end feels of joint motion that can indicate or rule out pathology.

Normal end feels

- **Bone-to-bone limitations** are hard end feels limited by one bone preventing further movement of another bone.
- **Soft-tissue approximation** occurs when the ROM ends with a soft, spongy end feel. Further movement is prohibited by soft-tissue mass (muscle, fatty tissue, etc.).
- **Tissue stretch** is a progressive tightening that has some give to it—usually a stretch feel but not painful.

Abnormal end feels

- **Bony or hard end feel** occurs where there should not be a bone-restricting motion.
- **Capsular limitations** produce an end feel that is a strong tightness before the expected tissue stretch, limiting the ROM. The tightness usually comes on abruptly.
- **Muscle spasm** causes an abrupt end in ROM due to muscle contraction/spasm brought on by pain.
- **Empty end feel** occurs when there is no feeling at the end of ROM because the patient's pain stops the examiner from continuing through the range.
- **Springy end feel** occurs when there is a rebound, or spring, during the range of motion but not at the end.

Capsular Patterns

Capsular patterns are patterns of restriction of joint motion that indicate the cause is an adhered joint capsule. The table below lists capsular patterns of joints with fibrous capsules.

Capsular Patterns

Temporomandibular	Jaw opening
Cervical spine	Side flexion and rotation > extension
Glenohumeral	External rotation > internal rotation > abduction
Humeroulnar	Flexion > extension
Radiohumeral	Flexion > extension > supination > pronation
Proximal/superior radioulnar	Supination > pronation
Wrist	Flexion and extension equally
Fingers	Flexion and extension equally
Thumb	Abduction
Hip	Internal rotation > flexion and abduction
Knee	Flexion > extension
Ankle	Plantar flexion > dorsiflexion, inversion > eversion
Foot (MTP joint)	Extension > flexion

This table was adapted from page 33 of *Orthopedic Physical Assessment*, 5th Edition, by David Magee with permission. Copyright Elsevier (2007).

Joint Play Assessment

Joint play is the accessory motion within the joint that occurs with passive, isolated movement done by the examiner. It is not controlled by the patient's volitional movement but must occur *with* active movements for smooth joint motion. Abnormalities in joint play will cause abnormal active/passive joint motion. During assessment of joint play, the patient should be in a resting position (see table below). Assessment is done bilaterally to feel for similarities and differences. The assessor should note the direction of any hyper- or hypomobility or coincident pain. Joint play movements include side glides, anterior/posterior glides, superior/inferior glides, and traction/distraction, translation, and rotation accessory movements.

Resting (Loose-Packed) Joint Positions

Facet of the spine	Neutral
Temporomandibular	Jaw slightly opened
Glenohumeral	55° abduction in scapular plane
Sternoclavicular and acromioclavicular	Arm in neutral
Elbow	70° flexion, 10° supination
Wrist	Neutral
MCP/IP	Slight flexion
Hip	30° flexion, 30° abduction, 5° ER
Knee	25° flexion
Ankle	10° plantar flexion, neutral inversion/eversion
Subtalar/midtarsal	Neutral

This table adapted from page 55 of *Orthopedic Physical Assessment*, 5th Edition, by David Magee with permission. Copyright Elsevier (2007).

Joint play assessment of individual joints

Each individual joint has accessory joint motion that allows physiologic motion to take place with action of the muscles that cross that joint. If there is dysfunction in the accessory joint motion, the physiologic motion will be restricted.

Temporomandibular joint

Assess anterior/posterior glide and medial/lateral glide.

Cervical spine

Assess anterior/posterior glide, side glides, and rotation and traction of the cervical spine as a whole. Assess segmental motion with passive accessory intervertebral movements (PAIVMs), posterior-anterior unilateral vertebral pressures (PAUVPs), and transverse vertebral pressures (TVPs). During assessment of the accessory movements of the vertebrae, there should be a spring back of the vertebrae with the posterior-to-anterior mobilization done by the examiner. Either excessive or nonexistent movement could indicate hyper- or hypomobility of that cervical vertebral segment.

Thoracic spine
Assess posteroanterior central vertebral pressures (PACVPs), PAUVPs, and TVPs of each segment.

Lumbar spine
Assess PACVPs, PAUVPs, and TVPs of each vertebral segment. With the patient in side-lying position, assess the whole lumbar motion of flexion, extension, and side-bending.

Sacral spine and pelvis
Assess cephalad/caudal glides (nutation/counternutation), anterior/posterior movement of the ilium on the sacrum, and superior/inferior movement of the ilium on the sacrum.

Glenohumeral joint
Assess anterior/posterior glide, superior/inferior glide, rotation, joint distraction with long arm traction, and lateral distraction.

Sternoclavicular joint
Assess anterior/posterior glide and superior/inferior glide.

Acromioclavicular joint
Assess anterior/posterior glide and superior inferior glide.

Elbow
Assess anterior/posterior glide of the radial head, radial/ulnar deviation at the elbow, and distraction at 90° flexion.

Wrist
Assess anterior/posterior glide, side glide, distraction at the distal radioulnar/metacarpal joint, and anterior/posterior glides at the midcarpal joints. Assess anterior/posterior and side glides of the PIP and DIP joints of the fingers.

Hip
Assess long-leg traction, anterior/posterior glide, lateral distraction, and compression, and scour the hip joint.

Knee
Assess anterior/posterior glide of the tibia on the femur, side glides of the tibia on the femur, and anterior/posterior glide of the fibular head on the tibia. Assess patellar mobility with superior/inferior and medial/lateral glides.

Ankle
Assess anterior/posterior glides of all joints, talocrural traction, subtalar lateral tilt, and rotation of the midfoot and forefoot. Assess intertarsal rigidity as well.

Component motions

Component motions are motions that occur at surrounding joints to allow motion at the joint being evaluated. Component mobility must also be assessed to provide adequate information about necessary joint mobilizations to surrounding joint impairments. An example of component motion would be the gliding of the superior tibia-fibula joint during ankle dorsiflexion and plantar flexion.

Functional Assessment

Assess the activities the patient wants or needs to be able to do that the current differential diagnosis is limiting. These are more true-to-life activities than those that have already been assessed. Some may be done in a clinical setting, some may be simulated, and some may need to be evaluated on-site (work, home, community). These tasks can be evaluated as "able/unable to do" for pre- and post-therapy comparison, or they can be used to provoke symptoms that were not seen on the previous examination. Functional assessment includes evaluation of self-care, home management, recreational activities/hobbies, sport-related activity, or work-related tasks.

Transfers

Transfers are assessed to determine the patient's ability to move from one area to another. The assessor should document the amount of assistance that the patient needs to transfer, as well as the type of transfer that is done and any assistive devices used. Transfers that should be evaluated, if necessary, include the following:

- **Bed mobility:** Assess the patient's ability to roll from prone to supine and to left and right side-lying; and to scoot up, down, left, and right in bed.
- **Sit-to-supine and supine-to-sit transfer:** Assess the patient's ability to move from lying down to sitting up, and reverse.
- **Sit-to-stand and stand-to-sit transfer:** Assess the patient's ability to get up and down from the chair or bed.
- **Bed-to-bed or chair-to-chair transfer:** Assess weight-bearing status and ability to transfer to both the left and right. This can include assessment of the patient's ability to perform a slide board transfer from bed-to-chair if appropriate.
- **Floor recovery:** Assess the ability to get up from and down to the floor either near furniture or in the middle of the room.

Levels of assistance

The examiner should also note how many people are providing assistance:

- Stand-by assistance or supervision only
- Contact guard assistance
- Minimal assistance
- Moderate assistance
- Maximum assistance
- Total assistance needed/unable to perform

Weight-bearing status

- Full weight-bearing (FWB)
- Partial weight-bearing (PWB) is usually 50 percent weight-bearing unless the percentage is otherwise indicated by the physician.
- Touch or toe-touch weight-bearing (TWB or TTWB) is very light weight-bearing ("on eggshells").
- Non-weight-bearing (NWB)

Functional mobility

Functional mobility should be assessed on level surfaces with the assistive device the patient currently uses, if appropriate, or with the examiner's assistive device of preference if the patient is not currently using one. If appropriate, mobility should be assessed going up and down stairs, going up and down a curb, or on a different surface. If those are situations the patient typically encounters, tests for functional mobility include the following:

- Timed up-and-go test
- Dynamic gait index
- Tinetti

Balance assessment and fall risk

Falls resulting from balance deficits are a major concern in the world of health care, as they are the major cause of hospitalizations and institutionalizations of otherwise independent individuals. Fractured hips, shoulders, and ankles can be the direct results of such falls. The examiner should screen each patient for fall risk by asking about recent falls or fall history and by quick assessment of balance if necessary. The following tests are designed primarily to screen for poor balance and subsequent fall risks. They also provide good direction for functional activities to retrain the balance systems:

- Tinetti
- Berg balance assessment
- Romberg/sharpened Romberg
- Single-leg stance

Special Tests

Special tests are used to give further support to a differential diagnosis that may already be indicated by previous evaluation tools. A positive special test gives credit to a diagnosis, but a negative special test does not completely rule out a specific pathology. Due to muscle guarding and pain-inhibiting behavior, it is sometimes difficult to get a good test measure when the patient is in the acute stages of injury. The following tables list common special tests and possible indications from a positive (+) test. For specifics of the techniques needed to perform the special tests, see your musculoskeletal evaluation textbook or the references listed at the end of the book. The techniques of performing these special tests may need to be modified if the patient is unable to get into the necessary test position. Keep in mind that this is a compilation of common special tests and is not inclusive of all special tests.

Cervical Spine

Spurling's test	For nerve-root irritation through compression of the spinal foramina
Distraction test	For relief of radicular symptoms caused by compression of structures
Sharp-Pursor test	For atlantoaxial instability and integrity of the transverse ligament
Bakody's sign	For C4-C5 pathology
Roos test	For thoracic outlet syndrome
Allen test	For thoracic outlet syndrome
Halstead maneuver	For thoracic outlet syndrome

Elbow

Varus stress test	For lateral collateral ligament
Valgus stress test	For medial collateral ligament
Tinel's sign	For ulnar nerve pathology
Tennis-elbow test	For pathology of the wrist extensors at the lateral epicondyle
Golfer's-elbow test	For pathology of the wrist flexors at the medial epicondyle

Wrist/Hand/Fingers

Phalen's test	For carpal tunnel or median nerve
Finkelstein test	For de Quervain's syndrome, thumb paratendinitis
Tinel's sign	For carpal tunnel or median nerve

Shoulder

Sulcus sign	For glenohumeral inferior subluxation
Step sign	For acromioclavicular joint sprain (3° also called tent-pole deformity)
Sprengel's deformity	For a congenital high-riding and poorly developed scapula
Load-and-shift test	For glenohumeral instability; greater than 25 percent humeral displacement in the glenoid fossa indicates multidirectional instability
Apprehension test	For anterior glenohumeral dislocation
Rockwood test	For anterior glenohumeral instability at various angles of abduction
Neer's impingement test	For impingement of the supraspinatus and/or biceps tendon
Hawkins-Kennedy test	For impingement of the supraspinatus tendon
Clunk test	For torn glenoid labrum or anterior glenohumeral dislocation
Crank test	For glenohumeral and posterior glenohumeral ligament pathology
O'Brien test	For superior labral anterior-posterior lesion (SLAP lesion)
Shear test	For AC joint pathology
Speed's test	For bicipital tendonitis or paratenitis
Empty-can test	For supraspinatus muscle or supraspinatus nerve pathology

Shoulder

Sulcus sign	For glenohumeral inferior subluxation
Drop-arm test	For rotator cuff tear
Abrasion sign	For rotator cuff tendonitis
Hornblower's sign	For teres minor pathology/tear

Thoracic Spine

Slump test	For dural tension, nerve-root irritation
Spring test for the ribs	For hyper- or hypomobility of the rib cage

Lumbar Spine

Slump test	For dural tension, nerve-root irritation
Straight leg raise test	For central disc pathology (back pain) or lateral disc protrusion (leg and back pain)
Quadrant test	For nerve-root irritation or facet pathology
Hoover test	For malingering

Sacral Spine and Pelvis

Gillet test	For hypomobility of the SI joint on the examined side
Gapping test	For anterior SI ligament sprain on the painful side
Approximation test	For SI ligament sprain
Supine-to-sit test	For functional leg-length discrepancy caused by a pelvic rotation

Hip

FABER test (Patrick's test)	For hip joint pathology (muscle tightness or joint)
Trendelenburg test	For gluteus medius weakness on the unilateral stance side
Ortolani's sign	For infant congenital hip dislocation
Leg-length test	For true leg-length discrepancy
Thomas test	For hip flexor tightness
Ober test	For iliotibial band tightness
Piriformis test	For piriformis syndrome (sciatic nerve may pass through the piriformis)
90-90 straight leg raise test	For hamstring tightness

Knee

Varus stress test	For lateral joint-line laxity, laxity of the lateral collateral ligament, posterolateral capsular laxity
Valgus stress test	For medial joint-line laxity, laxity of the medial collateral ligament, posteromedial capsular laxity
Lachman's test	For anterior cruciate ligament laxity or tear
Anterior drawer test for the knee	For anterior cruciate ligament laxity or tear
Sag test	For posterior cruciate ligament laxity or tear
Slocum test	For anteromedial or anterolateral instability (depending on test position)
Pivot-shift test	For anteriomedial capsular instability, anterior cruciate ligament laxity
McMurray's test	For medial/lateral meniscus tear
Apley's grind test	For medial/lateral meniscus tear
Hughston's test	For plica injury or tear
Active patellar grind test	For patellofemoral dysfunction
McConnell test	For patellofemoral dysfunction or chondromalacia
Q-angle	For increased probability of patellofemoral dysfunction

Ankle

Subtalar neutral test	For navicular drop or excessive pronation
Anterior drawer test	For anterior talofibular ligament laxity or tear
Talar tilt test	For calcaneofibular ligament laxity or tear
Thompson's test	For Achilles tendon rupture
Homan's sign	For deep vein thrombosis

Neural Tension Tests

Lower-limb tension testing	• Straight leg raise • Prone knee bend
Upper-limb tension testing	• Baseline test • Median nerve bias • Ulnar nerve bias • Radial nerve bias

Positive tests will reproduce symptoms or show limited excursion compared to the unaffected side. Limitations on ROM and location and intensity of the symptoms should be noted and compared with the unaffected side. If central neurologic system involvement is suspected, further neuromuscular assessment should be done. For further evaluation and treatment of the neuromuscular system, including reflexes, see the Nervous System chapter.

DIFFERENTIAL DIAGNOSIS AND PATHOLOGY

Based on the findings during the evaluation of the musculoskeletal system, a list of differential diagnoses is developed. Differential diagnoses represent all of the possible conditions or pathologies that could be causing the impairments found during the evaluation. Each condition or pathology of the musculoskeletal system is unique and will dictate what medical management is necessary and what physical therapy intervention is most effective. Comorbidities of conditions of other systems may play a role in the decision-making process when you are developing interventions, and may affect the rate or success of tissue healing as well.

Pathologies Specific to the Muscles and Tendons

Muscle tissue is unique in the fact that it is made up of contractile tissue. It has a different presentation than noncontractile tissue or joint impairment when being diagnosed. Contractile tissue involvement can be differentiated from noncontractile tissue pathology with strength testing and range of motion (both active and passive) assessments during the evaluation process.

Differential Diagnosis by Strength Testing

Strong and pain-free	No contractile tissue pathology
Strong and painful	First- or second-degree muscle or tendon strain, tendonitis
Weak and very painful	Fracture
Weak and pain-free	Third-degree muscle/tendon tear, neurologic

Differential Diagnosis by ROM Assessment

Pain and limited ROM in all directions	Capsulitis (capsular pattern), arthritis, osteophytes, joint pathology
Pain and ROM decreased or increased in some directions	Ligament sprain, capsular tightness on one side, internal derangement, bursitis, postsurgical scarring, joint pathology
No pain but limited ROM	Soft-tissue tightness, OA
No pain and no ROM limitation	No pathology

Muscle or tendon strain

Muscle or tendon strain happens when the load on the muscle is greater than the muscle can withstand. It is most typical over two-joint muscles such as the gastrocnemius or the hamstring near the musculotendinous junction. Normal tissue response after strain is activation of local edema followed by tissue repair beginning at around 5 days after injury and lasting up to 14 days. Following tissue injury there is a tendency for the replacement collagen to be weaker than that in normal muscle tissue. Medical management is usually not necessary unless there is a third-degree strain, which is synonymous with a muscle tear. In a complete tear there is no pain because the muscle disruption prevents any muscular contraction. Surgical intervention or immobilization may then be necessary. Physical therapy intervention can include controlled mobilization of a strained muscle to decrease scar formation and encourage collagen to orient in parallel with the myofibrils. Interventions after an acute injury include edema control and the management of range of motion and pain. Progression into strengthening should be gradual and specific to the muscle action desired. In the case of a sport-specific injury, strengthening should mimic the desired action needed for that sport.

Tendonitis, tendinosis, and tendinopathy

Tendonitis, tendinosis, and tendinopathy refer to injury and inflammation of a tendon or tendon sheath. The onset can be traumatic but is generally more chronic in nature. These conditions present with a gradual onset of pain and localized tenderness. Specifically, **tendonitis** is an inflammation of the tendon and **tendinosis** refers to the wearing down of a tendon that is not inflammatory. Examples of tendonitis injuries are rotator cuff (supraspinatus) tendonitis, lateral epicondylitis (tennis elbow), patellar tendonitis, and Achilles tendonitis. During the acute stage of inflammatory tendon injuries, inflammation is the primary concern. The term **tendinopathy** is a general term for any pathology of the tendon. Medical management may include drug therapy for anti-inflammatories and pain control. Physical therapy intervention is needed to manage pain and edema and can include ice, compression, activity modification or rest, and controlled mobilization. After day five, the inflammatory response has usually lessened and the proliferative response begins with tissue healing. At that point, ultrasound may help to increase tissue healing, with continued controlled mobilization progressing into resistive strengthening. Continued pain management and edema control should be done throughout treatment, if those impairments exist.

Paratenonitis

Paratenonitis is the inflammation of the paratenon or area surrounding the tendon (synonymous with tenosynovitis). In addition to pain and swelling, crepitus may be noted with movement to differentiate from tendonitis. Treatment of choice is anti-inflammatory drug therapy and rest and ice; progression is the same as with tendonitis.

Muscle contractures

Muscle contractures occur as a result of immobilization, peripheral or central nerve lesions, or general decreased mobility. Medical management of neurologic-based muscle contractures may include drug therapy for muscle relaxation. Physical therapy intervention includes the use of modalities to increase tissue extensibility, soft-tissue mobilization, stretching, range of motion exercise, and positioning to discourage the contracture.

Dupuytren's contracture

Dupuytren's contracture is specific to the palmar fascia, causing flexion of the metacarpal-phalangeal and proximal interphalangeal joints.

Torticollis

Torticollis is the shortening of the sternocleidomastoid (SCM) muscle of the neck, causing rotation to the opposite side and side-bending to the same side as the affected muscle. Congenital torticollis can occur with birthing trauma overstretching the muscle itself or with damage to the nerve. Acquired torticollis can result from a whiplash-type injury or a prolonged abnormal posture position. Medical management may include a local injection to relax the muscle spasm. Physical therapy intervention includes modalities to increase tissue extensibility, if appropriate; muscle stretching; and soft-tissue mobilization. Education on posture and positioning to maintain SCM length is recommended.

Contusion

A **contusion** is a hematoma from a direct blow or trauma. There is localized pain, ecchymosis, and inflammation. Physical therapy intervention is primarily to range of motion and functional mobility. Once initial pain and edema have decreased, progression to resistive strengthening is appropriate.

Muscle spasm

Muscle spasm is a continuous muscle contraction that can occur as a protective response to pain or overstretching. Protective muscle spasm stops the muscle from moving to attempt to prevent muscle strain or tear. Spasm can be caused by prolonged postures, stress, or trauma. Physical therapy intervention utilizes relaxation techniques: heat, ultrasound, ROM, stretching, biofeedback, postural education, soft-tissue mobilization, and progression into strengthening exercise to address muscle weakness.

Pathologies Specific to Connective Tissues

Connective tissue is noncontractile and, although stronger than contractile tissue, can be injured easily with overstretching. Connective tissues help to add stability to the joint to protect the joint, and they are often injured during joint trauma.

Ligament sprain

A **sprain** is the overstretching of a ligament beyond the limits of normal tissue length. Sprains are graded as first-, second-, or third-degree dependant on the amount of tissue injury and instability.

Grading of Sprains

First-degree (grade I)	A partial tear with no joint instability
Second-degree (grade II)	A partial tear with some joint instability
Third-degree (grade III)	A full-thickness tear causing significant joint instability

Ligament sprains, like muscle strains, go through stages of healing. There is an acute inflammatory response and localized pain response. Tissue healing takes place, but healthy tissue is replaced with scar tissue, not regenerated normal ligamentous tissue. Medical management of a torn ligament may involve arthroscopic surgery for ligament repair or grafting. Physical therapy intervention includes controlled mobilization to encourage proper alignment of scar tissue for eventual better tensile strength and stiffness. Icing immediately after acute injury controls the edema response. Low-load exercise can also improve the tensile strength of an injured ligament.

Plica syndrome

Plica syndrome is an abnormal folding of the joint capsule that can feel similar to a meniscus injury. Not all individuals have plicae, as they are typically resorbed into a smooth joint capsule at birth. Pain presentation is similar to patellofemoral syndrome (listed under pathologies specific to the bone or joint) but with some clicking or popping possible during activity. Physical therapy intervention includes pain and edema management, muscle strengthening, muscle stretching, and proprioceptive training. Patients also need education on squatting mechanics and activity modification to avoid irritating symptoms.

Plantar fasciitis

Plantar fasciitis is pain specific to the plantar surface of the foot. It can be from tissue tightness of the plantar fascia or from the Achilles tendon pulling on the attachment at the calcaneus. It presents as pain with direct pressure on the plantar fascia, either by palpation or by weight-bearing activity. Medical management can include drug therapy for anti-inflammatory benefits and pain management. Cortisone injections or a plantar fasciotomy can be done for more invasive treatment. Physical therapy management includes pain and edema management, soft-tissue stretching and mobilization, and patient education on activity modification and shoe wear. In some clinics the patient can be fitted for orthotics to improve plantar fascia support during weight-bearing.

Iliotibial band syndrome

Iliotibial (IT) band syndrome is an overuse injury to the IT band where it attaches to the lateral knee. The syndrome is most typical in runners and cyclists as repetitive flexion of the knee causes the IT band to rub over the femur. Pain is localized to the lateral knee. Physical therapy intervention is the same as for a sprain. Avoidance of irritating activity during healing is recommended. Ultrasound, cross-friction massage, and stretching can decrease the inflammation and pain.

Adhesive capsulitis (frozen shoulder)

Adhesive capsulitis (frozen shoulder) is capsular tightening of the glenohumeral joint causing decreased ROM and associated pain. Demographics are primarily middle-aged women, although both sexes are equally affected when diabetes is a comorbidity. The pattern of immobility is shoulder external rotation limited > abduction limited > internal rotation motion. Patients have difficulty reaching behind the back and overhead. Medical management may include drug therapy for pain management, and sometimes a steroid injection is given. In extreme cases, the physician does a manipulation under anesthesia. Physical therapy intervention is aggressive joint mobilization and ROM. Modalities may be used to allow greater tissue stretch, but some practitioners believe that ultrasound and heat do not penetrate to the capsule. Resistance exercise is usually not indicated, as the problem is hypomobility, not weakness.

Bursitis

Bursitis is an inflammation of the bursa sac, usually due to abnormal joint mechanics or overuse/repetitive injuries. It is a secondary condition that is usually the result of other pathology, such as tendonitis. The pain itself is most likely from the primary condition, not the bursae. Medical management is drug therapy for anti-inflammatory and pain-control effects. Physical therapy intervention is for edema control and pain management as in tendonitis treatment. Phonophoresis and iontophoresis are commonly used modalities. Joint impairments or abnormal mechanics should be evaluated and treated accordingly to address the primary pathology.

Meniscal tears

Meniscal tears occur most frequently as a direct result of contact or noncontact trauma to the knee. The medial meniscus has a greater incidence of injury than the lateral. Close-chained, rotational movement is the most typical mechanism of injury and may also affect the ACL and MCL (unhappy triad). Pain is usually deeper in the knee and may be accompanied by a clicking or even locking of the joint, depending on the size and location of the tear. Medical management may include arthroscopic surgical repair or resection of the tear. In the case of repair, the patient is usually non-weight-bearing for six to eight weeks after surgery. Physical therapy intervention, whether surgical or nonsurgical, includes progressive ROM, resistance exercise, proprioceptive training, pain management, and edema control. Postsurgically, gait training education with the appropriate assistive device and weight-bearing status is advised.

Pathologies Specific to the Bone or Joint

Bony tissue is much stronger than contractile tissue or connective tissue, but it does not allow the deformation that the other two allow. Injury to bone or articular surfaces can affect the surrounding soft tissues as well.

Arthritis

Arthritis is any disease process that destroys the articular surface of a joint. Presentations of arthritic joints can vary from asymptomatic to painful, and may include significant loss of motion and functional mobility. Severity of pain and limitation may also depend on whether the joint is weight-bearing or not. Specific types of arthritis are further discussed in chapter 7, Other Systems: Metabolic and Endocrine, Gastrointestinal, Genitourinary, and Multisystem Pathologies. Physical therapy intervention of arthritic conditions includes pain management and restoration of ROM to improve function. Strengthening of surrounding muscles is beneficial because they provide support and shock-absorbing protection to the joint surfaces.

Osteoarthritis (degenerative joint disease)

Osteoarthritis (OA) (**degenerative joint disease**) is a progressive degeneration of the articulating surfaces of synovial joints. It is nearly equal in prevalence among men and women but is most widely seen in those over the age of 60. Many factors contribute to the onset of OA, including activity level, anatomical structure and mechanics, nutrition, and weight. Muscle weakness and ligament laxity may also contribute to poor joint mechanics and thus the onset of OA. OA presents primarily in the weight-bearing joints of the knees, hips, and spine. Presentation of OA is increased morning stiffness that can improve or worsen with activity throughout the day. Crepitus and osteophytes may also be present. Noninvasive medical management of OA includes patient education on prevention and drug therapy for pain and inflammation. Injection of synthetic synovial substances, such as Synvisc to restore function and decrease pain, is a newer treatment. Surgical intervention can be for debridement, osteotomy, or arthrotomy. PT intervention begins with patient education on posture, body mechanics, use of assistive devices if necessary, and activity modification to avoid progression of the OA. Exercise for strengthening, and ROM or stretching activities to maintain joint lubrication and avoid excessive wear on portions of the joint, are also necessary.

Impingement

Impingement is the pinching or blocking of the movement of a joint, usually in one direction but not all directions. Inflammation or microscopic tears of a tendon, ligament, or articular cartilage can contribute to joint impingement, as there is active movement of the joint through its range. Impingement occurs most typically in the glenohumeral joint of the shoulder. Classically, it presents with a painful arc of motion and lessened pain during passive range of motion. Medical management may include drug therapy for pain management and control of inflammation. In some cases, surgical debridement of the injured tissues, subacromial decompression, or acromioplasty may be beneficial. Physical therapy intervention in nonsurgical conditions includes modalities to control pain and inflammation, activity modification to avoid overhead activity, rotator cuff strengthening, and stretching of tight surrounding soft tissues. Postsurgically, intervention includes restoration of full range of motion and progression of resistance exercise to strengthen the rotator cuff.

Subluxation/Dislocation

Subluxation/dislocation is the partial or complete displacement of a joint as a result of direct trauma or chronic instability. Soft-tissue damage, muscle spasm from pain, and inflammation accompany the joint disruption. The most common joints affected are the glenohumeral joint of the shoulder and the patellofemoral joint. The shoulder's position of vulnerability is external rotation in a position of 90° abduction. Medical management is reduction of the dislocation and controlled, temporary immobilization. Physical therapy intervention begins with gentle, progressive ROM and grade I/II accessory joint oscillations, isometric progressing to resistance strengthening to stabilize the joint, proprioceptive training, and pain management.

Fracture

A **fracture** is a break in the bony tissue. Fractures can be complete through the bone or just partial. They can remain closed, with no disruption of soft tissue or skin; or be compound, causing injury to surrounding soft tissue and breaking the skin barrier. Medical management of less severe fractures may be just simple immobilization or splinting and time for healing. More severe fractures (compound, comminuted, displaced, or through the growth plate of a child) may require surgical fixation and prolonged immobilization. General bone healing takes six to eight weeks and sometimes longer if there is nonhealing or other comorbidities. Physical therapy intervention during immobilization includes gait training with the appropriate assistive device and instruction in weight-bearing status. ROM of surrounding joints can be evaluated. After immobilization, treatment intervention should include ROM, edema control, pain management, and functional mobility.

Osgood-Schlatter's syndrome

Osgood-Schlatter's syndrome is a childhood disease of overgrowth of the tibial tuberosity, causing anterior knee pain. Pain is provoked with deep knee-bending and jumping activities. Medical management is X-ray confirmation of diagnosis based on the patient's complaints and pain location. PT intervention includes education in squatting mechanics and avoidance of irritating activities. General stretching of the lower extremities is recommended.

Patellofemoral syndrome (chondromalacia)

Patellofemoral syndrome (chondromalacia) occurs when there is degeneration of bony articulation between the back of the patella and the femoral groove. Pain typically increases with activity, such as going up and down stairs, rising from a chair, or deep squatting. Prolonged sitting with knees flexed may also elicit pain. There may or may not be crepitus in the joint. Incidence is higher in girls and women due to the Q-angle. Medical management is usually drug therapy for anti-inflammatory and pain management. Surgical intervention is sometimes used to realign the patella in the femoral groove with a lateral release of the retinaculum or transfer of the patellar tendon/tibial tubercle. Physical therapy intervention in nonsurgical situations includes strengthening, pain management, and edema control. Evaluation of the foot and hip are also necessary to assess biomechanical abnormalities that may contribute to poor patellar tracking. Strengthening of the weak muscles and stretching of the tight muscles are needed for a balance around the knee. Proprioceptive training for muscle reeducation in a dynamic situation is also recommended.

Temporomandibular joint syndrome

Temporomandibular joint (TMJ) syndrome is pain and dysfunction specific to the TMJ and surrounding musculature. TMJ syndrome can come from direct trauma to the jaw; from abnormalities with the joint mechanics involved in opening/closing the mouth; and/or from chewing or muscle dysfunction that results from forward head posture, tension, or injury. Physical therapy intervention is specific to the aggravating factor. Joint mobilization, soft-tissue mobilization, stretching, resistive strengthening, and postural/positioning education can address the causative factors.

Osteoporosis

Osteoporosis is a decrease in bone density that can put the individual at greater risk of multiple fractures. Patients present with low back pain and may have an increased thoracic kyphosis. Prevention of bone-density loss can include hormone replacement, calcium supplement, weight-bearing exercise (the National Osteoporosis Foundation says 45–60 minutes 4 times/week), calcium- and magnesium-rich foods, vitamin D (sunshine), and avoidance of alcohol and tobacco. Medical management includes diagnostic dual energy X-ray absorptiometry (DXA) to measure total-body bone density. Physical therapy intervention includes education in posture, body mechanics, fall prevention, balance retraining, assistive device training, weight-bearing exercise, and controlled resistance of muscles attached to affected bone. Isometric extension exercise, modalities for pain, and soft-tissue mobilizations can also decrease spasm. Return of functional mobility following fracture or immobilization may be necessary. These patients should avoid flexion, side-bending, or rotation of the spine. Caution should be used with mobilization techniques, especially in the thoracic spine, to avoid a fracture.

Congenital hip dysplasia

Congenital hip dysplasia (now called developmental dysplasia of the hip) is a hip instability defect that occurs developmentally or in infants. It is graded as unstable, subluxing, or dislocating. It is more dominant in females and may be related to fetal positions associated with birthing complications. Clinically, the infant may have decreased ROM, leg-length discrepancies, or asymmetries in skin folds. By the time the child is walking, s/he may present with a Trendelenburg gait. Medical management is bracing of the hips/legs in an abducted position, and extreme cases may require surgical intervention. Physical therapy intervention is necessary to assist in ROM and positioning before and after bracing and/or surgical intervention. Muscular strengthening with controlled-resistance exercise may help with hip stability. Mobility training with assistive devices, if necessary, may improve function. Caution should *always* be used with these patients during transfers and exercise, using care to maintain hip stability.

Legg-Calve-Perthes disease

Legg-Calve-Perthes disease is a congenital necrosis of the head of the femur in the hip joint. It is rare, but is seen primarily in boys age 3 to 12 years old. The extent of destruction of the femur is variable, but the prognosis is better for those who are younger. These patients present with hip pain that worsens with activity, and they demonstrate difficulty with functional mobility. There can be ROM, strength, and functional impairments, and a structural leg-length difference. Medical management of Legg-Calve-Perthes disease begins with diagnosis through radiologic examination and physical findings. Bracing in a position that prevents further deformity is sometimes necessary. Surgical intervention may be necessary to address soft-tissue and bony abnormalities. Physical therapy intervention may include ROM and functional training with appropriate assistive devices, if necessary.

Arthrogryposis multiplex congenita

Arthrogryposis multiplex congenita (AMC) is a congenital disease that can present in one of three forms: muscle contractures, lack of muscle development, or arthrogryposis of the hands and feet (clubfoot, specifically, is an arthrogryposis). It is thought that any of these three presentations is caused by inactivity of the fetus in the uterus. That inactivity can be caused by a number of things. AMC primarily affects functional mobility and positioning due to joint contractures, muscle weakness, and areas of fibrosis. Medical management may necessitate surgical intervention to correct contractures and joint deformities. PT intervention is necessary for positioning, fitting of orthoses, and instruction in the use of assistive devices to improve functional mobility. Techniques for ROM and stretching are beneficial, and strengthening of atrophied muscles is recommended.

Pathologies Specific to the Spine

The spine is comprised of all of the previously addressed tissues: muscle tissue, connective tissue, and bone. The spine is different from any other joint in that it contains nerve tissue. The spine has differential diagnoses that are specific to its components and function.

Accommodating and non-accommodating restrictions

Adaptive, or accommodating, restrictions occur in the spine as a response to some other factor. Side-bending of the affected spinal segment is primarily restricted. **Non-adaptive, or non-accommodating, restrictions** occur as reactions to a trauma or injury. Flexion and extension are restricted at the level of injury and may also be affected at the level above and below the injured segment.

Facet impingement syndrome

Facet impingement syndrome is an irritation of the facet joints of the cervical, thoracic, or lumbar spine. The mechanism of injury is usually a quick forward flexion coupled with rotation movement. Pain presents as aggravated by extension or return from flexion and is alleviated with flexion activity. There is stiffness and local tenderness that is better at rest and worse with activity. If there is actually subluxation or inflammation of the facet joint, there may be increased pressures on the nerve root that causes referral of pain. Pathologies of the facet joints usually follow degeneration of the disc as spacing between the vertebrae is decreased, causing initial hypermobility and eventual hypomobility of the altered joint.

Medical management of persistent facet pathologies may include a local steroid injection to decrease inflammation and pain. Physical therapy intervention should include intermittent traction, joint mobilization techniques to open the facet joint, pain management, and core stabilization once pain has diminished. Education on posture, body mechanics, lifting, and activity modification is recommended.

Spondylosis, spondylolysis, and spondylolisthesis

Spondylosis is degeneration of the intervertebral discs (patients are age >25 years; most prevalent in patients >65 years). **Spondylolysis** is a defect in the pars of the vertebrae.

Spondylolisthesis is the anterior slippage of one vertebra above another due to a bilateral pars defect. In all "spondy" pathologies, back pain is the primary symptom. In severe spondylolisthesis presentations, there may be a palpable or observed step-off deformity of the spine. Medical management is diagnostic with radiographs. Drug therapy may be necessary to control pain and inflammation. In severe cases of forward slippage, surgery may be indicated to fuse the segment to prevent further instability or compression of the spinal cord. PT intervention is necessary for core strengthening in a neutral spine position. There should be avoidance of painful end-range extension exercise. Lower-extremity stretching may also be indicated. It may be necessary to fit the patient with a Thoracic-lumbar-sacral orthosis if ordered by the physician.

Ankylosing spondylitis

Ankylosing spondylitis (AS) occurs predominantly in males ages 15–30 years and is characterized by morning stiffness and restricted ROM. AS is an inflammatory disease of the spine and pelvis and can be considered a systemic disease. Patients commonly have times of remission and exacerbation. There can be resultant postural abnormalities such as a flattened lumbar spine and increased thoracic kyphosis. In more progressed cases, there can be ossification of the joints, osteoporosis-associated fractures, spinal stenosis, and atlantoaxial instability. Although primarily a spinal disease, AS can affect the peripheral joints, causing stiffness and decreased ROM. Medical management of AS is primarily drug therapy to control inflammation and manage pain. Other drug therapy may be necessary if other systems are involved. Physical therapy intervention is similar to that needed with other inflammatory joint diseases. The same precautions should be taken as with patients who have osteoporosis. Emphasis should be on activities for ROM, stretching, and functional mobility. Modalities and soft-tissue mobilization can be used for pain and edema management. Low-intensity exercise on a regular basis and avoiding painful activities can help manage pain and maintain muscle strength.

Spinal stenosis

Spinal stenosis is the narrowing of the spinal canal that puts pressure on the spinal nerve roots. Pain is intermittent, is usually worse with standing, and may radiate down both legs at times. With stenosis, there may be no complaint of back pain but only leg symptoms. ROM is not necessarily restricted, but flexion may decrease symptoms, and extension may exacerbate symptoms. Physical therapy intervention can include spinal traction to decrease pressure on the spine or spinal nerve roots, joint mobilization and passive ROM to increase extension, and core stabilization exercises. Patient education on postures and activities to avoid and on positions of relief may be recommended.

Scheuermann's disease

Scheuermann's disease is first noted between the ages of 13 and 16 years and is excessive thoracic kyphosis. It is not a disease of symptoms but instead is one of spinal deformity. Medical management may include bracing to prevent further forward curvature of the spine and drug therapy to control inflammation, if needed. Physical therapy intervention emphasizes postural correction and postural strengthening. Stretching and soft-tissue mobilization of the anterior structures may help balance anterior and posterior muscles of the spine.

Scoliosis

Scoliosis is an abnormal lateral curvature of the thoracic or lumbar spine and is named for the side that has the convex portion of the curve. Curvature can be one-sided (C curve) or in two directions (S curve). Scoliosis is usually first diagnosed during childhood. It can cause pelvic and hip asymmetry and also functional leg-length differences. Medical management is screening for and monitoring the progression of scoliosis. Spinal bracing may be indicated to prevent further progression of the spinal deformity. Surgical intervention is usually not indicated unless the curvature is greater than 40°, when it begins to compromise lung or cardiovascular function. Surgical intervention with rod placement may then be necessary to prevent further curvature. Physical therapy intervention begins with screening for scoliosis. This can be done by visual inspection with the patient standing and in forward flexion. A "rib hump" is present during forward flexion on the convex side. Treatment intervention is primarily for pain management and dysfunction associated with muscle spasm using modalities, stretching, and soft-tissue mobilization. Postural and core strengthening are indicated to promote spinal stability. Use of a heel lift or recommendations for a buildup on the shoe itself may be necessary if the leg-length difference is significant. General postural strengthening is also recommended.

Disc protrusion and disc herniation

A **disc protrusion** is a bulge of the annular fibers of the disc from pressure by the nucleus. **Herniation** is the actual release of nuclear contents through the fibers of the annulus. Herniation is most common at the L4-L5 or L5-S1 level in a patient who is 30–40 years of age, but it can occur earlier or later in life depending on the mechanism of injury and integrity of the annulus. Generally, the water content of the nucleus decreases with age, so acute herniation is less common in those older than 50 years. The degree of herniation defines protrusion, extrusion, and free sequestration. Pain comes from pressure that the protrusion places on surrounding structures, not from the protrusion itself. It presents as back or neck pain that is worsened with flexion positions. Pain is usually localized to the back but can be radicular if the nerve root or spinal cord is being compressed with the herniation. It can be worse in the morning. Activities of lifting, twisting, prolonged postures (long duration sitting or standing), and moving from sit to stand increase pain. Pain is lessened with extension activities such as lying prone, walking, or standing. On examination, there may be a lateral shift away from the side of the herniation. There will be pain that worsens or moves down the leg with repeated flexion, and there may be pain with extension. Medical management becomes surgical if a disc herniation causes severe effects on surrounding tissues with secondary loss of strength or loss of sensation. A discectomy, laminectomy, or spinal fusion may be necessary to centralize the symptoms. Physical therapy intervention for nonsurgical treatment of disc herniation is to first centralize the symptoms with correction of a lateral shift and passive extension exercise. If symptoms are too severe and these treatments are not tolerated, a supine or 90/90 position with frequent position changes may initially be necessary. Once pain has decreased, core stabilization in a neutral position or extension exercises can be initiated. Repeated flexion exercises are avoided. Education on posture, body mechanics, and lifting technique is necessary to avoid re-injury. The patient should be taught activity modification and frequent positional changes to avoid irritating postures or activities.

Degenerative disc disease

Degenerative disc disease (DDD) is a breakdown of the fibers of the outer (typically posterolateral annular) layer of the disc. DDD can be chronic or acute and typically occurs in the 30-to-50-year-old population. Repetitive flexion and rotation of the spine are common mechanisms of injury. Severe degeneration of the annular fibers of the disc is what can lead to an increased incidence of disc herniation. Since the disc is avascular, tissue healing and surgical repair are not successful. PT intervention is core stability exercise to decrease accessory joint instability at the site of DDD. Accessory joint mobility should be evaluated at surrounding joints, as they may be hypomobile. A lower-extremity flexibility and stretching program may also be introduced to decrease excessive tension on the pelvis and paraspinal musculature. Modalities and soft-tissue mobilization may be needed to manage pain.

Nerve root irritation or compression

Nerve root irritation or compression occurs when there is pressure on the nerve root from the disc, from narrowing of the bony foramina of the spine, or from muscle spasm. Back pain is aggravated with extension activities and improves with flexion activities. Pain is usually accompanied by radicular symptoms to below the knee. Physical therapy intervention includes spinal traction.

Mechanical low-back pain

Mechanical low-back pain occurs as a result of injury to the muscles supporting the lumbar spine. Pain is aggravated with activity, particularly with repetitive movements, and is alleviated with rest. Pain is localized to the back. Other findings may include poor postural strength, decreased awareness of body mechanics, and lower-extremity muscular tightness. PT intervention includes modalities to manage pain, soft-tissue and joint mobilization if there is hypomobility, core stabilization/strengthening exercise, education in posture and body mechanics, and stretching of tight lower-extremity muscles. In cases of back pain as a work-related injury, it may be beneficial to progress to a work conditioning program that re-creates work-related activities for functional strengthening.

Pathologies of the Peripheral Nerve

A peripheral nerve consists of bundles of nerve fibers surrounded by connective tissue and blood vessels. Each axon is covered with endoneurium. Groups of these axons are called fascicles. Each fascicle is covered with perineurium. Groups of fascicles, blood vessels, and fat are called a nerve, and the nerve is covered by the epineurium. The epineurium normally glides smoothly along joints but can become restricted anywhere along its path.

Neurapraxia

Neurapraxia is a class 1 nerve injury. There is failure of nerve conduction where the axon remains intact, and injury is usually temporary.

Axonotmesis

Axonotmesis is a class 2 nerve injury. There is incomplete injury to the nerve with the connective tissue still intact. There is possible degeneration distal to the axonal injury, with possible axonal regeneration. Spontaneous recovery is possible.

Neurotmesis

Neurotmesis is a class 3 nerve injury. The entire nerve is severed. Spontaneous recovery is not possible.

Wallerian degeneration

Wallerian degeneration occurs when the peripheral nerve's axon dies distal to the site of injury, the myelin degenerates, and the Schwann cells phagocytize the area.

Specific Injuries to the Peripheral Nerves

Each peripheral nerve serves to provide sensation to a specific dermatomal area and innervation to a motor unit to allow muscle contraction. Any of the above pathologies can affect any one or more of the peripheral nerves with specific motor and sensory presentations. Medical management of any of the peripheral nerve injuries may include pharmacologic methods for neuropathic pain, such as opioids, anticonvulsants, and tricyclic antidepressants. Early surgical repair of nerve injury may be necessary. Later surgery includes sympathectomy or deafferentation to decrease pain; amputation; and/or tendon transfers for function or contracture management. Fabrication of orthotics may be recommended to treat the paralyzed extremity.

Brachial plexus (Erb-Duchenne syndrome)

Erb-Duchenne syndrome involves injury or pathology to the C5-C6 nerve roots of the brachial plexus as a compression or overstretch of the nerve bundle. Motor impairments affect the shoulder, elbow, and hand intrinsics. Sensory impairments are noted in the lateral forearm and the deltoid.

Burners or stingers

Burners, or **stingers**, are acute injuries to the brachial plexus that cause a burning or stinging sensation down the neck and sometimes into the arm.

Spinal accessory nerve (C3-C4)

Injury to the C3-C4 nerve root results from prolonged direct pressure or poor posture causing tension and trauma to the posterior angle of the neck. Motor impairments cause weakness or loss of the function of the trapezius, causing difficulty with abduction above the shoulder. No sensory impairments.

Axillary nerve (C5-C6)

Injury to the axillary nerve can result from anterior dislocation of the shoulder, fracture of the humeral neck, or trauma to the brachial plexus. Motor impairments include weakness or loss of shoulder abduction and external rotation. Sensory impairments are noted in the lateral deltoid.

Suprascapular nerve (C5-C6)

Injury to the suprascapular nerve can be caused by direct trauma to the scapula or overstretch of the supraspinatus muscle. Motor impairments include weakness or loss of shoulder scaption, external rotation, and abduction. No sensory impairments are noted.

Musculocutaneous nerve (C5-C6)

Injury to the musculocutaneous nerve is coincident with a brachial plexus compression, stretch or fracture/dislocation of the humerus, repetitive pronation, or elbow hyperextension. Motor impairments include weakness or loss of elbow flexion, shoulder flexion, and forearm supination. Sensory impairments are noted in the lateral forearm.

Long thoracic nerve (C5-C8)

Injury to the long thoracic nerve can be from a "backpacker's injury," causing compression of the nerve from direct pressure such as from a backpack or bag, or repetitive overhead activity. Motor impairments include weakness or loss of serratus anterior, causing winging and difficulty with abduction above the shoulder. No sensory impairments are noted.

Median nerve (C6-C8, T1)

Injury to the median nerve can come from compression or stretching, or from direct trauma to the elbow. Motor impairments include weakness or loss of wrist flexion, finger flexion, and forearm pronation. Sensory impairments are noted in the palmar surface of the hand over the thenar eminence.

Anterior interosseus nerve (C6-C8, T1)

Injury to the anterior interosseus nerve can result from a forearm fracture. Motor impairments include weakness or loss of index and thumb flexion. No sensory impairments are noted.

Ulnar nerve (C7-C8, T1)

Injury to the ulnar nerve can result from compression, arthritis, or repetitive trauma at the elbow or wrist at the hypothenar eminence. Motor impairments (usually delayed) include weakness of the hand intrinsics. Sensory impairments are noted along the medial elbow and the ulnar side of the forearm, or the little finger and ulnar half of the ring finger.

Radial nerve (C5-C8, T1)

Injury to the radial nerve is most often associated with a humeral fracture. Motor impairments include weakness or loss of the elbow and wrist extensors. No sensory impairments are noted unless the superficial branch is compressed. The superficial branch is only sensory, with no motor impairments and affects the dorsal wrist and thumb.

Carpal tunnel syndrome (median nerve)

Injury to the median nerve occurs with compression at the wrist from repetitive postures or from swelling, arthritis, or trauma. Motor impairments include weakness or loss of thumb flexion, abduction, and opposition. Sensory impairments are noted in the thumb, index finger, and radial half of the middle finger.

Ilioinguinal nerve

Injury to the ilioinguinal nerve occurs with compression at the transverse abdominus or external obliques. Sensory impairments are noted along the anterior thigh and genitalia. No motor impairments are noted.

Sciatic nerve (L4-S3)

Injury to the sciatic nerve can occur with traumatic dislocation of the hip, fracture, piriformis tightness, or any trauma along the posterior leg from the hip to the knee. Motor impairments include weakness or loss of hip extension, knee flexion, hip abduction, and hip external rotation. Sensory impairments are noted in the sacrum, buttock, posterior leg, lateral/posterior knee, and foot.

Femoral nerve (L2-L4)

Injury to the femoral nerve occurs with anterior hip trauma or as a secondary injury during surgery. Motor impairments include weakness or loss of hip flexion and knee extension. Sensory impairments are noted along the medial thigh, leg, and foot.

Obturator nerve (L2-L4)

Injury to the obturator nerve occurs with a hip or pelvic fracture or as a secondary injury in hip/pelvic surgery or pregnancy. Motor impairments include weakness or loss of hip adduction, knee flexion, and hip lateral rotation. Sensory impairments are noted along the medial thigh to the knee.

Thoracic outlet syndrome

Thoracic outlet syndrome (TOS) occurs when there is compression or overstretching of vessels and nerves as they move through the thoracic outlet. It presents as pain, numbness, and weakness in the neck and down the arm of the affected side. Compression can happen in the spinal foramina, or under the scalenes, first rib, or pectoralis minor. Overstretch of the brachial plexus can also trigger TOS. Physical therapy intervention must address the causative factors. It is valuable to identify the mechanism of injury (compression vs. overstretch) and, if appropriate, where the compression is occurring. Muscle stretching, soft-tissue mobilization, and neural gliding may be appropriate interventions. Education on postural correction and postural strengthening is also recommended.

Pathologies Specific to Pain

In musculoskeletal conditions where the primary impairment is related to pain, there are several considerations during evaluation that can assist with the differential diagnoses.

Description of Pain	Possible Cause
Aching/constant	Arthritis or degenerative joint disease
Sharp	Mechanical injury
Pain that lessens with activity	Arthritis
Pain that worsens with activity	Inflammatory condition

Referred pain

Cloward's areas are studied referral patterns from nociceptive input on the anterior portion of the affected intervertebral disc.

Cervical Level	Interscapular Referral Pattern
C3-C4	At the level of T1-T2 spinous processes
C4-C5	Between T4 spinous process and the scapular spine
C5-C6	At the level of T5-T6 spinous processes
C6-C7	At the inferior angle of the scapula

Common referred pain patterns

Site of Perceived Pain	Referred from (Site of Pathology)
Pelvis/lateral hip	Lumbar spine
Anterior/medial pelvis, groin	Hip joint
C5-C6 dermatome	Shoulder joint
Shoulder	C3-C4 or C4-C5 IV joints C4-C5 nerve root
Upper trap	Diaphragm
Shoulder/scapula	Gallbladder
Hand	C5-C6, C6-C7, C7-T1 IV joints C6, C7, C8 nerve roots
Foot	L4-L5, L5-S1 IV joints L4, L5, S1 nerve roots

In addition to the patient's general complaint of pain, the presence of other complications could indicate that what may initially be considered a local dysfunction may actually be more of a systemic pathology. The presence of any of the following systems in addition to other dysfunctions would indicate a need for a referral to a physician:

- Fever
- Fatigue
- Malaise
- 10-to-15-lb weight loss over two weeks
- Cardiac changes
- Pulmonary changes

Surgical Procedures of the Musculoskeletal System

Postsurgical physical therapy intervention must always follow the surgeon's instructions and restrictions. Early physical therapy intervention for mobility and positioning after surgery is important in preventing other complications, such as deep vein thrombosis, pneumonia, and pressure wounds. ROM for nonsurgical surrounding joints should be done to maintain good joint motion. Later, intervention techniques should include progressive ROM, strengthening, proprioceptive training, pain management, edema control, and restored functional mobility.

Arthroplasty

Arthroplasty is the use of synthetic materials to reconstruct a joint. Examples include total knee replacement (TKR), total hip replacement (THR), and total shoulder replacement (TSR). Arthroplasty can be used to replace either part or all of the joint for the purpose of decreased pain and increased function. Barring other complications, hospitalization is minimal and the patient is released to home or intermediate care for additional physical therapy. Some surgeons have restrictions on range of motion or weight-bearing status following surgery. Physical therapy intervention following TKR or TSR emphasizes ROM to make maximal use of the available joint surface, as well as strengthening to improve functional mobility. In all arthroplasties, pain management and edema control are goals during treatment intervention.

Laminectomy

Laminectomy is the removal of all or portions of the lamina of the vertebrae. In addition to bony removal, there may be excision of the ligamentum flavum and any disc fragments that are present. Physical therapy intervention begins almost immediately with instructions for the patient to begin a progressive walking program within 48 hours after surgery. Prolonged sitting is avoided. A core stabilization program with a neutral spine is initiated. Patient education on posture and body mechanics and lower extremity stretching is also necessary.

Bankart repair

Bankart repair is an arthroscopic approach that reattaches the glenoid labrum and the inferior glenohumeral ligament to the bone. The procedure is also referred to as capsulorrhaphy. Postsurgically and after initial immobilization, physical therapy intervention includes gradual progression of passive, then active, ROM. Scapular stabilization exercises progress to resistive rotator cuff strengthening for further glenohumeral joint stabilization. Proprioceptive retraining techniques will decrease the possibility of instability recurrence.

Soft-tissue repair

Examples of soft-tissue repair are Achilles tendon repair, rotator cuff repair, and ACL reconstruction. Initially, the repaired soft tissue is immobilized to allow tissue healing. Immobilization times vary depending on the degree of repair, the tissues used to repair (graft vs. no graft), and surgical techniques. ROM is often started early to decrease joint impairments caused by immobilization and to promote good alignment of collagen fibers. Special considerations for common surgical repairs include the following:

- **ACL reconstruction:** Avoid terminal knee extension in an open-chain position to avoid excess stress on healing graft. Use caution with overly aggressive functional progression, as the graft is at its weakest at four to six weeks postoperatively.
- **Rotator cuff repair:** Avoid repetitive overhead resistance exercise if painful, to avoid compression forces through the healing surgical site. Avoid overly aggressive joint mobilization or PROM to avoid tearing the surgical repair.

Amputation

Amputation (removal of a limb) can be either traumatic or surgical. In the case of a planned surgical amputation, special care is taken for the patient to retain as much viable tissue as possible. In the case of planned use of a prosthetic, amputation is done at a level that will allow the patient to function maximally. Often these patients have other comorbidities that may affect healing and function. Physical therapy intervention is extensive following amputation and includes wound care, the fitting of a prosthesis, and training and exercise for ROM and strengthening.

Diagnostic Testing and Radiologic Imaging

Many times, before being referred to physical therapy, the patient has already undergone some type of diagnostic testing or radiologic imaging. Although most imaging is not 100 percent accurate, it does help to drive treatment toward a specific differential diagnosis. Diagnostic testing and imaging can also help to rule out other suspected pathologies.

Plain film

Plain film (X-ray) is most effectively used to evaluate bone integrity and to identify structural abnormalities. Some soft-tissue and spatial abnormalities can also be identified, depending on the film quality and the patient's position.

Computed tomography

A **computed tomography** (CT) scan provides a cross-sectional picture of bone and soft tissues of the desired area in a high-resolution, computer-generated film.

Radionuclide scanning

Radionuclide scanning (bone scan) identifies areas of bone loss within skeletal structures. Radioactive isotopes are injected and taken up by the bone and show even minimal amounts of bone loss.

Magnetic resonance imaging

Magnetic resonance imaging (MRI) provides a detailed cross-sectional view of all anatomy (skeletal, soft tissue, etc.). As its name indicates, MRI uses magnetic field movement to provide a picture of the desired cross-sectional area.

Diagnostic ultrasound

Diagnostic ultrasound is used to evaluate circulation and specifically look for areas of decreased circulation or clots. It uses high-frequency sound waves to form an image on a screen to be read.

TREATMENT INTERVENTIONS

Once the evaluation is complete and the list of differential diagnoses is developed, it is necessary to choose the proper interventions to treat the impairments. Typically, physical therapy combines functional mobility, exercise, range of motion, mobilization, and modalities to work toward the patient's goals. (The use of assistive devices, implementation of orthotics and prosthetics, and the application of modalities are covered in their own chapters.)

Intervention Timeline

Treatment intervention differs depending on the amount of time that has passed since the onset of the impairment or injury.

Acute/inflammatory stage (0 to 4 days)

Goal: Decrease inflammation, control pain, protect the injured area

Intervention:

- The first 24 hours: rest or low-level activity that does not increase the pain, ice, compression, and elevation to decrease pain and inflammation
- Range of motion, either passive or active-assistive, to maintain joint mobility and encourage organized collagen formation in tissue healing
- May begin isometric strengthening if there is no coincident increase in pain
- Grade I/II accessory joint oscillations to increase movement of synovial fluid and manage pain
- Soft-tissue mobilization to stimulate blood flow and edema control and manage pain. Gentle cross-friction massage can be used to encourage collagen formation during tissue healing.
- Assistive device or bracing, if needed, to protect joint and to limit weight-bearing *Note:* The patient should be weaned from assistive devices and bracing/splinting as soon as able, to avoid impairments resulting from immobilization.
- Modalities as needed to manage pain and edema

Subacute stage (days 4 to 21)

Goal: Promote tissue healing, restore function, and control pain

Intervention:

- Progress to AROM and light resistance exercise as tolerated to limits of pain.
- Progress to soft-tissue stretching to increase ROM; may use PNF-based stretching techniques.
- Progress to joint mobilization, if necessary, to improve accessory mobility; continue grade I/II oscillations to manage pain.
- Continue soft-tissue mobilization and cross-friction massage more aggressively.
- Wean from any assistive device or bracing/splinting as soon as able.
- Modalities as needed to manage pain and edema

Chronic stage (>21 days, or recurrent)

Goal: Strengthening, full ROM, normal function, controlled pain

Intervention:

- Progress to resistive exercise program. Include proprioception training and functional activities to allow full return to sport, work, or prior level of activities.
- Continue with soft-tissue stretching and joint mobilization until full ROM is achieved.
- Continue with modalities as needed to manage pain and edema.

Exercise

The effects of exercise on the musculoskeletal system are numerous, and some are obvious. But exercise provides more physiologic benefits than being in good shape and losing weight.

Like nervous tissue, musculoskeletal tissue has a certain degree of plasticity—meaning it is able to adapt to the stresses put on it. There are primarily two types of exercise that have different effects on muscular tissue and muscular strength: resistance and aerobic training.

Resistance or strength training

Resistance or strength training uses weights, resistance bands, manual resistance, or mechanical resistance to build muscle. Changes are made to the oxygen capacity, muscle size, mitochondria volume within the tissue, and amount of muscle protein. There is an increase in the functional strength of the particular exercise performed. Well strengthened muscles can provide shock absorption to the joints. Low-resistance, high-repetition strength training can increase muscular endurance. This may be appropriate with strengthening of postural muscle, rotator cuff, and chronic knee impairments. Muscle power (the amount of work per unit of time) can be increased with high-resistance/low-repetition or low-resistance/high repetition to fatigue.

Isotonic exercise

Isotonic exercise involves constant or variable resistance given throughout the range of motion of the movement. It can be further broken down into two muscle actions:

- Concentric: the muscle is shortening during resistance.
- Eccentric: the muscle is lengthening during resistance.

Greater muscle tension occurs during eccentric exercise, but there is also greater muscle soreness and fatigue following eccentric exercise.

Isometric exercise

Isometric exercise involves a constant joint position with variable resistance and no change in muscle length. For strength gains, isometric contraction must last for at least six seconds. Even then, the strength gained is in that position only. Isometrics also include muscle-setting exercise in which the muscle is contracted but not against any resistance.

Isokinetic exercise

Isokinetic exercise involves a constant velocity of movement with variable resistance given throughout the muscle action. It can be concentric or eccentric. This allows maximum muscle tension throughout the range of motion to increase motor recruitment. Isokinetic strengthening must be done mechanically on a machine such as a Cybex or Dynatron.

Aerobic or endurance training

Aerobic or endurance training uses activity such as walking, jogging, bicycling, swimming, etc., to increase the muscles' ability to maintain a contraction or repeat a contraction over a period of time. This increases the actual number of type II muscle fibers, increases the cross-sectional area of all muscle fibers utilized, and increases the vascular support of the muscle fibers (capillaries). Aerobic/endurance training is also a source of increase in the number of mitochondria and protein within the muscle fibers.

In addition to muscle strength and cardiovascular health gains, low-intensity exercise can also increase flexibility and bone density, lessen body fat measures, improve balance and gait, and improve overall mental health. Specifically, combination of strength and aerobic training can increase bone mass and decrease the rate of osteoblastic activity. This appears to be especially important to postmenopausal women, who are at highest risk of osteopenia and osteoporosis. Exercise also plays a role in decreasing pain and increasing joint mobility and function in those patients who already have arthritic disease. As a preventive measure, exercise is known to prevent or delay diabetes, heart disease, and cancer.

> Caution must be used when performing exercise as a treatment intervention under the following conditions:
>
> - During acute, inflammatory impairments resulting from injury or flare-ups of inflammatory diseases such as arthritis
> - If there is a significant change in pain during the exercise
> - If the patient has compromised cardiovascular, pulmonary, or neurologic systems (see the appropriate chapters)
> - If the patient has a comorbidity of a fatiguing disease such as multiple sclerosis, lupus, etc.
> - Uncontrolled diabetes
> - Osteoporosis

Effects of Exercise as a Treatment Intervention

With both strengthening and endurance exercise, some effects can actually be seen as negative by the patient or the physical therapist. Delayed-onset muscle soreness, substitution patterns, and fatigue can result from exercise.

Delayed-onset muscle soreness

Delayed-onset muscle soreness (DOMS) usually occurs 24 to 48 hours after exercise, possibly as a result of lactic acid buildup or microscopic muscle tears during strengthening. DOMS should not necessarily be considered negative, but it is best to prepare the patient for some amount of muscle soreness (if appropriate) with certain exercise. There is not yet a definitive treatment for this, but the intensity, duration, and type of exercise may need to be adjusted to lessen the discomfort associated with DOMS.

Substitution patterns

Substitution patterns happen when a stronger muscle attempts to assist, or take over for, a weakened muscle or impaired joint during strengthening. This can be fixed by verbal and tactile cues to the patient to focus on the exercise or motion as described by the examiner. The use of a mirror or visual demonstration of the motion as feedback may be helpful in retraining the weakened muscle to function properly.

Fatigue

Fatigue can be good and bad. It is often necessary to exercise a muscle to the point of fatigue in order for the muscle to adapt and become stronger. Total body fatigue can have adverse effects on blood sugar, glycogen, and potassium levels. This is important to consider if the patient is diabetic or has diminished heart function. In all cases, the body must be given adequate time to recover from fatigue.

Exercise Prescription

The Centers for Disease Control (CDC) and the American College of Sports Medicine (ACSM) generally define moderate activity to be a duration of 30 minutes per day for five days per week. They also recommend combining aerobic exercise, strength training, and flexibility. Most of the published studies used exercise programs of 20–30 minutes' duration done two to three times per week for 12–16 weeks. Modifications to these recommendations are necessary for children and the geriatric population. Reevaluation of the patient's strength and assessment of pain periodically (typically, weekly) during an exercise regimen allows the examiner to determine if the exercises given are appropriate and if the muscle is responding as it should to strengthening. The following basic principles are implemented to maximize the effects of strength training.

Overload principle

In order to increase strength, the amount of resistance given to the muscle must exceed what that muscle can normally resist. The muscle must be exercised to fatigue to allow adaptation to occur.

Specificity of exercise

Muscular adaptations to exercise are specific to that particular exercise that is performed. Specificity of exercise refers to the type of muscle fiber recruited, the type of muscular contraction, the muscle action performed, and the joint at which the action takes place. Weakness of one particular muscle may indicate the need for a specific exercise to isolate that muscle, but functional goals steer exercise to be more functional for specificity.

Elements of exercise prescription

For the best results from exercise used as treatment intervention, there should be a specific and planned regimen for the patient to follow. Each element of the exercise prescription can be adjusted to best suit each patient's individual needs.

Type of resistance
This can be isometric, isotonic, or isokinetic. Not all resistance exercises are done through a full range of motion. Some muscles can be better isolated with movements through partial range. Some surgical procedures contraindicate strengthening in specific parts of the range of motion until the surgical site is fully healed.

Type of equipment
This includes (but is not limited to) free weights, resistive bands, manual resistance, isokinetic machines, pulleys, variable resistance equipment, hydraulic-based resistive equipment, and aerobic equipment (treadmill, stationary bicycle, upper-extremity ergometer, etc.).

Open- vs. closed-chain exercise
Open-chain exercise refers to movements in which the distal body part (foot, hand, etc.) moves freely and is not fixed. Long arc quads and biceps curls are open-chain exercises. **Closed-chain exercise** refers to movements in which the distal body part is fixed and the proximal body parts move around it. Squats and push-ups are examples of closed-chain exercises.

Amount of resistance
Amount of resistance can be determined using a ten-repetition maximum (10-RM) as described by any exercise schematic. A 10-RM is determined by the greatest amount of weight that a muscle can move through its full excursion of ten repetitions.

- **The DeLorme technique** uses the 10-RM to determine resistance, and then the protocol is to perform ten repetitions each at 50 percent, 75 percent, and 100 percent of the 10-RM with a brief rest between sets. The 10-RM is increased weekly.
- **The Oxford technique** also uses the 10-RM, but its protocol is to perform ten repetitions each at 100 percent, 75 percent, and 50 percent of the 10-RM with a brief rest between sets. A general warmup is done prior to exercise.

- **The daily adjustable progressive resistance exercise (DAPRE) system** uses four sets of exercise. The first set is ten repetitions at a resistance determined by the end resistance from the previous day. The second set is six repetitions at 75 percent of the first-set resistance. The third set uses the same resistance as the second but increases repetitions to the maximum number of which the patient is capable. The fourth set adjusts the resistance based on how many repetitions were completed in the third set, and also sets the starting resistance for the next day.

Speed of exercise

The exercise speed is slow to control the movement for safety and to maximally recruit muscle fibers. Slow speed also prevents momentum from assisting with the movement of the resistance. In isokinetic strengthening, the speed of exercise should eventually be comparable to the speed at which the goal activity or sport is done. Since the carryover of gains at one speed is minimal at other speeds, it is best to vary the speed of exercise.

Repetitions

Repetitions (reps) of exercise generally range from eight to ten if there is high resistance, such as strengthening type II fibers; or 20 to 30 if there is lower resistance, as in strengthening slow-twitch fibers. Multiple sets of exercise repetitions are done according to the number of reps in each set. Generally, higher reps are done for fewer sets (one or two sets of 20 reps) and lower repetitions are done for multiple sets (two or three sets of eight reps). This can also be determined by the exercise schematics described previously.

Frequency

Frequency of exercise is four or five days per week, preferably in a two-days-on/one-day-off pattern. In the geriatric population, exercise is done three days per week (i.e., every other day). In any case, the days off are to allow recovery and rebuilding of the muscle for further strength gains.

Duration

Duration is the total length of time the exercise program is to take place and must be at least eight to ten weeks to allow adaptation of the muscle to take place.

Range-of-Motion Exercise

Range-of-motion exercise more specifically refers to movement of the joint through the available range and potentially into a greater range for the purpose of improving joint mobility, improving synovial joint lubrication, and aiding in pain management. Range of motion is categorized as follows.

Passive range of motion (PROM)

In passive range of motion (PROM) the work is done by the examiner or another person or by a machine; the patient does no voluntary movement of the affected joint. PROM differs from stretching in that it is done only through the unrestricted available range. Indications for PROM include preventing contractures, improving circulation, improving joint lubrication, decreasing pain, improving proprioceptive input, and maintaining muscle and joint mobility. In acute settings, PROM can be used to prevent skin breakdown, clot formation, and bone loss, and can improve vascular function. A continuous passive motion (CPM) machine is an example of mechanical PROM.

Active-assistive range of motion (AAROM)

Active-assistive range of motion (AAROM) is done using part active motion by the patient and assistance by either the examiner, a machine, or the patient himself. AAROM is a progression from PROM to AROM. It is used on weakened muscle to move through ROM and to aid with pain or joint-limited ROM movements. Equipment used for AAROM may include overhead pulleys, a cane, or a wall ladder.

Active range of motion (AROM)

Active range of motion (AROM) is done by the patient moving through the available range and is a progression from AAROM to resistive exercises for strengthening. Along with the benefits of PROM and AAROM, AROM develops motor learning patterns.

ROM and mobilization as treatment interventions are contraindicated in the following situations:

- If it upsets the normal healing process of a joint or soft-tissue impairment (i.e., immediately postop, acute fractures, active bleeding)
- If the patient is in poor health or declining medical status (i.e., immediately following a stroke or heart attack)

Aquatic Exercise

In some cases the patient does not tolerate or respond well to conventional methods of strengthening. This may be due to pain or deconditioning or immobility. In these instances it may be appropriate to try aquatic exercise to achieve the treatment goals and improve the impairments. The recommended water temperatures for aquatic exercise are 78–82°F (25°–28°C) for high-intensity activity and 88–92°F (31–34°C) for low-intensity activity. It should be noted that water temperature over 94°F (34°C) might cause cardiac complications.

Indications for aquatic exercise

- Decreased range of motion
- Edema, muscle weakness, or pain
- Decreased weight-bearing status or balance deficits
- Impaired activity tolerance or breathing problems

Contraindications to aquatic exercise

- Infectious disease, infected open wound, or contagious skin rash
- Fever
- Diarrhea or bowel incontinence
- Uncontrolled seizures
- Unstable angina
- Severely decreased vital capacity (below 1 L)

Precautions for aquatic exercise

- Patient's fear of water
- Respiratory or cardiac disease
- Pregnancy
- Open wound, or tracheotomy, or chemical sensitivity
- Uncontrolled hypo- or hypertension or diabetes
- Autonomic dysreflexia
- Behavioral problems
- Multiple sclerosis patients tend to have symptom exacerbation in warm water.

Water depth

As water depth increases the pressure increases on the air-filled cavities of the body (lungs, respiratory passages, sinuses, and middle-ear space). As this pressure increases, volume inversely decreases. With breath-holding, carbon dioxide concentration increases, signaling the need for another breath. Even at a depth of one meter (about three feet), the compression forces on the thoracic cavity increase beyond the capacity of the inspiratory musculature. As the intensity of exercise with breath-holding increases, oxygen consumption and carbon dioxide production also increase, resulting in even greater need for respiration. Increased pressure can help compress tissue to eliminate edema.

Water buoyancy

As an object is immersed in fluid, there is an upward thrust that is equal to the weight of the fluid displaced. Water pressure increases as depth increases. Women are more buoyant than men, as higher body fat content is more buoyant. Body weight is off-loaded as water depth increases. For example, 50 percent of body weight is off-loaded when a person is immersed to the mid-pelvis line. Buoyancy can assist with range of motion, strength, gait training, and neuromuscular reeducation for balance.

- **Buoyancy-supported movement** is the equivalent of gravity-eliminated movement. The movement is horizontal.
- **Buoyancy-resisted movement** is the equivalent of gravity-resisted movement. Buoyancy resistance is created when movement is downward through water. Gravity resistance is upward movement against gravity.
- **Buoyancy-assisted movement** is the equivalent of gravity-assisted movement. Buoyancy assistance is created when movement is upward through water. Gravity assistance is downward movement with gravity.

Proprioceptive Training

Proprioceptive training teaches the neuromuscular system to receive and respond properly to information about the position of the musculoskeletal system. Injuries that involve joint mobility also affect the mechanoreceptors of that joint. Proprioception exercises are closed-chain exercises of the involved extremity. Proprioceptive training helps to fine-tune muscle response to activity. It is crucial to incorporate some proprioceptive training into all rehabilitation in which the goal is functional mobility. This is especially true in the rehabilitation of athletic injuries when the goal is return to play. Examples of proprioceptive training exercise include the following:

- **Upper extremity:** Push-ups on a Swiss ball against the wall or floor, weight-bearing activity through the upper extremity, scapular clock
- **Lower extremity:** Tandem stance, single-leg stance on level and unlevel surfaces, combined activities of upper extremity exercise in a tandem or single-leg position
- **Spinal (core) stabilization:** Seated or prone on a Swiss ball, seated on DynaDisc or foam

Manual Techniques

Manual techniques may be necessary when there is decreased ROM, pain, or inadequate function of the joint and surrounding soft tissues, including connective tissue and muscle. Manual techniques can be grouped into joint mobilization, stretching, and muscle energy techniques.

Joint mobilization

Joint mobilization is used to increase physiologic and accessory motions of the joint itself. It is considered a passive technique. After determining which joint motions or accessory motions may be limited during the joint-play portion of the evaluation, it can be determined which mobilization direction(s) will be most effective. Indications for the use of joint mobilization as a treatment intervention include pain, decreased joint mobility, or stiffness during movement. Along with improved joint mobility, joint mobilization improves joint proprioception and movement of synovial fluid to improve joint nutrition. Joint traction and joint oscillation are useful techniques in relaxation prior to stretching and pain management.

In the peripheral joints, the mobilization is named for the movement of the distal bone on the proximal bone. In the spinal joints, the mobilization is named for the superior or proximal bone. Following joint mobilization technique(s) and during follow-up visits, pain and mobility should be reevaluated. The amplitude and range of the oscillations may be adjusted to further increase range or lessened to treat pain. Similar to range-of-motion and stretching interventions, the use of heat, ultrasound, or light exercise may increase the mobility gained with mobilization techniques. Joint mobilization is contraindicated in an unstable or hypermobile joint, malignancy, or osteoporosis, or if there is significant joint swelling. Joint mobilization may not be appropriate immediately postoperatively on a joint or on an unhealed fracture. Oscillations may be used to increase movement of synovial fluid to aid in edema control. Joint mobilizations can be further categorized by grade according to the amplitude, range, and velocity of movement, outlined in the table below.

Grading Joint Mobilization

Grade I	• Small-amplitude, performed at the beginning of the range • Primarily used to manage pain and increase synovial joint lubrication
Grade II	• Large-amplitude, performed within available range • Used primarily to manage pain
Grade III	• Large-amplitude, performed up to end range • Used to increase joint mobility
Grade IV	• Small-amplitude, performed at end range • Used to increase joint mobility
Grade V	• Small-amplitude, high-velocity, performed at end range (also called manipulation or thrust) • Not as common • Used to reposition a joint or break up scar-tissue adhesions

Joint oscillations

Oscillatory techniques for accessory movement mobilization are grouped into glides (or slides), rolls, and spins.

Joint traction

Joint traction can be used for pain management, muscle relaxation, or decreased pressure on neurogenic tissues, or combined with glides to increase motion. Traction techniques separate joint surfaces.

Joint glides

Joint gliding techniques do not separate the joint but rather move in a direction parallel to the joint surfaces. Glides are done in the direction of the desired slide movement of the joint, following the convex-concave rule. This rule states that if the moving bone is the convex bone, joint slide is in the direction opposite to the motion. If the moving bone is the concave bone, joint slide occurs in the same direction as the motion.

Stretching

Stretching can be active or passive lengthening of the soft tissue itself, done in a slow, prolonged movement. (Specific active inhibition stretch techniques are discussed in the neuromuscular chapter.) During stretching, the soft tissue is moved into a lengthened position manually, mechanically, or by patient self-stretch or self-positioning. In this type of manual technique or exercise, there is no voluntary muscle contraction. Stretching has effects on contractile and noncontractile tissue.

- As a muscle is stretched, the sarcomeres are lengthened and the actin-myosin filament cross-bridges are broken, allowing the tissue to stretch. After muscle stretching, the sarcomeres return to their resting position. Immobilization in a shortened or lengthened position respectively decreases or increases the number of sarcomeres in series and temporarily changes the muscle fiber length.
- When noncontractile tissues are stretched, a certain amount of deformation occurs, known as strain. In noncontractile tissue there can be variable amounts of strain that cause elastic change (returns to original shape), plastic change (permanent deformation), or failure (total rupture) to occur.

Stretching is an indicated intervention for impairments such as contractures, adhesions, or soft-tissue tightness limiting function or causing pain. For adequate stretch to occur, the position must be held for at least 30 seconds or as tolerated for two to three repetitions with rest in between. For greatest flexibility gains, a stretching program may be implemented three to five days per week. Heat, ultrasound, massage, gentle oscillation, or low-intensity warm-up activity can be used prior to stretch to increase tissue extensibility. It is known that tissues made up of collagen have greater resistance to strain even with a 1°C (33°F) tissue temperature change. Contraindications to stretching are the same as those for range of motion. Under some conditions it may be appropriate to allow shortening or contractures of the muscle to aid in function; an example of this may be allowing contractures of the finger flexors in a patient with a spinal cord injury to facilitate a modified functional grip.

Soft-tissue mobilization

Soft-tissue mobilization (STM) uses manual techniques to stretch and mobilize the non-bony tissues. The benefits of STM can include increased blood flow, increased tissue extensibility, increased relaxation, decreased pain, and decreased spasm.

Massage

Massage of soft tissues is a general term for movement of the soft tissues with the physical therapist's hands. It is usually a precursor to other soft-tissue mobilization technique(s).

Myofascial release

Myofascial release is a group of techniques used to stretch and mobilize soft tissues. It can include J-stroking, strumming, and stripping. Some long-axis traction techniques are also considered myofascial release. The techniques vary in amounts of pressure used, and some are uncomfortable during application.

Cross-friction massage
Cross-friction massage (CFM) is a deep massage directly to the soft tissues involved. It is usually done perpendicular to the direction of the soft-tissue fibers. CFM can be useful in encouraging the laying down of collagen fibers in the proper direction for healing of soft tissues. It can also aid in increasing blood flow, decreasing pain, and improving ROM. Technique progresses from light to deep pressure across the intended soft tissue. No lotions are used with this technique.

Neural glides
Neural gliding is the movement of neuromusculoskeletal tissue through an area that may be impinging on the tissue. Neural glides can be done with the patient in the same position as for neural tension testing. Gliding is done up to the point of symptom production and should move into symptomatic range. It may be beneficial to glide at any one or combination of the joints through which the nerve passes. Gliding can also be done on the uninvolved side. Use care when mobilizing neural tissue, as symptoms can be worsened with too much mobilization.

Edema massage
Edema massage is a very light-pressure massage to encourage edema drainage and movement of fluid surrounding tissues. It is usually done proximally to drain lymph nodes, moving distally and then proximally again to encourage drainage and the direction of flow.

Muscle energy techniques

Muscle energy techniques (METs) use a submaximal muscle contraction in a contract-relax sequence coupled with segmental stabilization to move a joint to a desired position (active joint mobilization). Treatment with METs is determined by joint dysfunction, particularly with accessory joint motion. Muscle energy usually moves in the direction opposite to the restricted joint motion so as to pull the joint back into a more functional position. MET is most typically used on the spine and pelvis but can be used for some peripheral joint dysfunctions.

Pain Management

Pain can be managed through the use of exercise for range of motion and functional mobility and the manual techniques described above. The use of modalities (see modalities chapter) for tissue healing, edema management, and pain management can also be useful in breaking the pain cycle. Often drug therapy as prescribed by the physician is used in combination with physical therapy.

Home Programs

In most cases of PT intervention it is necessary to educate the patient on things to do at home and as a part of daily living. This instruction can include the following:

- Posture/ergonomics
- Body mechanics
- Home exercise (how to progress)
- Activity modification (when to return to activity, what to avoid)
- Home pain management (heat, ice)
- Home mobilization (stretching, joint mobilization, ROM, soft-tissue mobilization)
- Safety with mobility (transfers, ambulation)

A FINAL WORD

To adequately evaluate and treat a patient or client, the therapist must have a strong knowledge of the foundational sciences and background, evaluation, differential diagnoses, and treatment interventions of the musculoskeletal system. This chapter, which highlights each of these areas, along with your experience in lab practicals and clinical affiliations, will help prepare you to identify and treat impairments of these systems.

The following pages offer an end-of-chapter practice quiz to test your knowledge of some of the fundamentals of the musculoskeletal system. It is not necessary to time this, as it is a chapter review quiz.

Musculoskeletal System Chapter Quiz

1. A positive step deformity would indicate involvement of which joint of the shoulder?

   (A) Acromioclavicular

   (B) Sternoclavicular

   (C) Glenohumeral

   (D) Scapulothoracic

2. A physical therapist is performing manual muscle testing of a patient in acute care. What is the maximum grade the patient can receive for hip flexor strength if he is unable to sit up?

   (A) 0

   (B) 2

   (C) 3

   (D) 5

3. The following information is found during the patient interview. Which may be most indicative of a need to refer the patient back to the primary care physician?

   (A) Comorbidity of diabetes

   (B) A 10 lb weight loss in the last week

   (C) Pain at rest

   (D) Inability to get a shoe onto the swollen foot

4. A patient who has seen a physical therapist for three visits continues to have significant pain in the foot despite utilization of pain management techniques, light range-of-motion activity, and manual stretching and mobilization. What would be the *BEST* noninvasive diagnostic test for further radiological workup?

   (A) Plain film X-ray

   (B) Myelography

   (C) Computed tomography

   (D) Radionuclide scan

5. A college student presents with pain in the shoulder that began the week after finals, but she cannot recall any mechanism of injury. Upon inspection, the examiner notes scapular winging on the dominant side. During evaluation the patient has difficulty with elevation greater than 120°. She has normal scapular elevation. What would be the *BEST* differential diagnosis?

   (A) Acute rotator cuff tendonitis

   (B) Shoulder impingement

   (C) Long thoracic nerve lesion

   (D) Accessory nerve lesion

6. A patient presents with cervical pain that radiates down the right arm to just above the elbow. It is worse when he reaches overhead into his closet. It is better when he sits in the recliner with his hands on top of his head. What is the expected pathology?

   (A) C2-3 nerve root pathology

   (B) C4-5 nerve root pathology

   (C) Shoulder impingement

   (D) Cervical myopathy

7. During a patient interview, the patient states that he has been having pain down the arm and into the left shoulder blade. Which positive special test would *BEST* indicate the source of the symptoms?

   (A) Drop arm test

   (B) Spurling's test

   (C) Sharp-Pursor test

   (D) Neer's test

8. Which would be the *BEST* way to assess true internal rotation of the glenohumeral joint range of motion?
   (A) Have the patient reach his hands behind his back
   (B) Assess the motion at 90° abducted with the patient in supine position
   (C) Assess the motion with the arm by his side
   (D) Assess the motion with the patient reaching his hands behind his head

9. In which one of the following diagnoses would general spinal flexion exercises and spinal mobilization techniques be contraindicated as treatment interventions?
   (A) Spinal stenosis
   (B) Osteoporosis
   (C) L3 disc herniation
   (D) Degenerative disc disease

10. On examination of a patient's shoulder, clinical findings include glenohumeral joint hypomobility in all directions, pain with reaching overhead, and weakness of scapular stabilizers. During treatment intervention in the following weeks, the *BEST* order of addressing the problem list would be which of the following?
   (A) Strengthening the rotator cuff, followed by modalities to manage pain
   (B) Mobilize the glenohumeral joint, strengthen the scapular stabilizers, strengthen the rotator cuff
   (C) Modalities only
   (D) Strengthen the scapular stabilizers and rotator cuff together

11. Which one of the following exercise schematics uses sets of repetitions at 100 percent, 75 percent, and 50 percent of the ten-repetition maximum, in that order, for strengthening?
   (A) Oxford
   (B) DeLorme
   (C) DAPRE
   (D) DOMS

12. Which principle of exercise accounts for the fact that strengthening of the biceps with arm curls does not necessarily improve the biceps function during shoulder flexion?
   (A) Overload principle
   (B) Mode of exercise
   (C) Specificity of exercise
   (D) Principle of reversibility

13. Which one of the following has the greatest percentage composition of type I slow-twitch muscle fibers?
   (A) Gastrocnemius
   (B) Biceps femoris
   (C) Biceps brachialis
   (D) Supraspinatus

14. Which component of noncontractile tissue provides the greatest strength to the soft tissues?
   (A) Elastin
   (B) Collagen
   (C) Reticulin
   (D) Fascia

15. Which grade of joint mobilization would be *MOST* appropriate for improving joint motion using a large-amplitude movement into end range?
   (A) Grade I
   (B) Grade II
   (C) Grade III
   (D) Grade IV

Answers

1. A.

   The step deformity is indicative of acromioclavicular joint dislocation. With rupture of the acromioclavicular and coracoclavicular ligaments, the distal clavicle moves superiorly.
   (Magee, page 240)

2. B.

   A muscle strength grade of a 2 indicates the patient is able to move through complete range of motion in a gravity-eliminated position. To earn a 3 the patient must complete range of motion against gravity.
   (Magee, page 35)

3. B.

   An unexplained weight loss of 10 to 15 lb over a two-week period could be indicative of cancer. The other choices do necessitate extra attention to the systemic response to exercise but do not indicate the need for immediate referral.
   (Magee, page 2)

4. D.

   Radionuclide scan, or bone scan, can show a stress fracture at a much lower percentage of bone loss than a plain film. Myelography is invasive imaging for spinal soft tissues. CT scans are most expensive.
   (Magee, page 63)

5. C.

   The long thoracic nerve innervates the serratus anterior, a scapular stabilizer. The nerve can be compressed with a backpack strap as it lies along the chest wall. This patient will have scapular winging but good scapular elevation strength. Damage to the spinal accessory nerve will inhibit elevation of the scapula.
   (Magee, pages 241, 257)

6. B.

   Cervical nerve root pain increases with extension, such as looking up into the closet. It is also relieved with resting the hand on top of the head as it alters the position of the foramen. The patient's pain radiated to just above the elbow indicating C4–C5 involvement rather than C2–C3 pathology.
   (Magee, pages 139,140)

7. B.

   Spurling's test is for nerve root symptoms and is positive if the pain radiates down the arm and shoulder blade ipsilateral to the direction of cervical rotation.
   (Magee, page 163)

8. B.

   To truly assess internal rotation of the glenohumeral joint, the patient should have the arm abducted to 90°. True internal rotation is movement until the scapula begins to move.
   (Magee, page 253)

9. B.

   Due to the increased risk of fracture associated with osteoporosis and the increased pressures on the vertebral bodies with spinal flexion, flexion-based exercise and mobilization techniques are not appropriate for this patient.
   (Goodman/Pathology, page 883)

10. B.

    If there is hypomobility in the joint, it must first be addressed with mobilization. Strengthening of the supporting musculature without addressing the motion limitations will further tighten the joint, as the muscles shorten with strengthening.
    (Kisner, page 254)

11. A.

The Oxford technique uses the ten-repetition maximum (10-RM) and the protocol is to perform ten repetitions each at 100 percent, 75 percent, and 50 percent of the 10-RM with a brief rest between sets.
(Kisner, page 89)

12. C.

Specificity of exercise explains that muscular adaptations to exercise are specific to the particular exercise that is performed.
(Kisner, page 84)

13. D.

The supraspinatus is a phasic or postural muscle, which indicates it has higher composition of slow-twitch oxidative muscle fibers. It responds best to low-weight, high-repetition exercise.
(Kisner, page 63)

14. B.

Collagen provides tensile strength to the tissue and does not allow much for tissue lengthening without injury to the tissue.
(Kisner, page 118)

15. C.

Grade III joint mobilizations utilize a large-amplitude mobilization into the end range of accessory joint motion to improve range of motion.
(Kisner, page 158)

5

Nervous System

Communication and control are the main functions of the nervous system. These functions happen both within the nervous system and between other organ systems. The spinal cord contains ascending and descending tracts that send impulses both to the muscles, skin, and tissues and to the brain. A graduating physical therapy student should be familiar with the basic anatomy of this system, as it is involved in every movement of the body. Physical therapists routinely treat patients whose only diagnosis is a dysfunction of the nervous system, such as a brain injury or a cerebrovascular accident. However, a patient also cannot be categorized only as an "orthopedic patient" or a "cardiac patient"—the organ systems are interrelated and the examination and treatment techniques of other systems can directly affect the nervous or neuromuscular system. In providing treatment you must consider the patient as a whole and not just the injury or disability for which they are seeking physical therapy. To fully understand the nervous system, you must first know human anatomy and physiology, including the brain, spinal cord, and nerves. Examination of the nervous system may be appropriate even when you are evaluating a patient whose main medical diagnosis does not affect the nervous system. The patient's comorbidities, age, activity level, and psychology all play into the success of physical therapy as a treatment intervention. In this chapter you will delve a little deeper, beyond the basics, into the examination and treatment of this important system.

FOUNDATIONAL SCIENCES AND BACKGROUND

A strong understanding of the basic background and fundamental sciences of the nervous system is necessary before examination, evaluation, interpretation, and intervention can take place. It is necessary to understand how each component works, including the spinal cord tracts, specific areas of the brain, and the nerves, to be able to evaluate and treat a patient as a whole.

Anatomy and Physiology

Central nervous system

The central nervous system (CNS) consists of the brain and the spinal cord. The brain is further divided into several distinct areas, including the cerebrum, cerebellum, diencephalon, basal ganglia, and brain stem.

Cerebrum

The cerebrum is the large part of the brain that is divided into four lobes: the frontal lobe, parietal lobe, temporal lobe, and occipital lobe. Each lobe has different functions. The cerebrum contains ridges and fissures. Ridges are called **gyri** and the fissures are called **sulci**.

- The **frontal lobe** contains the **primary motor cortex**, which provides efferent control to the contralateral side of the body. Areas for higher cognitive functions and **Broca's motor speech area** are also found in the frontal lobe.
- The **parietal lobe** contains the **primary sensory cortex**, which works in the processing and perception of sensory information. Short-term memory and the **sensory homunculus** are also found in the parietal lobe. The sensory homunculus is a mapping of the sensory representation of the body.
- The **temporal lobe** contains the **primary auditory cortex**, which works in the processing and perception of auditory information. Long-term memory and **Wernicke's area** are also found in the temporal lobe. Wernicke's area provides us with the ability to hear and comprehend language.
- The **occipital lobe** contains the primary **visual cortex**, which works in the processing and perception of visual information.

Hemispheric control

The right hemisphere is the least common dominant hemisphere. Ninety-five percent of the population is left hemisphere–dominant. Each hemisphere is responsible for different functions, processes, and abilities.

Hemispheric Control

Left Hemisphere	Right Hemisphere
Analytical abilities	Artistic abilities
Verbal communication and interpretation	Nonverbal communication and interpretation
Reading	Processing and organizing information as a whole
Mathematical calculation	Mathematical and numerical processing
Sequencing of movements	Visual-spatial processing Organization and pattern recognition
Movement on command	Sustaining a movement or posture
Expression of positive emotions	Expression of negative emotions Perception of emotion

Cerebellum

The cerebellum is located posteriorly and inferiorly to the cerebrum. The cerebellum is involved in coordinated movement, initiation and timing of movement, and balance and posture.

Diencephalon

The diencephalon is composed of the **thalamus** and **hypothalamus**. This structure is found deep within the brain. The thalamus is a sensory integrative center. The hypothalamus helps to control the autonomic nervous system. Through its involvement in the autonomic nervous system, the hypothalamus helps to control body temperature, thirst, appetite, sleep, and emotion. The hypothalamus also releases hormones, thus also serving as an endocrine gland.

Basal ganglia
The basal ganglia are a group of nuclei that govern motor planning and motor control. Lesions of the basal ganglia result in rigidity; resting tremor; and meaningless, unintentional movements.

Brain stem
The brain stem is composed of three small structures: the **midbrain**, **pons**, and **medulla**. The brain stem is located at the superior end of the spinal cord. The brain stem controls basic life functions, such as breathing, blood pressure, and heart rate.

Spinal cord
The spinal cord meets the brain stem at the foramen magnum at the base of the skull. The spinal cord contains both gray matter and white matter. **Gray matter** is composed of neuronal cell bodies and synapses. **White matter** consists of tracts of ascending and descending pathways. The spinal cord has a series of nerve roots that either exit or enter, anteriorly or posteriorly. The anterior nerve roots contain motor neurons, and the posterior roots contain sensory neurons.

Blood supply to the brain

- The **internal carotid arteries** supply the anterior area of the brain. Each internal carotid artery branches into an anterior cerebral artery and a middle cerebral artery.
- The **vertebral arteries** supply the posterior area of the brain. Each vertebral artery becomes a posterior cerebral artery.
- **Cerebellar arteries:** The superior cerebellar artery, anterior inferior cerebellar artery, and posterior inferior cerebellar artery supply the cerebellum and parts of the brain stem.
- **Internal jugular vein:** The brain is drained via the dural sinuses that ultimately drain into the internal jugular vein.

Meninges
The meninges are three protective layers that cover the entire CNS. The **pia mater** is the thin covering of the CNS that directly covers the brain and spinal cord. The **arachnoid mater** is the middle layer. Finally, the **dura mater** is the outermost layer that contains the dural sinuses. The outer layer of the dura is termed **periosteum**.

Ventricles
Ventricles are spaces within the CNS. These spaces contain **choroid plexus** that secretes **cerebrospinal fluid (CSF)**, a clear fluid that protects and bathes the central nervous system.

Somatic motor and sensory tracts
The spinal cord contains main tracts that relay nerve impulses to and from the brain. Each tract has different functions and different starting and ending points. Some cross sides and some remain on the same side. Knowledge of these tracts can help you diagnose the source of your patient's neurologic problems.

- **Spinothalamic tract:** The spinothalamic tract carries information on pain, temperature, and light touch. This tract crosses to the contralateral side almost immediately after entering the spinal cord. Ultimately, this tract travels to the thalamus and the sensory area of the cerebral cortex.
- **Posterior columns:** The posterior columns include the **fasciculus gracilis** and **fasciculus cuneatus**. These tracts convey conscious proprioception, stereognosis, and light touch. These pathways cross to the opposite side at the junction of the spinal cord and brain stem. Like the spinothalamic tract, these tracts also travel to the thalamus and the sensory area of the cerebral cortex.

- **Spinocerebellar tract:** The spinocerebellar tract conveys unconscious proprioception and stereogenesis to the cerebellum. The spinocerebellar tract remains ipsilateral. Since this tract does not cross the midline, lesions of the cerebellum generally result in ipsilateral deficits of unconscious proprioception.
- **Corticospinal tract:** The corticospinal tract is the main motor pathway from the motor cortex. The corticospinal tract crosses over at the brain stem/spinal cord junction and synapses in the anterior horn of the gray matter. **Upper motor neurons** are neurons from the motor cortex to the anterior horn synapse. **Lower motor neurons** are motor neurons after the anterior horn synapse.
- **Rubrospinal tract:** The rubrospinal tract is the motor pathway from the red nucleus of the midbrain to the lower motor neurons of the upper extremities. This tract facilitates flexor musculature and inhibits extensor musculature.
- **Tectospinal tract:** The tectospinal tract controls orientation of the head toward a sound or a moving object.
- **Vestibulospinal tract:** The lateral vestibulospinal tract facilitates proximal extensor muscles to maintain posture. The medial vestibulospinal tract controls head and neck muscle tone to keep the head balanced over the trunk.

Peripheral nervous system

The peripheral nervous system (PNS) is divided into the cranial nerves and the peripheral nerves. There are 12 pairs of cranial nerves and 31 pairs of peripheral (spinal) nerves. Each peripheral nerve contains both a sensory and motor component.

Cranial Nerves

Nerve	Name	Function
Cranial nerve I	Olfactory	Sense of smell
Cranial nerve II	Optic	Sense of sight
Cranial nerve III	Oculomotor	Moves the eye superiorly, inferiorly, and medially; constricts the pupil
Cranial nerve IV	Trochlear	Moves the eyes superiorly and inferiorly
Cranial nerve V	Trigeminal	Chewing and sensation of the face
Cranial nerve VI	Abducens	Abducts the eye
Cranial nerve VII	Facial	Movements of the face; tastes, salivates, and tears
Cranial nerve VIII	Vestibulocochlear	Hearing and vestibular sense
Cranial nerve IX	Glossopharyngeal	Tastes, swallows, and salivates
Cranial nerve X	Vagus	Regulates viscera, speech, taste, and swallowing
Cranial nerve XI	Accessory	Innervates sternocleidomastoid and trapezius; turns head and elevates shoulders
Cranial nerve XII	Hypoglossal	Moves the tongue

Divisions of the PNS

The PNS is separated into divisions on the basis of physiology. First, it is divided into the **somatic** and **autonomic nervous systems.** The somatic nervous system includes the nerves and receptors of the skin and muscles. The autonomic nervous system includes the nerves and receptors of the viscera, glands, heart, smooth muscle, and blood vessels. The autonomic nervous system also includes the hypothalamus. The autonomic nervous system is further divided into the parasympathetic and sympathetic nervous systems.

- **Parasympathetic nervous system:** Uses acetylcholine as its neurotransmitter. This system works to decrease heart rate and increase blood flow to the digestive system.
- **Sympathetic nervous system:** Our fight or flight response system, it uses norepinephrine and epinephrine as its neurotransmitters. Sympathetic impulses increase the heart rate and shunt blood to the heart and muscles, away from the abdominal viscera.

Neuron

A neuron is a nerve cell that contains a cell body, an axon, and dendrites. The axon carries impulses away from the cell body, while dendrites carry impulses toward the cell body. Neurons synapse with other neurons or an effector cell. **Neurotransmitters** are chemical messengers that transmit impulses across the synapse.

Sensory neurons are termed **afferent neurons.** Motor neurons are termed **efferent neurons. Myelin** is the white substance that covers axons. The function of myelin is to increase the speed of nerve impulse transmission. A group of neurons outside the CNS is called a nerve. A group of neurons within the CNS is called a tract.

Upper motor neuron lesion symptoms

- Spastic paralysis
- Hyperreflexia
- Positive Babinski reflex
- Clonus

Lower motor neuron lesion symptoms

- Flaccid paralysis
- Hyporeflexia
- Negative Babinski reflex
- Muscle atrophy
- Muscle fasciculations

Neuronal physiology

Surrounding a neuron, the extracellular space is higher than the intracellular space in concentration of Na+ ions; the intracellular space is higher in concentration of K+ ions. This allows for passive diffusion of Na+ into the cell and K+ out of the cell. The resting membrane potential of a neuron is −70 to −90 mV. During an action potential, the membrane potential decreases (or becomes more positive). This is called **depolarization.** Depolarization is excitatory to the neuron. An action potential starts due to ion channels that are activated to change the resting membrane potential. Threshold level must be reached for depolarization to occur. The sodium-potassium pump opens and allows Na+ ions into the cell. Depolarization occurs, and the membrane potential changes to +30 mV. Following depolarization, repolarization occurs, allowing K+ ions out of the cell. Action potentials occur down the membrane of the neuron in only one direction. Myelin that covers the axons and nodes of Ranvier allow for saltatory conduction. Following an action potential, there is a brief refractory period when the neuron cannot respond to another stimulus.

Synapses

Synapses are the space between neurons. Human synapses are predominately chemical; few are electrical. At a chemical synapse, the presynaptic neuron releases neurotransmitter into the synaptic cleft (the space between neurons) that is either excitatory or inhibitory to the postsynaptic neuron.

Neuroglia

Neuroglia are the support cells of the nervous system.

Astrocytes are mostly in the gray matter of the central nervous system.

Oligodendrocytes are mostly in the white matter of the CNS; these cells produce myelin.

Schwann cells are in the peripheral nervous system; these cells also produce myelin.

Microglia have a phagocytic function.

Peripheral nerves

There are 31 pairs of peripheral (spinal) nerves. There are eight cervical nerves, 12 thoracic nerves, five lumbar nerves, five sacral nerves, and one coccygeal nerve.

Naming of spinal nerves

Cervical nerves exit the spinal column above the vertebrae. Spinal nerve C1 exits above the C1 vertebra. Cervical nerve C8 exits below the C7 vertebra. There is no such thing as a C8 vertebra. Thoracic and lumbar nerves exit the spinal column below the corresponding vertebrae. Spinal nerve T1 exits below the T1 vertebra. The spinal cord ends at approximately L2. Below L2, the nerves continue and are referred to as the cauda equina.

Networks of nerves

There are three complicated networks of nerves: the cervical plexus, brachial plexus, and lumbosacral plexus. These include branches from several spinal nerves.

- **Cervical plexus:** The cervical plexus is the network of C1 through C4 spinal nerves that supply the neck and upper shoulder. The cervical plexus includes the phrenic nerve, which contains branches from C3 through C5, innervating the diaphragm.
- **Brachial plexus:** The brachial plexus is the network of C5 through T1 spinal nerves that supply the upper extremity, upper chest, and back. The brachial plexus includes the musculocutaneous, axillary, radial, median, and ulnar nerves.
- **Lumbosacral plexus:** The lumbosacral plexus is the network of L1 through S3 spinal nerves that innervate the lower extremity. This plexus includes the obturator, femoral, superior and inferior gluteal, common peroneal, and tibial nerves.

Receptors of the neuromuscular system

Afferent impulses convey sensory information to the CNS. **Receptors** are stimulated by mechanical, chemical, or thermal stimuli and are converted to a generator potential which, if sufficient, will cause depolarization of the afferent axon. Receptors provide information about the external environment, the internal environment, and the position of the musculoskeletal system. Receptors include the special sense receptors (for taste, smell, vision, hearing, and the vestibular system). Cutaneous receptors provide information on touch, pressure, temperature, stretch, and pain.

Proprioceptors provide information on a person's position. Muscle spindles and Golgi tendon organs are two types of proprioceptors.

Muscle spindles

Muscle spindles are found in between muscle fibers and sense change in the length of a muscle. If the change in length is sufficient, depolarization of an afferent sensory nerve occurs. Muscle spindles are involved in the stretch reflex. This reflex arc occurs at the level of the spinal cord, without cerebral involvement. The muscle spindle regulates reciprocal innervation, stimulating the agonist muscle to contract and the antagonist muscle to relax.

Golgi tendon organs

Golgi tendon organs are encapsulated nerve endings found in the musculotendinous junction. These receptors sense the change in tension and the level of fatigue of muscle fibers. Golgi tendon organs mediate non-reciprocal innervation wherein the agonist is inhibited and the antagonist is facilitated.

Joint receptors

Joint receptors are found in the joint and sense joint position.

Free nerve endings

Free nerve endings are also called naked nerve endings. These are found in the skin and mucosa and work to sense pain, touch, and temperature.

Meissner corpuscles

Meissner corpuscles are found in the skin and sense fine touch and low-frequency vibration.

Ruffini corpuscles

Ruffini corpuscles are found in the skin and sense touch and pressure.

Pacini corpuscles

Pacini corpuscles are found in subcutaneous, submucous, and subserous tissues. They are also found around joints and in mammary glands and external genitalia. Pacini corpuscles sense pressure and high-frequency vibration.

Krause-end bulbs

Krause-end bulbs are found in the skin, mucosa, subcutaneous tissue, and external genitalia. These receptors sense touch.

Dermatomes and cutaneous distribution of peripheral nerves

A dermatome is a specific area of the skin that is innervated by a single, specific spinal nerve. A **myotome** is a group of muscles innervated by a single, specific spinal nerve. Later in this chapter is a diagram depicting the location of dermatomes. Refer to "Standard Neurological Classification of Spinal Cord Injury" on page 150.

Neuromuscular Pharmacology

Disorder or Problem	Drugs Commonly Used (followed by common brand name)
Spasticity	• Baclofen (Lioresal) • Botulinum A toxin (Botox) • Dantrolene (Dantrium) • Diazepam (Valium)

Disorder or Problem	Drugs Commonly Used (followed by common brand name)
Parkinson's disease	• Amantadine (Symmetrel) • Bromocriptine (Parlodel) • Levodopa with dopa-decarboxylase inhibitor carbidopa (Sinemet) • Selegiline HCl (Eldepryl) • Pramipexole (Mirapex) • Entacapone (Comtan) • Antimuscarinic antiparkinsonian drugs
Movement disorders (e.g., chorea, essential tremor)	• Botulinum A and B toxins (Botox) • Haloperidol (Haldol) • Clonidine (Catapres)
Multiple sclerosis	• Corticosteroids • Amantadine (Symmetrel) • Beta-1a-interferon (Rebif, Avonex) and beta-1b-interferon (Betaseron) • Glatiramer acetate (Copaxone) • Mitoxantrone (Novantrone) • Natalizumab (Tysabri) • Clonazepam (Klonopin) • Modafinil (Provigil) • Methylphenidate hydrochloride (Ritalin) • Carbamazepine (Tegretol) • Diazepam (Valium) • Cannabis
Cerebrovascular accident and head and spinal cord injury	• Anticoagulants • Antispasticity drugs • Antidepressants • Antiplatelet drugs (e.g., aspirin) • Nimodipine (Nimotop) • Analgesics • Diuretics • Antihypertensives • Thrombolytics
Trigeminal neuralgia	• Carbamazepine (Tegretol) • Gabapentin (Neurontin)

Disorder or Problem	Drugs Commonly Used (followed by common brand name)
Epilepsy	• Carbamazepine (Tegretol) • Clonazepam (Klonopin) • Gabapentin (Neurontin) • Phenobarbital • Phenytoin (Dilantin)
Phenobarbital	• Levetiracetam (Keppra) • Divalproex (Depakote) • Lamotrigine (Lamictal) • Topiramate (Topamax) • Tiagabine (Gabitril) • Oxcarbazepine (Trileptal)
Guillain-Barré syndrome	• Immunoglobulins

Responses to Exercise and Inactivity

Immobility and specific pathologies affecting the neuromuscular system can result in atrophy of muscle. As a result of this atrophy, the cross-sectional area of the muscle decreases and weakness occurs.

Exercise affects both the physiology and anatomy of a muscle. Exercise can increase muscle strength, coordination, and range of motion. Motor units are increasingly recruited and demonstrate improved timing and sequencing. Agonist and antagonist coordination is improved. Muscle length and muscular endurance are increased. Fluency, fluidity, and coordination can be improved due to improved motor neuron activation.

Neuroplasticity

Neuroplasticity is the ability of the nervous system to change in response to repeated stimuli. Developmentally (from childhood), the CNS grows and subsequently exhibits cell death and projection withdrawal. In the adult, neuroplasticity is more limited. During childhood development, the changes in the nervous system are anatomical due to cell growth, axon and dendrite formation, and routing. In the adult, nervous system changes are linked to the strength and efficiency of synapses. Repetitive stimulation of a neural pathway is key in strengthening neural connections in the child and the adult.

Motor Control

Motor control is the ability to maintain and change posture and movement due to neurologic, physical, and behavioral processes. Motor control is largely due to the interaction and development of the nervous and muscular systems and involves neural pathways and physiologic interactions. The nervous system directs what muscles should be utilized and the force, speed, and order in which they should be activated. Motor control is environmental and task-dependent. This evolves over the course of the lifespan and is integral in motor development.

Motor control refers to quick physiologic changes in the body and occurs in milliseconds. Sensation plays a dominant role in the development of control of movement, beginning with infantile reflexes and progressing through development of motor skills and, later, refinement of advanced motor skills. Sensory feedback is required for smooth, coordinated movements. Impairments of motor control result in timing and sequencing errors.

There are varying theories of motor control. These include the hierarchic theory and systems models.

Hierarchic theory of motor control

The cerebral cortex is the highest level of motor control and directs subcortical areas to produce coordinated, voluntary movement. The hierarchic theory of motor control states that a hierarchy of reflexes exists. These reflexes include spinal cord reflexes, tonic reflexes, and postural responses. **Spinal cord reflexes** are the most primitive. **Tonic reflexes** reach the level of the brain stem and produce muscle tone and posture. Finally, **postural responses** reach the level of the midbrain and the cortex and include righting, equilibrium, and protective reactions. Higher structures of the nervous system influence and inhibit lower reflexes.

Stages of motor control

- **Mobility**: Beginning random movements that are often reflex-based
- **Stability**: Maintenance of posture in weight-bearing and antigravity positions
- **Controlled mobility**: Movement within a posture
- **Skill**: Movement from one posture to another posture

Postural control

- **Righting reactions**: Include head and trunk righting
- **Protective reactions**: Extremity movement to protect balance in higher postures
- **Equilibrium reactions**: Maintain center of gravity over the base of support

Systems models of motor control

There are various systems models of motor control that have similar characteristics. Systems models purport that it takes a combined effort of all of the body's organ systems to produce smooth, coordinated movement; it is not solely the responsibility of the nervous system. For example, the musculoskeletal system, the cardiopulmonary system, and the special senses all make contributions to the production of movement. Posture and movement are organized by the mastery of movement patterns.

Feedback is necessary in the mastery of movement patterns. Feedback is supplied both by sensory information and from the external environment. An absence of movement can be due to problems in any system or a problem in the environment. Systems of movement change, evolve, and mature due to growth, aging, disease, and environmental changes.

Balance, movement, and postural control

- **Postural control:** Postural control is the relationship between stability and mobility.
- **Limits of stability:** Limits of stability are the boundaries of the base of support. A person must keep the center of gravity over the base of support in order to maintain stability.
- **Cone of stability:** A person's cone of stability is the limit of their stability in standing. These standing limitations are cone-shaped, as the boundaries are wider toward the head and narrower toward the feet.

- **Predictive central set:** The predictive central set is the readiness to support posture and mobility. This predictive set can also be anticipatory in nature.
- **Degrees of freedom:** The degrees of freedom are all of the possible movement combinations that are available to an individual.

Nashner's Model of Postural Control

The maintenance of posture is controlled by three strategies that occur in a specific order when standing balance is challenged.

1. **Ankle strategy:** First, movement at the ankles occurs as the first defense in postural control.
2. **Hip strategy:** Second, if the ankle strategy is insufficient, muscles at the hip are activated to maintain posture.
3. **Stepping strategy:** As a final strategy to maintain posture, a person must take a step to prevent a fall.

Motor Learning

Motor learning is the process of eliciting a permanent change in motor performance as a result of experience and practice. Acquisition of new skills, retention of skills, and transfer of skills to new environments are included. During infancy and childhood, motor learning occurs as the infant progresses through new postures and motor milestones. As we progress though adolescence and adulthood, motor learning involves more difficult and refined motor tasks.

Fitts and Posner's Phases of Motor Learning

Cognitive phase

During the cognitive phase, as a person is learning a completely new task, cognition is paramount. Concentration and focus on the task are needed to master the task. Those with decreased cognitive abilities need longer times for motor learning. Children with cognitive impairments require a longer time to reach developmental milestones.

Associative phase

The associative phase of motor learning is the process of learning through many trials and is focused on error detection and correction. During the associative phase, movements are perfected and made more efficient.

Autonomous phase

The autonomous phase is the final phase of motor learning. This occurs when the task is carried out with relative autonomy, without conscious feedback.

Feedback

Motor learning requires feedback. **Intrinsic feedback** is generated from within the human body and involves how a particular movement feels and compares it to the reference of how that movement *should* feel. **Extrinsic feedback** is necessary to evaluate the performance of the movement. Extrinsic feedback is also called the knowledge of results. Once a movement is learned, a motor program is developed. The motor program is then used and requires little to no feedback. Feedback that is ongoing throughout a task can result in increased immediate performance yet decreased retention. Feedback that is given at the completion of the task can decrease immediate performance yet increase long-term retention.

- **Intrinsic feedback:** Internal sensory feedback that comes from joint receptors, special senses, and skin receptors
- **Extrinsic feedback:** External feedback provided to the person; examples include verbal, tactile, and biofeedback
- **Knowledge of results:** Information given on the outcome of the movement
- **Knowledge of performance:** Information given on the details of the performance that resulted in the outcome
- **Timing of feedback:** Can be frequent initially; as learning increases, feedback should decrease in amount and frequency

Practice

Motor learning relies on practice. Practice and motor learning are heavily environment- and task-dependent. The transfer of learning is increased when the motor task is learned in the environment in which the task will actually be carried out. Even a seemingly insignificant change (i.e., getting dressed while sitting on the side of the bed versus getting dressed while sitting in a chair) may result in difficulty in the transfer of learning.

Motor Development

Motor development is defined as the changes of movement performance that occur throughout the lifespan. Motor development tends to occur in the sequence of cephalic to caudal, proximal to distal, mass movements to specific movements, and gross movements to fine movements.

Motor control is the ability to perform quality and effective movements.

Motor learning is the process used to learn new motor skills.

Motor development is the age-related progression of change in motor behavior.

Motor milestones

Motor milestones provide a developmental timeline for the appearance of motor skills. Motor milestones can vary by two to four months in normal infants.

Gross-Motor Milestones

Age	Gross-Motor Milestone
4 to 5 months	Head control
4 to 5 months	Supported sitting
6 to 8 months	Unsupported sitting
8 to 9 months	Crawling
10 to 11 months	Cruising
12 months	Walking

Primitive Reflexes

Tonic labyrinthine reflex

The tonic labyrinthine reflex (TLR) is normally present from birth to six months. Presentation of this reflex in the prone position is increased flexor tone of all extremities. In the supine position, increased extensor tone of all extremities is exhibited.

Asymmetric tonic neck reflex

The asymmetric tonic neck reflex (ATNR) is normally present from birth to age four to six months. The stimulus for this reflex is rotation of the head. The extremities on the side toward which the head is rotated extend, while the extremities on the opposite side flex.

Symmetric tonic neck reflex

The symmetric tonic neck reflex (STNR) is normally present starting at 4–6 months of age and continues to age 8–12 months. The stimulus for this reflex is flexing the neck: flexion of the arms and extension of the legs occur. The opposite is also true: with neck extension, extension of the arms and flexion of the legs occur.

Palmar grasp reflex

The palmar grasp reflex is normally present from birth to age four months. Presentation of this reflex is strong finger flexion in response to pressure applied on the palm of the hand.

Rooting reflex

The rooting reflex is normally present from 28 weeks' gestation to age three months. Stimulus is touching the infant's cheek. The response is the head turning ipsilaterally and the mouth opening.

Moro reflex

The Moro reflex is normally present from 28 weeks' gestation to age six months. The stimulus is a sudden change in head position. The response is mass extension and abduction, followed by flexion and adduction.

Startle reflex

The startle reflex is normally present from birth onward. The stimulus is a sudden loud noise, and the response is mass extension and abduction of arms.

Positive support reflex

The positive support reflex is normally present from 35 weeks' gestation to age two months. The stimulus is placing weight on the ball of the infant's foot when the infant is in an upright position. The infant then extends the lower extremities.

Stepping reflex

The stepping reflex is normally present from 38 weeks' gestation to age two months. The stimulus is to place weight on the infant's foot on a firm surface while the infant is upright. The infant then reflexively and alternately flexes and extends the lower extremities in a walking manner.

Flexor withdrawal

The flexor withdrawal reflex is normally present from 28 weeks' gestation to age one month. To elicit, apply a noxious stimulus to the plantar surface of the infant's foot. The infant then withdraws from the stimulus with lower extremity flexion, dorsiflexion, and toe extension.

Crossed extension

The crossed extension reflex is normally present from 28 weeks' gestation to age one month. A noxious stimulus is applied to the plantar surface of the infant's foot. The response is extension and adduction of the opposite lower extremity.

Neurologic Functioning

Cognition

Cognition is defined as the mental activities of thinking, learning, memory, reasoning, perception, and language.

Affect

Affect is the emotional tone, mood, and presentation of emotion.

Arousal

Arousal is the level of alertness or consciousness of the cerebral cortex. Sleeping is a lower level of arousal than awakening.

Attention

Attention is the capacity to process cues and information from the environment and retrieve information from memory. Attention also entails the ability to focus on task, disregarding irrelevant stimuli while responding to relevant stimuli. Switching attention between tasks is also important.

Selective attention

Selective attention is the ability to focus on one selected task and related stimuli, ignoring nonrelated stimuli.

Sustained attention

Sustained attention is attention that is maintained for an appropriate length of time for the task being performed.

Divided attention

Divided attention is the ability to multitask—to do several tasks at the same time.

Memory

Memory is the mental information processing system that encodes, stores, and retrieves information.

Long-term memory

Long-term memory is the permanent storage of information for future retrieval.

Short-term memory

Short-term memory is information that is registered and stored only briefly, generally only for seconds.

Motivation

Motivation is the internal force that guides task initiation and continual involvement. Motivation is goal-dependent and can be increased with positive reinforcement.

Neurologic Terminology

- **Agnosia:** Inability to recognize common objects
- **Akinesia:** Absence of voluntary movement or difficulty initiating movement
- **Aphasia:** Deficit of language caused by brain damage
    - **Broca's aphasia:** Expressive aphasia
    - **Global aphasia:** Both expressive and receptive aphasia
    - **Wernicke's aphasia:** Receptive aphasia
- **Apraxia:** Loss or impairment of the ability to plan complex coordinated movement
- **Ataxia:** Uncoordinated movement
- **Ballismus:** Involuntary movement of proximal limb musculature that results in large, flinging motions of the extremity
- **Bradykinesia:** Decrease in spontaneity and movement, or a slowness of movement
- **Chorea:** Irregular, involuntary, excessive movements of the extremities or face
- **Clonus:** Alternating contractions of antagonistic muscle groups in response to passive stretch
- **Conjugate eye gaze:** Movement of the eyes in parallel
- **Diplopia:** Double vision
- **Dysarthria:** Difficulty forming words
- **Dysesthesia:** Abnormal burning or aching
- **Dyskinesia:** Difficulty with voluntary movement
- **Dysphagia:** Difficulty swallowing
- **Dystonia:** State of abnormal tone
- **Flaccidity:** Muscle weakness and decreased tone
- **Hemiplegia:** Paralysis of muscles on one side of the body
- **Homonymous hemianopsia:** Loss of the contralateral half of each visual field; the temporal half of one eye and the nasal half of the other
- **Hydromyelia:** Accumulation of CSF in the central canal of the spinal cord that can cause rapidly occurring scoliosis, upper extremity weakness, and increased tone
- **Hypesthesias:** Abnormal sensitivity to touch
- **Hypokinesia:** Slowness of movement
- **Hypometria:** Ataxia that results in under-reaching of a target
- **Locked-in syndrome:** Patient is alert and oriented but has weakness of all muscles, with the exception of the eyes
- **Myoclonus:** Shocklike contractions of a group of muscles, with variable regularity
- **Neglect:** Neglect of the affected side of the body
- **Nystagmus:** Rhythmic oscillation of the eyeballs
- **Paresthesia:** Pins-and-needles feeling
- **Perseveration:** Repetition of verbal or motor response
- **Proprioception:** Perception of where limbs and body are positioned
- **Pusher syndrome:** With right CVA, patient tends to push and lean toward the affected side

- **Rigidity:** Increased resistance to passive movement
- **Spasticity:** Hyperreflexia of deep tendon reflexes and increased muscle tone
- **Synergy:** Stereotypical patterns of movement that do not change in response to task or environment
- **Tethered spinal cord:** Adhesions of the spinal cord coupled with bony growth that causes rapidly progressing neurological signs and symptoms
- **Tic:** Habitual, repeated contractions of certain muscles
- **Thalamic pain syndrome:** Intolerable, intense burning pain even after removal of the stimulus
- **Tremor:** Repetitive oscillatory movements caused by alternate contraction of antagonist muscle groups

EVALUATION

During the evaluation process it is important for the examiner to make decisions on what tests and measures are appropriate in order to establish a good list of differential diagnoses to treat the injury or disability. Again, during the examination process the patient must be viewed as a whole. The examination may take place in a hospital room, a home setting, an outpatient setting, a long- or short-term care facility, or another setting. In all cases, each part of the examination process must be considered, although it is known that some portions of the examination are more appropriate for certain settings. Special tests may be more appropriate in an outpatient setting, mobility evaluation may be more appropriate in a home setting, and a chart review of labs and medical tests may be more appropriate for the acute-care setting.

Cranial Nerve Testing

Cranial Nerve	Test
I. Olfactory	Smell familiar odors with the eyes closed
II. Optic	Visual acuity, visual fields
III. Oculomotor	Elevate, depress, adduct the eye
IV. Trochlear	Depress and adduct the eye
V. Trigeminal	Sensation of face, corneal reflex, jaw reflex
VI. Abducens	Abduct the eye
VII. Facial	Facial expression imitation, eye closure with manual resistance, sense of taste to anterior tongue
VIII. Vestibulocochlear	Hearing, patient index finger to examiner's index finger to test past-pointing
IX. Glossopharyngeal	Sensation portion of test for vagus nerve
X. Vagus	Touch side of pharynx with stick to elicit gag reflex; note rise of uvula when stroked
XI. Accessory	Resisted shoulder shrug and neck side-bending
XII. Hypoglossal	Protrude tongue to the midline

Deep Tendon Reflexes (Muscle Stretch Reflexes)

To perform a test of a deep tendon reflex, strike the tendon with a reflex hammer while the muscle is on slight stretch. Test bilaterally, testing the unaffected side first.

Reflex	Nerve Level	Stimulus	Normal Response
Jaw	Cranial nerve V	Tap mandible when half open	Jaw closes
Biceps	C5-C6, musculocutaneous nerve	Tap biceps tendon	Biceps contracts
Brachioradialis	C5-C6, musculocutaneous nerve	Tap styloid process of radius	Elbow flexes and pronates
Triceps	C6-C8, radial nerve	Tap triceps tendon	Elbow extends
Wrist extension	C7-C8, radial nerve	Tap wrist extensor tendons	Wrist extends
Wrist flexion	C6-C8, median nerve	Tap wrist flexor tendons	Wrist flexes
Patellar	L2-L4, femoral nerve	Tap patellar tendon	Knee extends
Tendocalcaneus	S1-S2, tibial nerve	Tap Achilles tendon	Ankle plantar flexes

Grading of Deep Tendon Reflexes

Grade	Response
0	Areflexia (no response)
1	Hyporeflexia (minimal response)
2	Average
3	Hyperreflexia (exaggerated response)
4	Clonus

Modified Ashworth Scale for Grading Spasticity

Score	Appearance of Spasticity
0	Normal muscle tone
1	Slightly increased muscle tone noted at the end of the ROM
1+	Slightly increased muscle tone noted through less than half of the ROM
2	Obvious increase in muscle tone through most of the ROM; however, the affected segment is still movable
3	Substantial increase in muscle tone; passive PROM is challenging
4	Affected segment is rigid in position of flexion or extension

Glasgow Coma Scale

The Glasgow Coma Scale score is obtained by totaling the three subsection scores of eye opening, motor response, and verbal response. A score of less than 8 indicates that the person is in a coma and has a severe brain injury.

Glasgow Coma Scale

Eye Opening	**Score**
Spontaneous	4
To speech	3
To pain	2
No eye opening	1

Motor Response	**Score**
Obeys commands	6
Localized (moves a limb to remove stimulus)	5
Withdraws from pain	4
Decorticate posture	3
Decerebrate posture	2
No response	1

Verbal Response	**Score**
Oriented	5
Conversationally confused	4
Inappropriate; speech is intelligible but conversation is not possible	3
Incomprehensible and unintelligible sounds	2
No response	1

Rancho Los Amigos Cognitive Functioning Scale

Level	Description
Level I No response: Total assistance	No response to stimuli
Level II Generalized response: Total assistance	Inconsistent and nonpurposeful response to stimuli. Responses are often the same regardless of stimuli. Responses include physiologic changes, gross body movement, and vocalizations.
Level III Localized response: Total assistance	Specific but inconsistent response to stimuli. Reactions are related to the stimuli. May follow simple commands inconsistently and in a delayed manner.
Level IV Confused-agitated: Maximal assistance	Heightened state of activity with bizarre, non-purposeful behavior. Indiscriminate among people and objects. Unable to cooperate directly with treatment. Inappropriate or incoherent verbalizations. Gross attention is very limited; selective attention can be nonexistent. Lacks recall ability.
Level V Confused-inappropriate-non-agitated: Maximal assistance	Fairly consistent in ability to respond to simple commands. Without structure or with complex commands, responses are nonpurposeful and random. Highly distractible; cannot focus attention to specific task. Verbalizations are mostly inappropriate and confabulated. Severely impaired memory. Can perform previously learned activity with structure, but unable to learn new information.
Level VI Confused-appropriate: Moderate assistance	Goal-directed behavior, yet dependent on input or direction. Simple commands followed consistently; demonstrates carryover for relearned task. Past memories better than recent memory.
Level VII Automatic-appropriate: Minimal assistance for daily living skills	Appropriate and oriented. Able to complete daily activities automatically with some confusion. Shallow recall of activities. Demonstrates some recall of new learning. Structure is needed to begin social activities. Judgment is impaired.
Level VIII Purposeful-appropriate: Standby assistance	Oriented; able to recall and integrate past events; uses lists and schedules for use with standby assistance. Completes familiar tasks with standby assistance; needs minimal assistance to change plan. Able to think about consequences with minimal assistance. However, over- or underestimates abilities. Can be depressed, irritable, confrontational, and easily disturbed.

Level	Description
Level IX Purposeful-appropriate: Standby assistance on request	Able to complete tasks and alternate between tasks for at least two hours. Uses lists and schedules with assistance upon request. Completes familiar tasks with assistance upon request. Aware of abilities but may require standby assistance to change tasks, depending on complexity. May have depression, irritability, and frustration.
Level X Purposeful-appropriate: Modified independent	Independent in different environments; independent with lists and schedules; and independent with activities of daily living, with compensatory strategies. Aware of abilities, socially appropriate, and aware of others' feelings and needs, and can respond independently. May continue to battle periods of depression and frustration.

Permission granted by Rancho Los Amigos National Rehabilitation Center Downey, CA.

Brunnstrom's Stages of Recovery from Hemiplegia

Stage	Spasticity	Movement Pattern
One	None	None
Two	Emergent	Weak associated movements, minimal active finger flexion
Three	Marked	Mass synergy movement patterns, maximal grasp
Four	Decreasing	Beginning to deviate from synergies
Five	Decreasing additionally	Nearly clear of synergy patterns
Six	Minimal except during rapid movement	Free of synergy, but awkward

Pediatric Motor Assessment Tests

Peabody Developmental Motor Scales

The Peabody Developmental Motor Scales test reflexes and gross motor and fine motor abilities. It is useful for patients age 0 to 83 months.

Gross Motor Function Measure

The Gross Motor Function Measure (GMFM) is used to measure motor skills of children with cerebral palsy. Generally, this measure is useful for ages two to five years.

Movement assessment of infants

The movement assessment of infants (MAI) tests neurologic function, specifically tone, automatic reactions, reflexes, and voluntary movement. It is used for ages 0 to 12 months.

Bayley Scales of Infant Development II

The Bayley Scales of Infant Development II are used to test the realms of cognition, behavior, and motor activity of children 0 to 42 months.

Pediatric Evaluation of Disability Index

The Pediatric Evaluation of Disability Index (PEDI) is functionally based with evaluation of self-care, social function, and mobility. It is useful for ages six months to seven and a half years.

Alberta Infant Motor Scale

The Alberta Infant Motor Scale (AIMS) is a tool for evaluating motor abilities, including postures and skills in a variety of positions. This test is used for ages 0 to 18 months.

Tests for Balance

Timed up-and-go test

In the timed up-and-go test, the patient is asked to stand up from a chair, ambulate three meters (about ten feet), and return to the chair. The therapist times how long this takes.

Berg balance test

The Berg balance test is a 14-item test for balance, with a possible score of 56. This test includes tasks such as standing on one leg, sit-to-stand without the use of the hands, tandem standing, and static stance.

Tinetti balance test

The Tinetti, a 16-item test for balance, includes tasks such as transfers, turning the head, and picking up an item from the floor.

Functional reach test

The functional reach test measures the distance that a person can reach in an upright position with an outstretched arm.

Upper Limb Function Tests

Nine-hole peg test

To perform the nine-hole peg test, the patient is timed on how long it takes to place nine wooden pegs into a wooden base.

Frenchay arm test

To perform the Frenchay arm test, the patient is asked to perform five specific tasks with the affected hand.

Mini-Mental Exam

The mini-mental exam tests cognitive functions such as orientation, attention, recall, and language.

Muscle Tone Evaluation

To evaluate a patient's muscle tone, move the patient's extremities and trunk through passive range of motion.

Evaluation of Coordination

Finger-to-nose test

The patient uses his index finger to touch the therapist's index finger, then his own nose, then the therapist's index finger, alternately. If the patient is able to do this, the therapist asks him to increase the speed of motion. This test can show intention tremor or dysmetria.

Heel-shin test

When positioned in supine, the patient actively runs the heel of one leg down the opposite shin from the knee to the foot. This test can show ataxia.

Tests for Proprioception

Joint position test

To perform this test, the patient is asked to close her eyes. The therapist then places the patient's distal joint into a specific position (i.e., flexion or extension) and asks the patient to identify the position of the joint.

Romberg test

In this test the patient stands with his feet together, and the therapist instructs him to close his eyes. A loss of balance with the eyes closed indicates loss of proprioception.

Evaluation of Light Touch

To evaluate a patient's ability to sense light touch, start distally and test the dermatomes. There are several components of light touch that can and should be tested. The basic test assesses the patient's ability to identify light touch. The pinprick test is used to identify a patient's sensitivity to sharp and dull, using a pin's point versus a dull end. Other tests include testing for pressure sense, tactile localization, and two-point discrimination.

Evaluation of Temperature Sensation

To evaluate sensation to temperature, the patient is asked to identify if she is being touched with a tube of hot water or tube of cold water.

Evaluation of Gait

The physical therapist should evaluate each patient's gait for level of assistance needed, safety, and gait deviation. Possible gait deviations that are common to the neurologic population are hip retraction, hip hiking, circumduction, inappropriate knee flexion and extension, foot drop, and ankle inversion or eversion.

DIFFERENTIAL DIAGNOSIS AND PATHOLOGY

On the basis of the findings obtained during the evaluation of the nervous system, a list of differential diagnoses can be made. Each pathology or condition of the nervous system is unique and will dictate the medical management and treatment intervention choices made by the physical therapist. Each differential diagnosis and pathology of the nervous system can have its own wide range of problems and impairments it causes, based on the location and severity of the injury. This information also helps to drive treatment intervention decisions.

There are several treatments, techniques, and interventions that can be performed by the medical team in the treatment of patients with nervous system impairments. Since medical management is highly dependent on and specific to the type of injury or pathology of the nervous system, this information is included with each pathology. This section discusses some of the more common methods of medical management according to specific pathologies.

Injury to the Central Nervous System

Obstruction of blood supply to the CNS can result in cell death in minutes. These oxygen-deprived neurons cannot be regenerated. Cells that are near the injured cells are at risk of glutamate toxicity and possibly death. Glutamate is a neurotransmitter that, at high levels, can promote neuronal death. The necrotic tissue becomes soft and edematous and eventually becomes a cyst. Ultimately, a glial scar forms around this cyst.

Four or five days after the neuronal injury, axonal collateral sprouting occurs. Examples of CNS injury are cerebrovascular accident, traumatic brain injury, and spinal cord injury. An overview of these injuries is presented in the following sections.

Transient Ischemic Attack

A transient ischemic attack (TIA) is a temporary reduction in blood supply to the brain. The patient can experience neurologic deficits but have no lasting brain damage or neurologic dysfunction. By definition, effects of a TIA disappear within 24 hours. Diagnosis is made by examination of sensory and motor function, reflex testing, onset of symptoms, CT scan, and MRI.

Cerebrovascular Accident

Cerebrovascular accident (CVA) is due to a disruption of the blood supply to the brain that causes neurologic signs and symptoms. Two types of cerebrovascular accident are ischemic and hemorrhagic.

Ischemic CVA

An ischemic CVA is caused by hypoxia to brain tissue from poor blood supply. Ischemic CVAs can be divided into two causes: thrombosis and embolus.

Thrombosis

A thrombosis is an atherosclerotic lesion that completely occludes a cerebral vessel. A cerebral infarct is the necrosis of brain tissue.

Embolus

An embolus is a blood clot from another blood vessel that is carried to the brain, where it occludes an artery.

Hemorrhagic CVA

A hemorrhagic CVA is caused by abnormal bleeding from the rupture of a cerebral vessel. Common hemorrhages are intracerebral and subarachnoid hemorrhages. An **arteriovenous malformation** is a congenital malformation of the blood supply.

Risk factors for CVA

- Hypertension
- Heart disease
- Diabetes
- Smoking
- Hyperlipidemia
- Male gender
- African American
- Family history
- Alcohol intake
- Low activity level
- Obesity
- Age
- Use of oral contraceptives
- History of prior CVA

Signs and symptoms of CVA

The typical signs and symptoms of a CVA vary widely and depend greatly on the location and the severity of the accident. One common impairment following a CVA is shoulder subluxation, due to flaccid paralysis of one shoulder girdle. Another common impairment is foot drop, or decreased active dorsiflexion. Often an orthotic must be used to accommodate for this muscular weakness. Listed here are other common signs and symptoms, based on the location of the cerebrovascular accident.

Anterior cerebral artery

- Contralateral motor loss of lower extremities
- Contralateral sensory deficits of lower extremities
- Aphasia
- Memory and behavioral deficits
- Incontinence

Middle cerebral artery

- Contralateral motor loss of face and upper extremity
- Contralateral sensory loss of face and upper extremity
- Homonymous hemianopsia
- Global aphasia
- Conjugate eye gaze

Vertebrobasilar artery

- Cranial nerve impairments (dysphagia, dysarthria)
- Ataxia and incoordination
- Dizziness and headaches
- Locked-in syndrome

Posterior artery

- Visual deficits
    - Homonymous hemianopsia
    - Visual agnosia
    - Cortical blindness
- Contralateral sensory loss
- Memory deficits
- Thalamic pain syndrome

Lacunar infarct

- Contralateral motor loss
- Contralateral sensory loss
- Ataxia
- Dysarthria

Brain-stem CVA

- Affected vital signs
- Paralysis (contralateral or bilateral)
- Dysphagia
- Decreased consciousness
- Cranial nerve palsy

Cerebellar CVA

- Poor posture
- Impaired balance
- Nystagmus
- Ataxia
- Incoordination
- Nausea
- Tremor
- Decreased tendon reflexes

Right hemispheric CVA

- Paralysis of the left side of the body
- Left hemianopsia
- Left neglect
- Impaired memory and reasoning
- Unrealistic expectations
- Denial of disability

- Unrealistic body image
- Emotional lability
- Sluggishness
- Pusher syndrome

Left hemispheric CVA

- Paralysis of the right side of the body
- Right hemianopsia
- Impaired right and left discrimination
- Apraxia
- Akinesia
- Difficulty with sequencing
- Aphasia
- Anxiousness
- Perseveration

Brunnstrom's synergy patterns

Brunnstrom's classification of synergies can be used to describe and direct treatment of a patient who has experienced a CVA. Typically, the flexion synergy is more dominant in the upper extremity and the extension synergy is more dominant in the lower extremity.

Upper-extremity flexion synergy

- Scapulothoracic retraction and/or elevation
- Shoulder abduction, external rotation
- Elbow flexion
- Forearm supination
- Wrist flexion
- Finger extension

Upper-extremity extension synergy

- Scapulothoracic protraction
- Shoulder adduction, internal rotation
- Elbow extension
- Forearm pronation
- Wrist extension
- Finger flexion

Lower-extremity flexion synergy

- Hip flexion, abduction, external rotation
- Knee flexion to 90°
- Ankle dorsiflexion and inversion
- Toe extension

Lower-extremity extension synergy

- Hip extension, adduction, and internal rotation
- Knee extension
- Ankle plantar flexion and inversion
- Toe flexion

Associated reactions

Associated reactions are involuntary movements of a body part that occur with voluntary movement of another body part. These can be seen in patients who have experienced a CVA.

Souques' phenomenon
During Souques' phenomenon, flexion of the involved arm above 150° is accompanied by finger extension and abduction.

Raimiste's phenomenon
With Raimiste's phenomenon, resisted hip abduction or adduction of the unaffected leg elicits comparable response in the affected leg.

Homolateral limb synkinesis
During homolateral limb synkinesis, flexion of the affected upper extremity elicits flexion of the affected lower extremity.

Medical management of CVA

- Hospitalization with regulation of the patient's vital signs, intracranial pressure, and cerebral perfusion
- Thrombolytic pharmaceuticals given within three hours of CVA decrease potential neurologic injury
- Surgery to remove or repair aneurysm, or remove hematoma or abnormal vessel

Traumatic Brain Injury

A traumatic brain injury (TBI) is trauma to the brain from an external force that causes neurologic impairment. Traumatic brain injuries may be open or closed.

Open TBI

The skin is penetrated during an open TBI. This causes focal injury and a high risk of infections. The skull may or may not fracture.

Closed TBI

The skin remains intact and there is no skull fracture with a closed TBI.

Concussion

A concussion is a momentary loss of consciousness and reflexes. The brain is not structurally damaged. Symptoms are dizziness, disorientation, blurred vision, difficulty concentrating, nausea, headache, and impaired balance. The patient may also have pre- or posttraumatic amnesia.

Contusion

A contusion happens when there is bruising on the surface of the brain at the time of impact. Contusions can be coup or countercoup.

Coup
A coup is a contusion on the same side of the brain as the impact.

Countercoup
A countercoup is a contusion on the side of the brain opposite the impact.

Hematoma

An epidural hematoma is the rupture of a meningeal artery that results in initial unconsciousness followed by alertness. As the hematoma continues to hemorrhage, the patient rapidly declines. Surgical intervention is then required to remove the hematoma.

Subdural hematoma is the rupture of a vein between the dura and the arachnoid. Bleeding occurs slowly, and thus symptoms fluctuate.

Acquired brain injury

An acquired brain injury diffusely affects cell physiology and metabolism through the entire brain. Anoxic injuries result from a disruption of adequate perfusion to brain tissue, resulting in diffuse neuronal injury. Common causes of acquired brain injuries are near-drowning, CVA, toxins, electrical shock, and lightning strike. Anoxic injuries are often caused by myocardial infarction.

Signs and Symptoms of TBI

- Decreased level of consciousness
- Cognitive deficits
- Motor deficits, including hypertonicity, ataxia, weakness, difficulty initiating movement, dyskinesia, and/or dyspraxia
- Sensory deficits
- Communication deficits
- Behavioral deficits

The signs and symptoms of a TBI vary widely, based on the location and severity of the injury. Many problems can occur following an insult to the nervous system. Common post-TBI problems are described here.

Increased intracranial pressure

Increased intracranial pressure (ICP) can occur due to a traumatic brain injury. The skull does not accommodate increases in volume from edema or hemorrhage. Increased pressure can compress the brain, decrease blood supply to the brain, and lead to herniation. Normal ICP is 5 to 10 mm Hg, and >20 mm Hg is abnormal. Cervical flexion, percussion and vibration techniques to assist pulmonary function, and coughing can increase ICP.

Signs and symptoms of increased ICP are:

- Decreased responsiveness
- Impaired consciousness
- Severe headache
- Vomiting
- Irritability
- Papilledema
- Changes in vital signs

Posttraumatic epilepsy

Following a traumatic brain injury, seizures often occur. Therapists should be aware of this potential and ready for management of a patient who is experiencing a seizure. Avoid vestibular stimulation techniques for patients with history of seizure.

Locked-in syndrome

Locked-in syndrome can occur after a TBI and consists of paralysis of all voluntary muscles except for the eye musculature. The patient is "locked in" because he is alert and oriented but cannot move. This is associated with a poor prognosis.

Vegetative state

A patient who exhibits brain-stem reflexes and sleep/wake cycles but is unconscious is in a vegetative state. If the patient remains in a vegetative state for more than one year, it is termed persistent vegetative state.

Coma

A coma is a state of unconsciousness. The patient is unresponsive and not arousable.

Confabulation

A patient who fills in lapses of memory with made-up stories and out-of-place words is confabulating.

Decerebrate rigidity

The posture of decerebrate rigidity is: lower extremity extension, hip adduction and internal rotation, shoulder internal rotation and extension, elbow extension, forearm pronation, and wrist and finger flexion.

Decorticate rigidity

The posture of decorticate rigidity is: shoulder adduction and internal rotation, elbow flexion, forearm pronation, wrist flexion, and lower-extremity extension.

Heterotopic ossification

Heterotopic ossification is abnormal bone growth in the soft tissue surrounding joints.

Retrograde amnesia

Retrograde amnesia is memory loss for events prior to the injury.

Posttraumatic amnesia

Posttraumatic amnesia is the inability to remember new information following the brain injury.

Spinal Cord Injury

Each spinal cord injury (SCI) is identified by the last spinal nerve root segment that is preserved. For example, a C7 spinal cord injury signifies that the C7 spinal nerve and above are intact. Quadriplegia and tetraplegia are terms that indicate that all of the extremities and all of the extremities plus the trunk, respectively, are affected. The term paraplegia indicates that only the trunk and lower extremities are affected.

In a complete SCI, there is total loss of motor and sensory function below the level of the lesion. With an incomplete SCI, there is partial preservation of motor and sensory function below the level of the injury and in S4 and S5. Sacral sparing is a phenomenon seen with an incomplete SCI. Perianal sensation is spared, as sacral tracts are located medially in the spinal cord and therefore may be unaffected. Spasticity and abnormal muscle tone are also seen in an incomplete SCI.

Spinal shock

Immediately following a spinal cord injury, spinal shock occurs. This is a period of profound weakness and flaccidity, areflexia, loss of bowel and bladder function, and autonomic deficits. Spinal shock normally lasts 24 to 48 hours.

Spinal cord syndromes

Spinal cord syndromes are based on the location of injury, and they demonstrate predictable signs and symptoms. These syndromes include:

Brown-Sequard syndrome

Brown-Sequard syndrome is due to injury of half of the spinal cord. Symptoms are ipsilateral loss of motor function, vibration, and proprioception, and contralateral loss of pain and temperature sensation.

Anterior cord syndrome

Anterior cord syndrome is injury to the anterior portion of the spinal cord. Symptoms are bilateral loss of motor function and loss of pain and temperature sensation. Proprioception and vibration are preserved.

Central cord syndrome

Central cord syndrome is due to injury to the central portion of the spinal cord. Weakness results, more in the upper extremities than the lower extremities. Sensory deficits vary with each injury, depending on the extent of injury.

Dorsal cord syndrome

Dorsal cord syndrome is due to damage to the posterior portion of the spinal cord. Symptoms are a loss of proprioception and vibration sense.

Cauda equina injuries

Injury to the cauda equina results in signs and symptoms of flaccid paralysis, areflexia, and loss of bowel and bladder function.

Signs and symptoms of spinal cord injury

The signs and symptoms of a spinal cord injury vary, based on the location and extent of the injury. Many problems can occur following an insult to the nervous system. Common post-SCI signs and symptoms are:

- Paralysis below the level of the injury
- Loss of sensation two spinal levels below the injury
- Cardiopulmonary dysfunction
- Autonomic nervous system disruption
- Spasticity
- Bladder and bowel dysfunction
- Sexual dysfunction
- Pressure ulcers
- Autonomic dysreflexia
- Postural hypotension
- Pain
- Contractures
- Heterotopic ossification
- Deep vein thrombosis

Autonomic dysreflexia

Autonomic dysreflexia is a medical emergency experienced by patients with a spinal cord injury above T6. In response to noxious stimuli, the patient may experience abnormal sympathetic response. If left untreated, autonomic dysreflexia may lead to seizure, hemorrhage, renal failure, and/or death. The treatment of autonomic dysreflexia is to remove the noxious stimulus and to lower the blood pressure by upright positioning or pharmaceutical intervention. Signs and symptoms of autonomic dysreflexia include:

- Vasoconstriction below the lesion
- Vasodilation above the lesion
- Immediate and large increase in blood pressure
- Severe headache
- Profuse sweating
- Blurred vision
- Constricted pupils

Postural hypotension

Postural hypotension is also a common problem of patients with spinal cord injury. Postural hypotension is decreased blood pressure with progressively upright postures. Use of an abdominal binder to increase intra-abdominal pressure is one treatment that can be used to counteract this drop in blood pressure.

Pain

Pain is common in patients with spinal cord injuries, for different reasons. Dysesthetic pain is poorly localized pain below the level of the injury. Musculoskeletal pain is often experienced due to overuse injuries; an example of this is musculoskeletal pain of the shoulder due to manual wheelchair propulsion.

Contractures

Patients with spinal cord injuries are at risk of developing contractures due to prolonged sitting in a wheelchair and lack of positional changes. The prone position should be assumed daily to prevent hip flexion contractures. Daily stretching is important to the prevention of contractures.

Medical management of SCI

- Methylprednisolone given within eight hours of injury decreases the extent of injury.
- Stabilization of the spine prevents further neurologic injury and includes:
  - Surgical fusion of bony fracture
  - Bone grafting
  - Internal fixation
  - External fixation with orthoses
- Presurgical traction improves bony alignment

Standard Neurological Classification of Spinal Cord Injury

The American Spinal Injury Association publishes the "International Standard for Neurological Classification of Spinal Cord Injury" which includes motor levels and dermatomes associated with spinal cord injury. These dermatomes and key muscles can also be used to evaluate peripheral nerve injuries.

American Spinal Injury Association: "International Standards for Neurological Classification of Spinal Cord Injury", revised 2002; Chicago, IL.

Patient Name ______________________

Examiner Name ______________________ Date/Time of Exam ______________________

ASIA AMERICAN SPINAL INJURY ASSOCIATION

STANDARD NEUROLOGICAL CLASSIFICATION OF SPINAL CORD INJURY

ISCOS

MOTOR

KEY MUSCLES
(scoring on reverse side)

	R	L	
C5			Elbow flexors
C6			Wrist extensors
C7			Elbow extensors
C8			Finger flexors (distal phalanx of middle finger)
T1			Finger abductors (little finger)

UPPER LIMB TOTAL (MAXIMUM) ☐ + ☐ = ☐
(25) (25) (50)

Comments:

	R	L	
L2			Hip flexors
L3			Knee extensors
L4			Ankle dorsiflexors
L5			Long toe extensors
S1			Ankle plantar flexors

Voluntary anal contraction (Yes/No) ☐

LOWER LIMB TOTAL (MAXIMUM) ☐ + ☐ = ☐
(25) (25) (50)

SENSORY

KEY SENSORY POINTS

	LIGHT TOUCH R	LIGHT TOUCH L	PIN PRICK R	PIN PRICK L
C2				
C3				
C4				
C5				
C6				
C7				
C8				
T1				
T2				
T3				
T4				
T5				
T6				
T7				
T8				
T9				
T10				
T11				
T12				
L1				
L2				
L3				
L4				
L5				
S1				
S2				
S3				
S4-5				

0 = absent
1 = impaired
2 = normal
NT = not testable

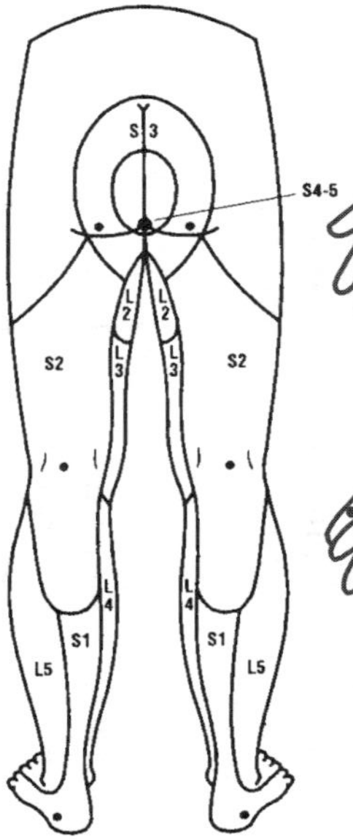

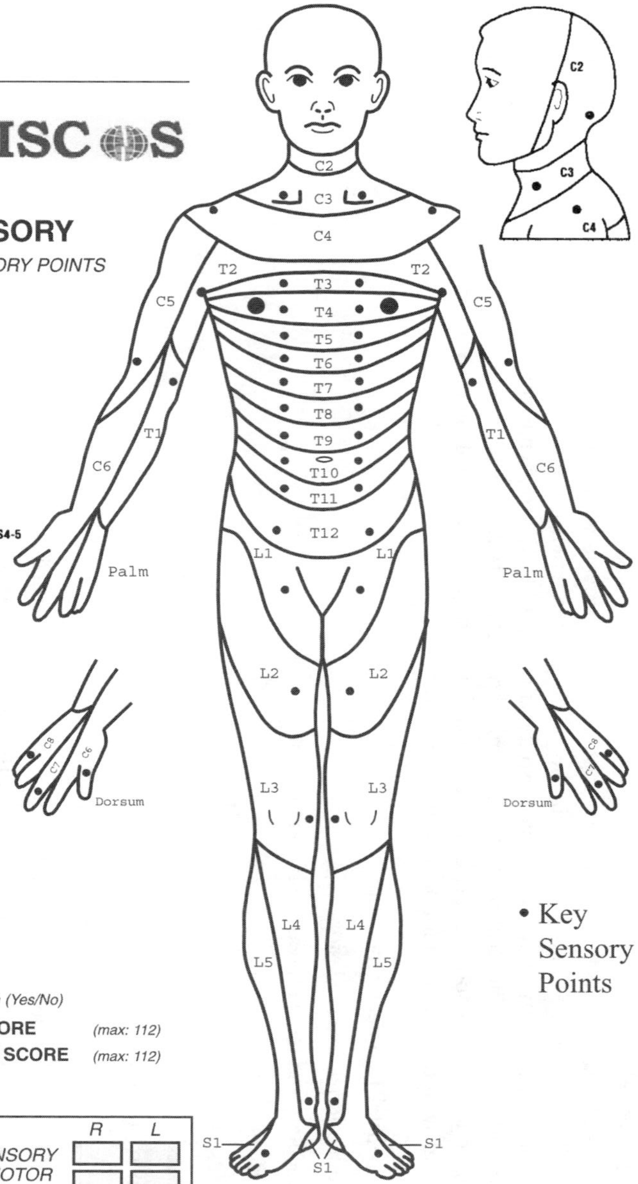

• Key Sensory Points

Any anal sensation (Yes/No) ☐

TOTALS { ☐ + ☐ → ☐ + ☐ = PIN PRICK SCORE (max: 112)
= LIGHT TOUCH SCORE (max: 112)

(MAXIMUM) (56) (56) (56) (56)

NEUROLOGICAL LEVEL The most caudal segment with normal function		R	L	COMPLETE OR INCOMPLETE? ☐ Incomplete = Any sensory or motor function in S4-S5 ASIA IMPAIRMENT SCALE ☐	ZONE OF PARTIAL PRESERVATION Caudal extent of partially innervated segments		R	L
	SENSORY					SENSORY		
	MOTOR					MOTOR		

REV 03/06

MUSCLE GRADING

0 total paralysis

1 palpable or visible contraction

2 active movement, full range of motion, gravity eliminated

3 active movement, full range of motion, against gravity

4 active movement, full range of motion, against gravity and provides some resistance

5 active movement, full range of motion, against gravity and provides normal resistance

5* muscle able to exert, in examiner's judgement, sufficient resistance to be considered normal if identifiable inhibiting factors were not present

NT not testable. Patient unable to reliably exert effort or muscle unavailable for testing due to factors such as immobilization, pain on effort, or contracture.

ASIA IMPAIRMENT SCALE

☐ A = **Complete:** No motor or sensory function is preserved in the sacral segments S4-S5.

☐ B = **Incomplete:** Sensory but not motor function is preserved below the neurological level and includes the sacral segments S4-S5.

☐ C = **Incomplete:** Motor function is preserved below the neurological level, and more than half of key muscles below the neurological level have a muscle grade less than 3.

☐ D = **Incomplete:** Motor function is preserved below the neurological level, and at least half of key muscles below the neurological level have a muscle grade of 3 or more.

☐ E = **Normal:** Motor and sensory function are normal.

CLINICAL SYNDROMES (OPTIONAL)

☐ Central Cord
☐ Brown-Sequard
☐ Anterior Cord
☐ Conus Medullaris
☐ Cauda Equina

STEPS IN CLASSIFICATION

The following order is recommended in determining the classification of individuals with SCI.

1. Determine sensory levels for right and left sides.
2. Determine motor levels for right and left sides.
   Note: In regions where there is no myotome to test, the motor level is presumed to be the same as the sensory level.
3. Determine the single neurological level.
   This is the lowest segment where motor and sensory function is normal on both sides, and is the most cephalad of the sensory and motor levels determined in steps 1 and 2.
4. Determine whether the injury is Complete or Incomplete (sacral sparing).
   If voluntary anal contraction = **No** *AND all S4-5 sensory scores =* **0** *AND any anal sensation =* **No***, then injury is COMPLETE. Otherwise injury is incomplete.*
5. Determine ASIA Impairment Scale (AIS) Grade:

Is injury Complete? If **YES**, AIS=A Record ZPP (For ZPP record lowest dermatome or myotome on each side with some (nonzero score) preservation)

NO ↓

Is injury motor incomplete? If **NO**, AIS=B (Yes=voluntary anal contraction OR motor function more than three levels below the motor level on a given side.)

YES ↓

Are at least half of the key muscles below the (single) neurological level graded 3 or better?

NO ↓ AIS=C

YES ↓ AIS=D

If sensation and motor function is normal in all segments, AIS=E
Note: AIS E is used in follow-up testing when an individual with a documented SCI has recovered normal function. If at initial testing no deficits are found, the individual is neurologically intact; the ASIA Impairment Scale does not apply.

Cerebral Palsy

Cerebral palsy (CP) is a nonprogressive disorder of motor function that results from damage to the immature brain before, during, or after birth. CP is due to birth asphyxia in only 10 percent of cases. The incidence of CP increases with decreased birth weight of the infant. CP is also caused by prenatal, perinatal, and postnatal factors. Postnatal factors are factors seen in the first year of life.

Prenatal factors related to CP

- Maternal infections
- Placental malformation
- Genetic influences
- Brain malformation
- Maternal diabetes
- Rh incompatibility

Perinatal factors related to CP

- Asphyxia/anoxia
- Low birth weight
- Breech presentation
- Prematurity
- Prolonged labor
- Prolapsed cord
- Placenta previa or premature separation

Postnatal factors related to CP

- Cerebral infection
- Cerebrovascular infection
- Head trauma
- Seizures
- Intraventricular hemorrhage
- Near-drowning

Classification of CP

Cerebral palsy can be classified by type, distribution, and severity.

CP classification by type

Spastic CP: Spastic CP is the most common type of CP. **Spasticity** is defined as a velocity-dependent increase in muscle tone. **Hypertonia** is defined as an increased resistance to passive ROM that is not velocity-dependent. A typical problem list for patients with spastic CP is as follows:

- Poor head and neck control
- Dominant, persistent tonic reflexes (ATNR, STNR, TLR)
- Difficulty with transitional movements
- Decreased ambulation skills
- Contractures due to spasticity

Dyskinetic CP: Patients with dyskinetic CP present with disordered movement. **Athetoid CP** is the most common form of dyskinetic CP. A patient affected with athetoid CP displays disordered movement in the mid-range of the affected extremities. Tone often fluctuates from low to high to normal. Poor postural control and stability are seen in this type of CP. The patient with dyskinetic CP often performs large, uncontrolled movements of the extremities.

Ataxic CP: Patients with ataxic CP demonstrate decreased coordination and low postural tone. Ataxic CP is usually diplegic. Due to poor postural control, a child with ataxic CP adopts a wide base of support in standing and walking.

Hypotonic CP: Patients with hypotonic CP demonstrate decreased muscular tone and weakness. This type is also known as flaccid CP.

CP classification by distribution

- **Hemiplegia:** One side of the body is affected.
- **Diplegia:** The lower half of the body is affected, often including the trunk.
- **Quadriplegia:** The whole body is affected; often the upper extremities are affected more than the lower extremities.

CP classification by severity

According to the **Gross Motor Classification Scale** (**GMCS**), the child with CP is ranked on a five-level system according to the severity of involvement.

Complications of CP

- Epilepsy
- Visual impairments
- Sleep disorders
- Feeding and speech impairments
- Mental retardation
- Decreased life expectancy
- Musculoskeletal defects

Medical management of CP

- Orthopedic surgery to offset musculoskeletal defects
- Surgical release of tendon or muscle to decrease contracture
- Spinal curvature correction for curves greater than 35°
- Selective dorsal rhizotomy

Treatment intervention for CP

Treatment of patients with CP starts at infancy and continues throughout the lifespan. A child with CP often experiences incorrect motor learning. The child performs an incorrect movement and subsequently repeats the movement, thereby learning an abnormal movement. Physical therapy interventions focus on motor learning of normal, purposeful movement. The physical therapist should keep in mind the developmental sequence in the treatment of a patient with cerebral palsy.

Developmental sequence

- Supine
- Rolling

- Prone
- Quadruped
- Sitting
- Scooting
- Sit to stand
- Standing
- Pre-gait activities
- Gait

Parkinson's Disease

Parkinson's disease (PD) is a chronic progressive neurologic condition caused by the decrease of the neurotransmitter dopamine in the substantia nigra. The diagnosis of PD is based on the signs and symptoms. No definitive diagnostic tests exist for PD. The cardinal signs of PD are bradykinesia, rigidity, tremor, and postural instability.

Signs and symptoms of PD

- Bradykinesia
- Rigidity
    - Lead-pipe rigidity: constant resistance to PROM in any direction and at any speed
    - Cogwheel rigidity: ratchety, alternating resistance with relaxation throughout PROM
- Tremor
- Postural instability
- Akinesia
- Festinating gait
- Masked facies
- Freezing
- Flexed posture
- Dysphagia
- Decreased arm swing
- Difficulty stopping a motor program once it has begun
- Falls
- Incoordination
- Dysarthria
- Kyphosis
- Fatigue
- Dementia

Medical management of PD

- Surgical destruction of thalamus to decrease tremor
- Pallidotomy (removal of globus pallidus) to improve cardinal symptoms
- Implantable deep brain simulator

Multiple Sclerosis

Multiple sclerosis (MS) is a chronic progressive neurologic disease caused by demyelination of the CNS. The diagnosis of MS is made by laboratory studies, MRI, and correlation of signs and symptoms. The symptoms of multiple sclerosis tend to be exacerbated by hot and cold temperatures.

Types of MS

Relapsing remitting MS

The course of relapsing remitting MS is one of recurrent relapses and remissions. Symptoms may disappear completely or partially during remission. This is the most common type of MS.

Secondary progressing MS

The course of secondary progressing MS is one of initial periods of exacerbations and remissions, followed by progressive deterioration without substantial remissions.

Primary progressing MS

The course of primary progressing MS is one of progressive exacerbations without any remission.

Progressive relapsing MS

The course of progressive relapsing MS is one of progression throughout the course of the disease without exacerbations and remissions.

Signs and symptoms of MS

- Paresthesias
- Dysesthesia
- Visual symptoms
    - Visual loss, due to optic neuritis
    - Diplopia
    - Nystagmus
- Weakness
- Ataxia
- Impaired balance
- Scanning and slurred speech
- Intention tremor
- Trigeminal neuralgia
- Fatigue
- Spasticity
- Bowel and bladder dysfunction

Medical management of MS

The medical management of MS involves pharmaceutical agents to treat symptoms and to alter the course of disease, alternative treatments, and symptom management. Acute exacerbations are normally treated with corticosteroids.

Guillain-Barré Syndrome

Guillain-Barré syndrome (GBS) is a lower motor neuron disorder. It is an acute inflammatory demyelinating polyneuropathy. Usually the patient experiences a respiratory tract or gastrointestinal infection in the weeks prior to the onset of the illness. GBS is an autoimmune reaction that causes demyelination of axons, which results in acute paralysis. The symptoms begin distally and progress proximally to include the trunk and face. **Flaccid paralysis** is a hallmark sign. Sensation is often less impaired than strength. Patients afflicted with GBS may require mechanical ventilation if the diaphragm is affected.

Most GBS patients see resolution of their symptoms within one year. Some patients may have residual neurologic dysfunction after recovery. Return of strength is in a proximal-to-distal pattern.

Signs and symptoms of GBS

- Weakness
- Sensory loss
- Flaccid paralysis
- Areflexia
- Paresthesias and hyperesthesias
- Autonomic dysfunction
- Myalgia
- Dysarthria
- Dysphagia
- Cranial nerve involvement

Three phases of GBS

Acute phase

The acute phase is the initial phase in which the symptoms of GBS appear. The acute phase lasts up to four weeks. Maximizing pulmonary function, prevention of contractures, and prevention of skin breakdown are keys to treatment. The patient's pain should also be addressed with possible treatment via modalities and massage. Splinting and passive ROM are techniques that can be used to prevent contractures.

Plateau

The plateau is the period of time when the symptoms are present yet stable. The plateau generally lasts up to four weeks. During the plateau phase, the patient's tolerance to upright posture can be increased. Strengthening and continuation of acute-phase interventions are utilized.

Recovery

The recovery is the period of time in which the symptoms improve; it can last for months or years. Therapeutic activities and exercise are used to address the patient's impairments. Care should be taken to avoid muscle fatigue, as overworking a muscle that is partially denervated can result in decreased muscle strength and endurance. Therefore, begin with low repetitions of gravity-eliminated exercise.

Medical management of GBS

- Plasmapheresis to stimulate new plasma production
- Intravenous immunoglobins

Post-Polio Syndrome

Poliomyelitis (polio) is caused by a virus that attacks the anterior horn cells of the spinal cord and causes paralysis. Poliomyelitis is all but eradicated today, however polio patients are now experiencing **post-polio syndrome** (PPS). PPS is the late effects of poliomyelitis. The severity of PPS matches the severity of the original case of polio. Medical management of PPS includes lifestyle changes to accommodate for the signs and symptoms.

Signs and Symptoms of PPS

- Fatigue with minimal exertion
- New weakness that is usually proximal, progressive, and asymmetrical
- Myalgia and joint pain
- Cold intolerance
- Impaired functional activities and deconditioning due to other symptoms

Myelomeningocele

A **myelomeningocele** (MMC) is caused by the failure of the neural tube to close before the 28th day of gestation. Prenatal diagnosis of this condition is made by a lab test for high levels of alpha-fetoprotein. High-resolution ultrasound confirms the presence of a defect. Medical treatment prenatally includes both intrauterine surgery to repair the bony defect and delivery of the baby by induction or cesarean section. The treatment of MMC varies with the level of involvement and the stage of intervention (newborn vs. later life). A child with MMC should avoid positions such as frog-leg, w-sitting, ring-sitting, heel-sitting, and crossed-leg sitting.

Signs and symptoms of MMC depend on the level and severity of the malformation.

Spina bifida occulta

Spina bifida occulta is a vertebral abnormality without abnormality of the spinal cord or meninges. Often the skin is covered with a tuft of hair or a dimple.

Spina bifida cystica

Spina bifida cystica (or spina bifida aperta) presents as a cyst over the spinal defect. The cyst can be made of skin or meninges. Spina bifida cystica can be classified as a meningocele of myelomeningocele.

Meningocele
A meningocele is a cyst that contains only cerebrospinal fluid and meninges.

Myelomeningocele
A myelomeningocele (MMC) is a cyst that contains abnormal spinal cord. This cyst can be covered with meninges or skin. The most commonly affected area is the lumbar region.

Anencephaly

Anencephaly is a condition in which the brain does not develop. Anencephaly is incompatible with life.

Encephalocele

Encephalocele is a condition in which the brain projects from the skull. Chance of a live birth is greatly reduced with presence of encephalocele.

Causes of MMC

- Genetic predisposition
- Fetal alcohol syndrome
- Irish ethnicity
- Lack of folic acid intake by the mother

Signs and symptoms of MMC

- Motor impairments
- (Incomplete) sensory impairments
- Upper motor neuron and lower motor neuron symptoms
- Flaccid paralysis
- Spasticity
- Congenital musculoskeletal deformities
- Clubfoot, if there is involvement of L4 or L5
- Muscle imbalances and subsequent abnormal positions of the lower extremity
- Osteoporosis and associated increased risk for fracture
- Congenital or acquired scoliosis
- Arnold-Chiari type II malformation: causes hydrocephalus and bulbar palsies
- Hydrocephalus
- Hydromyelia
- Tethered spinal cord
- Bowel and bladder dysfunction
- Latex allergy
- Upper-extremity motor control dysfunction
- Cognitive impairment

Medical management of MMC

- Ventriculoperitoneal shunt
- Surgical closure or removal of MMC within 24 hours of birth
- Serial casting to manage contractures

Down Syndrome

Down syndrome is a genetic disease that causes mental retardation. Down syndrome is caused by an extra 21st chromosome in all or most of the body's cells. The major risk factor for the development of Down syndrome is higher parental age. Surgical fixation of an unstable atlantoaxial joint is a common medical treatment for this population.

Signs and symptoms of Down syndrome

- Hypotonicity
- Joint hypermobility
- Stereotypical facial abnormalities, upward-slanting eyes, and flat facial features
- Developmental delay
- Motor control deficits
- Congenital heart disease
- Musculoskeletal deficits
  - Pes planus
  - Scoliosis
  - Patellar instability
  - Atlantoaxial instability
- Visual disturbances
- Hearing deficits
- Mental retardation
- Decreased endurance

Osteogenesis Imperfecta

Osteogenesis imperfecta is a congenital autosomal dominant disease that impairs bone metabolism. Patients with osteogenesis imperfecta have an increased risk of fractures. A key to treatment of osteogenesis imperfecta is early family education and later patient education on activities to be avoided due to risk of fracture, such as proper patient handling and protective positioning.

Signs and symptoms of osteogenesis imperfecta

- Fractures
- Ligamentous laxity
- Kyphoscoliosis
- Decreased height
- Long-bone bowing

Spinal Muscular Atrophy

Spinal muscular atrophy (SMA) is a progressive neurologic disease caused by an autosomal recessive trait. Anterior horn cells and lower motor neurons are destroyed. There are three types of SMA.

Type I SMA: Acute infantile SMA

The typical onset of Type I SMA (acute infantile SMA) is between birth and two months of age. Normal survival is typically two to three years. Death is due to respiratory involvement.

Signs and symptoms of Type I SMA

- Weak cry
- Frog-leg posture
- Areflexia
- Tongue weakness

Type II SMA: Chronic SMA

The typical onset of Type II SMA is between 2 and 18 months. Weakness of proximal musculature and scoliosis are normally seen in this chronic form of SMA.

Kugelberg-Welander SMA

The typical onset of Kugelberg-Welander SMA is after 18 months of age. Weakness of proximal musculature is seen. As a consequence, developmental activities are delayed.

Duchenne Muscular Dystrophy

Duchenne muscular dystrophy (DMD) results from an X-linked recessive gene. Because it is X-linked, only males exhibit symptoms; but females can be carriers. The patient does not produce the muscle protein dystrophin, which leads to the destruction of muscle fibers. Muscle contractions are inefficient and uncoordinated.

Signs and symptoms of DMD

- Progressive weakness, most profound in the shoulder and pelvis and progressing distally
- Decreased range of motion
- Cardiac and respiratory muscle weakness
- Contractures

Medical management of DMD

- Gene therapy
- Myoblast transplantation
- Tendon surgery

Amyotrophic Lateral Sclerosis

Amyotrophic lateral sclerosis (ALS) is a chronic and progressive motor neuron disease that affects both upper and lower motor neurons. This disease is also called Lou Gehrig's disease and is most commonly seen in older men. Weakness appears first in the hands and progresses proximally.

Signs and symptoms of ALS

- Muscle fasciculations
- Weakness
- Flaccidity
- Spasticity
- Cranial nerve impairments
- Incoordination

Alzheimer's Disease

Sixty to 70 percent of cases of senile dementia are of Alzheimer's type. Forgetfulness is the earliest symptom of Alzheimer's disease. Progression of Alzheimer's disease results in decreased mathematical abilities, word-finding difficulties, concentration problems, and impaired activities of daily living. At end stages, severe memory loss, disorientation, and social withdrawal are common. The diagnosis of Alzheimer's disease is based on history and physical, mental status evaluation, and ruling out other disease processes that cause dementia. Conservative treatment includes careful management of the patient's comorbidities, involvement of home health services, and caregiver training and support. Ensuring the patient's physical safety is of paramount importance.

Polyneuropathies

Polyneuropathy is a broad term that includes peripheral nerve disorders that result in motor, sensory, and/or autonomic deficits. Polyneuropathies primarily affect the distal musculature. Sensation impairment may include loss of sensation, dysesthesia, or numbness and tingling. Autonomic deficits can be seen in vital sign changes. Diabetic neuropathy is the most common neuropathy. Diabetic neuropathy presents as weakness and sensory loss in the feet and ankles.

Huntington's Disease

Huntington's disease is a genetic disease linked to an autosomal dominant gene. It is caused by neuronal loss, particularly in the basal ganglia but also in other areas of the brain. The typical age of onset is between 35 and 55 years of age.

Signs and symptoms of Huntington's disease

- Chorea
- Dystonia
- Bradykinesia
- Rigidity

- Dysarthria
- Dysphagia
- Cognitive impairment
- Depression
- Incontinence

Medical management of Huntington's disease

- Behavioral modifications and training
- Dopamine blocking agent decreases large-amplitude chorea
- Antidepressants
- Genetic counseling

Myasthenia Gravis

Myasthenia gravis is a disorder of the neuromuscular junction. It can be inherited or acquired.

Signs and symptoms of myasthenia gravis

- Muscle fatigue, worse at the end of the day
- Ptosis, diplopia
- Cranial nerve impairments
- Proximal weakness

Complex Regional Pain Syndrome

Complex regional pain syndrome (CRPS) is neuropathic pain caused by a lesion to the nervous system.

CRPS Type 1

CRPS Type 1 (formerly reflex sympathetic dystrophy) is usually associated with a crushing trauma of the hand or foot or with surgery at one of the large joints of the body. Pain is more severe than expected following the given trauma. Symptoms are inflammation, pain, decreased range of motion, sweating, trophic skin changes and discoloration, and joint stiffness. Pain is worse at night and diffuse. Early medical treatment is key.

CRPS Type 2

CRPS Type 2 occurs after a proximal injury to a major nerve trunk. This injury results in neuropathic pain. Pain is severe, spontaneous, unrelenting, and burning. The skin is hyperesthetic. Nonpainful stimuli are perceived as painful (allodynia). Change in circulation and sweating are present. Pain begins in the affected nerve supply but also continues past its borders into unaffected nerve distribution.

Medical management of CRPS

- Early motion and functional activities
- Forceful range of motion is not contraindicated.
- Protection of painful area from stimuli
- Analgesics
- Surgical repair of nerve injury or sympathetic block
- Implantable stimulators

Trigeminal Neuralgia

Trigeminal neuralgia, also called tic douloureux, is more common in middle-age to later life and more common in women than in men. When seen in a younger patient, MS or tumor should be ruled out. The presentation of trigeminal neuralgia is pain in the trigeminal nerve root distribution. The complaints are of sudden severe facial pain that typically starts out on one side of the mouth and shoots toward the ipsilateral nostril, eye, or ear. Pain can be triggered by touch or movement of air flow or can be spontaneous in nature. Remissions may occur for months, but as the disorder progresses, attacks become more frequent and remissions become shorter. As the disorder progresses, a dull ache may persist in between the attacks of pain. CT scans are usually normal and do not reveal a cause. One possible cause is a structural malformation such as an anomalous artery or vein on the trigeminal nerve root. Surgical separation or radiofrequency rhizotomy may give relief. Conservative treatment uses pharmaceutical agents such as carbamazepine, phenytoin, or baclofen.

Bell's Palsy

Bell's palsy is an idiopathic inflammatory process of the facial nerve that results in facial paresis. The paralysis is sudden and is often preceded by pain around the ear. Patients may have difficulty with complete eye closure, eating, and fine facial movements. In some cases, taste is impaired. Sixty percent of cases resolve completely without treatment, and most have substantial improvement in symptoms over time. Prognosis is based on the severity of the initial paresis. If paresis is complete, prognosis is poor. Corticosteroids are used in the medical management of Bell's palsy.

Arthrogryposis Multiplex Congenital

Arthrogryposis multiplex congenital is also known as multiple congenital contractures. This is a nonprogressive neuromuscular syndrome that causes multiple joint contractures. Medical management of arthrogryposis multiplex congenital includes surgery to align joints. Also, fracture treatment, including casting and surgical fixation, is often required.

Birth Injury of the Brachial Plexus

Birth injury of the brachial plexus (obstetric brachial plexus palsy) is any trauma to the infant's brachial plexus during the birthing process. Risk factors include breech delivery and disproportionate relationship between birth canal size and the size of the baby.

Headaches

There are several types of headaches, including migraines, tension headaches, sinus headaches, and hypertension headaches. Acute headaches can be warning signals of head trauma, infection, impending CVA, or subarachnoid hemorrhage. Severe and intense headaches can be warning signs of meningitis, aneurysm, or brain tumor.

Migraine headaches

Migraines are intense, severe headaches. Pain may be described as throbbing or pulsating. Most commonly, migraine pain is located on one side of the head. Typically, migraines are chronic, recurrent, and more common in the morning. Migraine headaches may be accompanied by nausea, vomiting, photophobia, and pallor.

Sinus headaches

Sinus headaches are dull and persistent. Pain is located in the forehead or face and is worsened by bending and straining. Sinus headaches are caused by infection and inflammation of the sinuses.

Tension headaches

Tension headaches are constant, daily headaches. The pain is often described as tightness. Tension headaches are intense and are located at the back of the head and neck. Stress, fatigue, and noise may worsen tension-headache symptoms. Analgesics and relaxation therapy are conservative treatments. Elimination of stress and anxiety are also effective in the treatment of tension headaches.

Hypertension headaches

Hypertension headaches are dull and poorly localized. Any activity that increases blood pressure can cause hypertensive headaches.

Vestibular System Anatomy and Physiology

The vestibular system senses position and movement of the head. Along with the visual system and the somatosensory system, the vestibular system receives sensory input to create balance. Cilia line the walls of the semicircular canals of the ear and are sensitive to movement in any direction. If the head turns to the right, then the cilia move right with the head, and the fluid stays because of inertia and the cilia are bent. Incorrect sensory inputs can cause problems, with the sensations of vertigo, dizziness, and balance problems. The evaluation and treatment of vestibular impairments are quite different from those of other nervous system dysfunctions and are specific to vestibular dysfunction. Vestibular system disorders can be classified as central or peripheral in origin.

Central vestibular disorders

Examples of vestibular disorders of a central origin are TBI, CVA, degeneration, MS, and overlapping diagnoses. Intervention is primarily symptom management with vestibular suppressants, antinausea medications, and hydration. Habituation and adaptation techniques may be appropriate.

Peripheral vestibular disorders

Benign paroxysmal positional vertigo

Benign paroxysmal positional vertigo (BPPV) is a peripheral vestibular disorder. Symptoms tend to occur within two to six seconds after position change and last less than 30 seconds. The irritating position change is often a change from supine to sit or sit to stand. Symptoms improve with repetition.

Labyrinthitis

Labyrinthitis (also vestibular neuronitis) is another peripheral vestibular disorder. Symptoms tend to onset gradually, in minutes to hours, and peak at 24 hours. Resolution of symptoms occurs within days or weeks. Full recovery takes one to three months. The source of the infection should be treated first.

Migraine-associated vertigo

To treat migraine-associated vertigo, the risk factors of migraines should be controlled. These risk factors include stress, alcohol intake, caffeine, aged cheese, chocolate, and MSG.

Ménière's disease

Ménière's disease produces a vestibular component and is accompanied by tinnitus and hearing loss. This type of vertigo lasts 30 minutes to four hours. Ménière's disease is idiopathic. Vestibular rehab is effective to control symptoms.

History and physical examination

Patient interview

Very specific information is needed when interviewing a patient with vestibular system impairments. Necessary information includes: the date and circumstances of onset; duration, intensity, and frequency of symptoms; aggravating and alleviating factors; recent trauma or ear/sinus infection; and recent medicine changes or eye examination. A history of motion sickness and recent falls should be considered. The patient should also be asked if the symptoms occur in the shower, with reading, and/or at the grocery store. If the patient has seen a physician, the physical therapist should inquire about the results of caloric testing.

Oculomotor exam

Resting nystagmus indicates a problem of central origin.

AROM

Test the range of motion by having the patient move his eyes through the six directions of left, right, superior, inferior, convergence, and divergence.

Smooth pursuit

If a patient demonstrates problems with smooth pursuit, a problem of central origin is indicated. Asking the patient to follow a pen tip left, right, superior, and inferior tests smooth pursuit. Pause at the end of each movement to look for gaze nystagmus. This can be turned into a treatment intervention. To use it as a treatment, the patient holds a target and follows it with her eyes. The target is then progressed from small to large, and background changes are added. Watching tennis or traffic can be one form of practice.

Saccades

A problem with saccadic eye movement indicates a problem of central origin. Saccadic eye movements are tested by asking the patient to perform eye movements (left, right, superior, and inferior) between two targets. Possible treatments are reading and word-finding games.

Vestibulo-ocular reflex

If a patient presents with an impaired vestibulo-ocular reflex (VOR), a problem of peripheral origin is suspected. Tilt the patient's head forward 30° and ask him to keep his eyes focused on a target while he is turning his head left, right, superior, and inferior. This may also be performed passively. Normally, a person should be able to maintain focus on the target with head movement without onset of symptoms. The treatment is similar to the test. With the patient's head forward flexed 30°, have the patient focus his eyes on a stationary point and turn his head left and right repeatedly.

VOR cancellation/suppression

Vestibulo-ocular reflex cancellation or suppression impairments indicate a central problem. Having the patient fixate on a target that is rotating with him tests cancellation of the VOR. If suppression is abnormal, the eyes will move off-target.

Dix-Hallpike maneuver

To perform the Dix-Hallpike maneuver, the patient long-sits on a table with pillows set to be under the patient's shoulders when she is lying down. Instruct the patient to turn her head 45° to the left or the right and to lie back quickly, allowing the head to move back into extension and remain rotated 45°. The patient should keep her eyes open and report any symptoms of vertigo. Keep the patient in this position for 30 seconds. Return the patient to upright, wait for the symptoms to subside, and then repeat in the opposite direction. Treatment interventions include the Epley maneuver (canalith repositioning technique) and the home-modified Epley.

Roll test

To perform the roll test, the patient lies with the head flexed 20° (on a pillow) and quickly turns the head to the left or the right. Wait 30 seconds, have the patient turn his head back to midline, and then repeat in the other direction.

Vestibular system treatment theories

There are many treatment theories used in the treatment of vestibular system impairments. The **canalith repositioning technique** attempts to move otoconia, or "rocks," out of the semicircular canal to a benign area. The **adaptation theory** relies on the ability of the nervous system to make long-term changes to reset the system. **Habituation** is used to decrease responses by the nervous system to repeated, nonpainful stimuli. **Substitution theory** is a method of using other strategies or senses to fill in for missing or problematic senses. Finally, the **compensation theory** emphasizes substitution and changing the environment and often utilizes assistive devices to compensate for impairments.

Vestibular System Diagnoses and Treatments

Diagnosis	Treatment
BPPV	CRT
Unilateral vestibular hypofunction	Adaptation, substitution
Motion sensitivity	Habituation
Bilateral vestibular loss	Substitution, adaptation, habituation
CNS problem	Habituation

Treatment techniques

- Cawthorne exercises
- Brandt-Daroff exercises
- Canalith repositioning techniques
    - Epley maneuver
    - Liberatory maneuver

After use of these techniques, follow-up is usually in seven to ten days if there are no concurrent balance deficits. If symptoms are heightened for longer than 30 to 60 minutes after treatment, then have the patient *stop* the exercise and reassess the symptom origin.

Medical and Diagnostic Imaging

There are a multitude of diagnostic tests and imaging that can be used to diagnose dysfunctions, conditions, and diseases of the neuromuscular system. Included here are highlights of the most common tests and imaging techniques.

Neuroimaging

- X-ray (radiograph)
- CT scan
- Magnetic resonance imaging (MRI)
- Angiography, which outlines the blood flow through the cerebral blood vessels
- Positron emission tomography (PET scan)

Electrodiagnostic tests

Electrodiagnostic tests record the electric activity of the brain and peripheral nerves.

Electroencephalography
Electroencephalography (EEG) records spontaneous electrical activity of the brain.

Evoked potentials
Evoked potentials (EPs) are timed electrical activations of specific areas of the brain in response to specific stimuli.

Electromyography
Electromyography records and studies the spontaneous and voluntary electric activity of muscle. Electromyography is also known as nerve conduction studies.

Nerve conduction velocity
Nerve conduction velocity studies measure the velocity of action potential in a specific peripheral nerve. Both the sensory and the motor components of the nerve can be measured.

Lumbar puncture

A lumbar puncture is a procedure to extract cerebrospinal fluid from the spinal column for examination.

TREATMENT INTERVENTIONS

Once the evaluation is completed and the differential diagnosis is listed, it is necessary to choose the proper interventions to treat the patient's impairments. Typically, functional mobility, exercise, range of motion, mobilization, and modalities are combined to work toward the patient's physical therapy goals. Specific methods of proprioceptive neuromuscular facilitation and neurodevelopmental treatment are used to treat dysfunctions of these systems. The use of assistive devices, the implementation of orthotics and prosthetics, and the application of modalities are listed here as treatment interventions but are covered in chapter 8, Equipment and Devices, and Therapeutic Modalities.

Proprioceptive Neuromuscular Facilitation

Proprioceptive neuromuscular facilitation (PNF) was established by Dr. Herman Kabat and physical therapists Margaret Knott and Dorothy Voss. The essential components of PNF are aimed at facilitating proper movement patterns. The patterns of movement that are used in PNF are diagonal. Timing and sequencing of movement are stressed. During performance of the desired movements, physical therapists provide visual and verbal cues.

Manual contact

Manual contact with the patient provides sensory feedback about the preferred direction of movement.

Body position and body mechanics

For the movement to be effective, the physical therapist must be aligned in the desired direction of movement.

Stretch

Stretch of an elongated muscle facilitates muscle activity.

Manual resistance

The therapist should provide manual resistance leading to the desired outcome of either mobility or stability.

Irradiation

Irradiation refers to the spread of muscle activity due to resistance or overflow.

Joint facilitation

Joint facilitation techniques include traction and approximation.

Patterns of movement

Upper extremity

D1 flexion starts in shoulder abduction, extension, and internal rotation; elbow extension and pronation; and ulnar deviation. It ends with shoulder flexion, adduction, and external rotation; elbow extension; wrist supination; and radial deviation with the fisted hand. **D1 extension** is the reverse of D1 flexion.

D2 flexion starts with the arm down and across the body with forearm pronation, wrist flexion, and ulnar deviation with the fisted hand. It ends with the arm up on the same side of the body in shoulder flexion, abduction, and external rotation; forearm supination; wrist extension; radial deviation; and finger extension. **D2 extension** is the reverse of D2 flexion.

Lower extremity

D1 flexion starts with hip extension, abduction, and internal rotation; knee extension; and ankle plantar flexion and eversion. It ends with hip flexion, adduction, and external rotation; knee flexion; and ankle dorsiflexion and inversion. **D1 extension** is the reverse of D1 flexion.

D2 flexion starts with hip extension, adduction, and external rotation; knee extension; and ankle plantar flexion and inversion. It ends with hip flexion, abduction, and internal rotation; knee flexion; and ankle dorsiflexion and eversion. **D2 extension** is the reverse of D2 flexion.

PNF techniques

Rhythmic initiation

During rhythmic initiation, motion is first passive then progresses through active assisted, active, and resisted components. Passive motion is used for relaxation.

Rhythmic rotation

Rhythmic rotation uses slow, rhythmic, passive rotation to encourage relaxation and tone reduction.

Hold-relax active movement

The first step of the hold-relax active movement technique is an isometric contraction of the agonist in a shortened range. This is followed by relaxation and movement of the agonist into a lengthened position. This technique is used to increase range of motion.

Hold-relax
Hold-relax utilizes an isometric contraction at the end of the antagonist's available range of motion. The anticipated response is relaxation of the antagonist and passive movement through an increased range of motion.

Contract-relax
Contract-relax is similar to the hold-relax technique; however, rotation is allowed. The isometric contraction is held for five seconds or longer. Contract-relax can be used to increase range of motion.

Alternating isometrics
To use alternating isometrics, isometric resistance is provided to both the agonist and antagonist muscles. Alternating isometrics is used to increase stability.

Rhythmic stabilization
Rhythmic stabilization is similar to alternating isometrics but with a rotational component. The therapist provides two manual contacts to resist motion. Rhythmic stabilization is also used to increase stability.

Slow reversal
To perform the slow reversal technique, first a concentric contraction of an agonist is performed with manual contacts. At the end of the range of motion, the manual contacts change to facilitate the antagonist concentric contraction. This resistance can vary from light to maximal resistance. Slow reversal is used to increase strength, ROM, and coordination.

Slow reversal hold
Slow reversal hold is performed like slow reversal, but at the end of the range of motion an isometric contraction is held. This technique is used to increase strength, balance, and endurance.

Agonistic reversal
To perform the agonistic reversal technique, first the therapist provides resistance to the patient's concentric movement. At the end point of the motion, the patient holds an isometric contraction and then eccentrically resists the reversed motion to the starting point. Agonistic reversals can be used to increase functional stability, strength, endurance, and eccentric control.

Resisted progression
Resisted progression is performed by providing manual resistance to crawling, creeping, or walking. The resistance is provided to the trunk, extremities, pelvis, or scapula. Resisted progression is used to improve skill, strength, endurance, and sequencing.

Neurodevelopmental Treatment

Neurodevelopmental treatment (NDT) was developed by Kal and Berta Bobath. The goal of treatment is to facilitate normal postural control and provide the sensation of normal movement while inhibiting abnormal posture and muscle tone. Directing basic components of movement is the center of treatment. Components of movement include head and trunk control, midline orientation, weight-shifting over the base of support, balance, and control of the extremities. The therapist guides and facilitates movement by key points of control. Proximal key points of control (shoulder and pelvis) control distal movements of the extremities. Distal key points of control (the extremities) control trunk movements. Once muscle tone is normalized, functional activities and movements are added. Key diagnoses that benefit from NDT are cerebrovascular accident, traumatic brain injury, and cerebral palsy.

Treatment Interventions for Neurological Impairments

It is difficult to list treatment interventions for each neurologic pathology. Signs and symptoms of each pathology vary widely, and there is a wide range of treatment techniques available to the physical therapist. Instead, it is important to establish a problem list for the patient and to choose treatment interventions based on the patient's problems. For example, if a patient's problem list includes weakness and postural instability, the physical therapist should choose treatment interventions to address these problems. The following sections provide an overview of treatment options available to the physical therapist.

Approximation

To provide approximation, the therapist provides compression of joint surfaces. Approximation activates joint receptors and facilitates postural responses. One application is to apply compression at the knees during bridging to increase weight-bearing through the feet.

Facilitation techniques

Facilitation techniques facilitate movement and functional activities. Facilitation techniques include quick stretching, tapping, vibration, weight-bearing, and approximation.

Inhibition techniques

Inhibition techniques are used to decrease tone. Inhibition techniques include rhythmic rotation, weight-bearing, and icing.

Gait training

Gait training with an appropriate assistive device and appropriate level of assistance is often necessary in the neurologic population. Elimination of gait deviations while maximizing safety and efficiency is important. The physical therapist should consider a patient's stride length and efficiency and velocity of gait when training a patient in ambulation.

Prescription of an appropriate assistive device should be completed by the physical therapist. Chapter 8, Equipment and Devices, and Therapeutic Modalities, includes information on assistive device options.

Pre-gait activities include lower-extremity weight-bearing and acclimation to upright postures. Other options for gait training include variance of the walking path with obstacles, and alternate walking patterns (i.e., side-stepping, retro-walking, and marching). Levels of ambulation include therapeutic ambulation, household ambulation, and community ambulation.

Wheelchair prescription

Wheelchair prescription, training, and positioning are integral parts of physical therapy intervention for patients with neurologic impairment. This includes power mobility prescription, as needed. Chapter 8, Equipment and Devices, and Therapeutic Modalities, discusses specific wheelchair options.

The physical therapist not only helps to prescribe the wheelchair, but also trains the patient and/or family on the use and benefits of the wheelchair. Wheelchair skills such as "wheelies," ascending/descending ramps, and managing curbs should be taught to wheelchair-dependent patients.

Wheelchair cushions also need to be prescribed for the neurologically involved patient. These cushions need to maximize optimal positioning while providing adequate pressure relief. Again, refer to chapter 8 for specific wheelchair cushion options.

Therapeutic exercise

There are a multitude of exercises that can be utilized for the neurologically impaired patient. For the comatose patient, passive range of motion is needed to preserve sufficient muscular length. Stretching exercises are used to decrease stiffness, tone, and spasticity. Strengthening exercises are used in the treatment of muscular weakness. Fine motor exercises are used to improve fine motor skills. Coordination exercises such as Frenkel exercises can improve muscular incoordination. Aerobic exercise can prevent deconditioning and improve aerobic capacity. Exercises performed bilaterally can help to avoid muscular imbalances. Postural exercises and education to improve postural stability and balance can be prescribed.

Patients with spinal cord injury have special considerations for exercise. A patient with a spinal cord injury must maintain functional lengths of key muscles (hamstrings, gluteus maximus, hip musculature, gastrocnemius, and soleus). These patients should be proficient at self-ROM of these muscles. Also, one contraindication to active exercise is an unstable fracture of the spine, which may occur with a spinal cord injury.

Balance exercises

A wide range of balance exercises is available. Lower-level patients may need to work on static sitting balance, whereas more advanced patients can work on dynamic standing balance. Higher-level dynamic balance treatment techniques can utilize equipment such as Swiss balls, balance boards, and alternate weight-bearing surfaces. Eliminating visual input by closing the eyes adds another challenge to maintaining balance. Neuromuscular reeducation for balance retraining and postural training is a common treatment intervention in the neurologic population.

Orthotic prescription

Orthoses are commonly required in the neurologic patient population. Orthotic prescription is based on muscular weakness, tightness, and functional abilities. Gait in a spinal cord injured patient can even be performed through the use of appropriate orthoses, such as a hip-knee-ankle-foot orthosis or a reciprocating gait orthosis. Orthotic training must include training in donning/doffing, a schedule for wearing the orthosis, and details of proper skin inspection. Refer to chapter 8 for the specifics of orthoses.

Forced use

Forced use of an affected extremity is a treatment intervention that is useful for patients with hemiplegia. The unaffected extremity is not allowed to be used functionally, which forces the use of the hemiplegic extremity.

Home evaluation

Prior to a patient's being discharged home from an inpatient stay, a home evaluation can be performed to ensure the functional appropriateness of the patient's home environment. Home physical therapy is an important aspect in improving a patient's functional abilities at home.

Positioning

Proper bed and wheelchair positioning is essential in the treatment of a patient with neurologic impairments. Goals of positioning are the prevention of contractures, the prevention of skin breakdown, and maximizing the patient's functional abilities.

Patients who present with decerebrate and decorticate postures need to be positioned out of these postures and into **reflex-inhibiting postures**. These reflex-inhibiting postures are positions that are in the opposite pattern of the reflexive position and can decrease abnormal tone.

Prevention and treatment of contractures include therapeutic exercise, passive range of motion, and proper daytime and nighttime positioning. The physical therapist should provide the patient, family, and caregiver with education on postures and movement patterns to avoid and to encourage. Proper seating and positioning to allow independence while maintaining posture is also necessary.

For a child or dependent adult, the family or caregiver needs to be trained in proper pressure-relief techniques. If able, the patient should be taught independent pressure-relief techniques.

Sensory stimulation

Sensory stimulation is a systematic technique of providing sensory stimuli to the patient who has impaired sensation. The length of time that the patient is stimulated should be limited. Only one stimulus should be used at a time. The physical therapist should monitor the patient for responses to the stimuli. Responses include changes in vital signs, changes in muscle tone, head movement, wincing, eye movement, and vocalizations.

Sensory stimuli

- Auditory
- Olfactory
- Tactile
- Kinesthetic
- Oral

Functional mobility training

Functional mobility training is the training of patients to perform safe transfers, bed mobility, and postural readjustments. Safety and efficiency of functional mobility must be considered. Functional activities include self-care and activities of daily living.

There are special considerations for the patient with a spinal cord injury. Rolling into and out of the prone position should be emphasized to utilize the prone position in the prevention of contractures. Long sitting is an important functional position for patients with SCI. The patient with an injured spinal cord needs adequate hamstring ROM (90 to 100°) to tolerate long sitting. Persons with C1 to C4 spinal cord injuries are dependent for transfers.

Therapeutic activities and functional mobility can be used in the developing child to teach head and trunk control and to encourage righting and equilibrium reactions. In general, pathologies that affect children can be partially addressed with therapeutic activities to develop head and trunk control.

Patient, family, and caregiver education

After a diagnosis of a neurologic impairment, the patient and the family or caregiver may make major life changes. One of the physical therapist's most important treatment interventions is education. Education must be given on pathology, prognosis, evaluation, and treatment intervention. For patients with sensory impairments, the patient, family, and caregiver require education for safe handling and positioning in order to avoid accidental injury to the patient.

Tilt table

A tilt table can help with strengthening, range of motion, and acclimation to an upright posture. The physical therapist must monitor the patient for signs of orthostatic hypotension by taking blood pressure readings in supine, sitting, and standing positions. Other vital signs such as respiratory rate, pulse oxygen saturation, and pulse should also be monitored.

Therapeutic standing

Weight-bearing through the lower extremities has many benefits. Therapeutic standing is particularly useful for patients with SCI or traumatic brain injury and can prevent future complications. Therapeutic standing can be accomplished through the use of a standing frame, parapodium, or other orthoses. Body-weight-supported treadmill training can also be used for the neurologically impaired patient.

Goals of therapeutic standing

- Decrease abnormal muscle tone and spasms
- Improve bowel and bladder function
- Strengthen lower-extremity musculature
- Prevent osteoporosis
- Improve circulation
- Improve reflexes
- Improve emotional status

Air splints

Air splints to the extremities can be used to position, reduce tone, and increase sensory awareness. Air splints are applied to the patient's arm or leg and filled with air to 38–40 mm Hg. Air splints can be worn for up to one hour at a time.

Cardiopulmonary treatment

The cardiopulmonary system is also compromised when the nervous system is impaired. Decreased muscular tone and nervous input have detrimental effects on the cardiopulmonary system. Breathing and diaphragmatic exercises to retrain the muscles of respiration are useful. Aerobic exercise can maintain or improve the aerobic capacity of the neurologic patient.

Special cardiopulmonary considerations must be made for a patient with SCI. After an SCI, sympathetic nervous system input is decreased. This decreased sympathetic input results in a distorted cardiovascular response to exercise. The physical therapist should use the Borg Rating of Perceived Exertion scale as well as the patient's complaints and symptoms to evaluate the patient's exercise tolerance. To improve abdominal tone, an abdominal binder can support the abdominal contents. Elastic stockings and wraps can be used to help increase venous return.

Airway clearance techniques can be used if there is inadequate secretion clearance. Cardiopulmonary considerations are key in the treatment of the unconscious patient.

All medical personnel must work together to maintain respiration and airways of the unconscious patient.

Aquatic therapy

Exercise in water eliminates gravity and helps to support the body. Water can also provide resistance to movement. Generally, aquatic therapy is performed in warm water, 92–96°F (33.3°–33.6°C).

Goals of aquatic therapy

- Increase circulation
- Increase the heart rate
- Increase the respiration rate
- Decrease the blood pressure
- General relaxation

Benefits of aquatic therapy

- Decreases muscle tone
- Increases strength and ROM
- Improves pulmonary function
- Provides opportunity to stand and to bear weight
- Decreases spasticity

Contraindications to aquatic therapy

- Fever
- Infection
- Tracheostomy
- Uncontrolled blood pressure
- Abnormally low vital capacity
- Bowel and bladder incontinence
- Open wound

Neuromuscular stimulation

Neuromuscular stimulation (NMS) is an electrotherapeutic modality that increases the strength and endurance of muscular contraction. NMS also decreases spasticity. Refer to chapter 8 for more information on therapeutic modalities.

Icing

Icing a hypertonic muscle tends to decrease abnormal tone.

Spasticity management

Techniques to inhibit spasticity include weight-bearing, weight-shifting, rocking, and trunk rotation.

Energy conservation

Prevention of fatigue through energy conservation techniques is another treatment intervention used in the neurologic population. Energy conservation techniques include the use of assistive devices and/or wheelchairs and scheduling of appropriate amounts and times of rest and activity. Patients are taught to avoid muscular fatigue; and when exercising, they should use low repetitions of submaximal exercise.

Pain-relieving techniques

Many neurologic disorders are accompanied by pain. Modalities, massage, positioning, and relaxation are techniques used to reduce pain. Reduction of the painful process (i.e., improving tight, painful musculature through stretching) is also indicated. See the chapter 8 section on pain in the therapeutic modalities for further information on pain relief.

A FINAL WORD

To adequately evaluate and treat a patient or client, the therapist must have a strong knowledge of the foundational sciences and the background, evaluation, differential diagnoses, and treatment interventions of the nervous system. This chapter, which highlights each of these areas, along with your experience in lab practicals and clinical affiliations, will help prepare you to identify and treat impairments of these systems.

The following pages offer an end-of-chapter practice quiz to test your knowledge of some of the fundamentals of the nervous system. It is not necessary to time this, as it is a chapter review quiz.

Nervous System Chapter Quiz

1. A patient with a vertebrobasilar artery infarct is alert and oriented but is unable to move or speak. He is only able to move his eyes. What syndrome is this patient demonstrating?

    (A) Thalamic pain syndrome

    (B) Pusher syndrome

    (C) Locked-in syndrome

    (D) Homonymous hemianopia

2. An infant is receiving physical therapy. The physical therapist notices that the infant tends to put her extremities out to try to maintain her balance after a challenge in her balance. What level of postural control is this infant demonstrating?

    (A) Righting reactions

    (B) Protective reactions

    (C) Equilibrium reactions

    (D) Tonic reflexes

3. A five-year-old child with cerebral palsy receives physical therapy. The physical therapist uses multiple treatment interventions for this child. In one treatment session, the therapist has the child sit on a stability ball, weight-shift in multiple directions with unsupported sitting, and play catch while sitting on the floor. What treatment goal is the therapist *MOST* likely addressing with these treatment interventions?

    (A) Increase lower extremity strength

    (B) Increase upper extremity strength

    (C) Improve seated and standing balance

    (D) Improve gait

4. In what way does motor development tend to occur?

    (A) Cephalic to caudal, distal to proximal, and fine to gross movements

    (B) Cephalic to caudal, distal to proximal, and gross to fine movements

    (C) Cephalic to caudal, proximal to distal, and gross to fine movements

    (D) Caudal to cephalic, proximal to distal, and gross to fine movements

5. A physical therapist evaluates a three-month-old infant. The therapist elicits the symmetrical tonic neck reflex. When the head is flexed, what does the therapist expect to see?

    (A) Flexion of upper and lower extremities

    (B) Extension of upper and lower extremities

    (C) Flexion of upper extremities and extension of lower extremities

    (D) Extension of upper extremities and flexion of lower extremities

6. A newborn infant demonstrates physiological flexion. What is the next normal kinesiological movement that a physical therapist should expect the infant to develop?

    (A) Antigravity flexion

    (B) Antigravity extension

    (C) Rotation

    (D) Lateral flexion

7. Following a traumatic spinal cord injury, a patient receives physical therapy at an inpatient rehab unit. The physical therapist examines the patient and determines that his C7 level is the most caudal level that is intact. What key muscle group is maintained in a C7 spinal cord injury?

   (A) Elbow flexors
   (B) Elbow extensors
   (C) Wrist flexors
   (D) Wrist extensors

8. Following a cerebrovascular accident, a patient ambulates with an equinus gait pattern. What is most likely *NOT* the cause of this gait deviation?

   (A) Weakness of the dorsiflexors
   (B) Excess activity of the dorsiflexors
   (C) Excess activity of the plantar flexors
   (D) Plantar flexion contracture

9. An 80-year-old patient sustains a L2 compression fracture. The patient begins to complain of poor sensation of the lower extremities, and her lower-extremity strength begins to deteriorate. What intervention by the physician is *MOST* likely?

   (A) Surgical stabilization of the vertebral fracture
   (B) Cervical collar
   (C) Prescription of pain pills
   (D) Recommendation of sustained flexion position

10. Following a crushing injury to his hand, a patient complains of pain that is more severe than expected. The pain is described as burning and fluctuating. The hand is discolored and inflamed, and the knuckles are stiff. The patient complains that the pain gets worse at night. The patient is demonstrating signs and symptoms of what pathology?

   (A) Myasthenia gravis
   (B) Complex regional pain syndrome
   (C) Trigeminal neuralgia
   (D) Huntington's disease

11. Following a traumatic brain injury, a patient is in a coma. A physical therapy referral is made to increase the patient's level of arousal. What treatment technique could the therapist use to increase the patient's level of arousal?

   (A) Sensory stimulation
   (B) Relaxation techniques
   (C) Therapeutic positioning
   (D) Vestibular training

12. A physical therapist asks a patient to actively flex her upper extremity to full end range of motion. Upon moving the upper extremity into this position, facilitation of the finger extensors and abductors is noted. The physical therapist recognizes this as Souques' phenomenon. What type of sign is Souques' phenomenon?

   (A) Associated reaction
   (B) Brain-stem reflex
   (C) Deep tendon reflex
   (D) Spasticity

13. A patient with multiple sclerosis is receiving physical therapy for strengthening and symptom management. The patient is seen in the outpatient clinic by a physical therapist. The patient performs all of the therapeutic exercise the physical therapist asks her to do and does not complain about pain or fatigue during the treatment session. However, when the patient returns to the clinic two days later, she tells the physical therapist that she was unable to get out of bed the day after the exercise due to extreme fatigue, and that she took increased amounts of pain pills due to the increased pain and needed her husband's help with tasks with which she is ordinarily independent. Today she feels back to normal. What should the therapist do?

   (A) Explain to the patient that this is normal and exercise should be maximal if it is working
   (B) Modify the exercise program and ask the patient throughout the treatment session about levels of fatigue and pain
   (C) Discharge the patient from physical therapy because she is too weak to continue
   (D) Cancel today's treatment session and reschedule to next week to allow the patient to rest

14. Following a cerebrovascular accident, a patient receives physical therapy at a skilled nursing facility. The patient demonstrates pusher syndrome. The patient has weakness, impaired sensation, and neglect all on the left side of her body. She is able to ambulate with a wheeled walker with moderate assistance and verbal cues. The physical therapist gives the patient a visual target to place the left foot near the front left wheel of the walker. This treatment intervention is focused on what problem?

    (A) Impaired weight-shifting during gait
    (B) Left ankle weakness
    (C) Hypertonicity
    (D) Left leg contracture

15. A physical therapist is testing a patient's postural control. The patient stands, and the physical therapist provides challenges to the patient's balance. With the first challenge to balance, the patient leans posterior and then moves her right foot to maintain balance. From Nashner's Model of Postural Control, what strategy did the patient use?

    (A) Ankle strategy
    (B) Hip strategy
    (C) Stepping strategy
    (D) Balance strategy

Answers

1. **C.**

   Locked-in syndrome occurs with a vertebrobasilar artery infarct. Locked-in syndrome presents as lack of active movement and speech, except for eye movement. The patient is alert and oriented.
   (Martin, page 285)

2. **B.**

   The development of postural control is a part of motor control. Righting reactions include head and trunk righting. Protective reactions include extremity movements to protect balance. Equilibrium reactions are the most advanced level of postural control that maintain the center of gravity over the base of support. Tonic reflexes are reflexes that produce muscle tone and posture.
   (Martin, page 34)

3. **C.**

   These are techniques used to improve balance. Balance in a seated position can prepare the child for balance in standing.
   (Campbell, page 52)

4. **C.**

   Motor development tends to progress cephalic to caudal, proximal to distal, mass to specific, and gross to fine movements.
   (Martin, page 52)

5. **C.**

   In the symmetrical tonic neck reflex, head flexion is accompanied by flexion of the upper extremities and extension of the lower extremities. If the head is extended, the response is extension of the upper extremities and flexion of the lower extremities.
   (Rothstein, page 689)

6. **B.**

   Infants progress from physiological flexion at birth to antigravity extension, antigravity flexion, lateral flexion, and then rotation.
   (Martin, page 54)

7. **B.**

   The neurological level is the most caudal segment of the spinal cord with normal sensation and motor function bilaterally. In a C7 spinal cord injury, the elbow extensors (the triceps) are intact.
   (Martin, page 379)

8. **B.**

   Excess activity of the dorsiflexors may cause a varus foot during gait. Weakness of the dorsiflexors, excess activity of the plantar flexors, and plantar flexion contracture can all cause an equinus gait pattern.
   (Rothstein, page 460)

9. **A.**

   A vertebral fracture that begins to show signs of progression of neurological signs may need surgical fixation.
   (Umphred, page 481)

10. **B.**

    Complex regional pain syndrome is often associated with a crushing injury to a body part. It presents as pain that is worse than is expected. The skin is discolored, and there are signs of inflammation, trophic changes, and decreased range of motion.
    (Umphred, page 892)

11. **A.**

Sensory stimulation is a controlled treatment intervention that systematically stimulates auditory, olfactory, gustatory, visual, tactile, kinesthetic, and vestibular systems. Sensory stimulation can help to improve the level of arousal and produce movement.
(O'Sullivan, page 909)

12. **A.**

Associated reactions are involuntary movements that happen due to active or resisted movements at another body part. Examples of associated reactions are Souque phenomenon, Raimiste phenomenon, and homolateral limb synkinesis.
(Martin, page 290)

13. **B.**

Exercise is patient-dependent and you, as the therapist, must listen to the symptoms the patient reports. A patient with multiple sclerosis tends to benefit from submaximal exercise every other day. Progression is slower in patients with multiple sclerosis.
(O'Sullivan, page 795)

14. **A.**

Impaired weight-shifting during gait is a common problem and can be addressed in many ways. In this example, a visual target is used to improve weight-shifting during gait.
(Lewis, page 396)

15. **C.**

The stepping strategy is a final strategy to avoid falling. Ankle strategy is the first strategy and includes movement at the ankles. Hip strategy is the second strategy and uses hip musculature to maintain balance.
(Martin, page 38)

Integumentary System

6

The integumentary system protects and affects the body as a whole, and every graduating physical therapy student should be familiar with the basic anatomy of this system. Physical therapists often treat patients who have the sole diagnosis of dysfunction of the integumentary system. However, a patient also cannot be narrowly defined as simply an "orthopedic patient" or a "neurological patient"—the organ systems are interrelated, and the examination and treatment techniques of other systems can directly affect the integumentary system. In providing treatment you must consider the patient as a whole, and not just as the injury or disability for which they are seeking physical therapy.

To fully understand the integumentary system, you must first know human anatomy and physiology, including the skin and accessory organs. Examination of the skin may be necessary when evaluating a patient whose main medical diagnosis does not include the integumentary system. The patient's comorbidities, age, activity level, and psychology all play into the success of physical therapy as a treatment intervention. In this chapter, you will move beyond the basics into the examination and treatment of this important system.

FOUNDATIONAL SCIENCES AND BACKGROUND

A strong understanding of the basic background and fundamental sciences of the integumentary system is necessary before examination, evaluation, interpretation, and intervention can take place. It is necessary to understand how the skin is organized and to know the essential functions of the skin and its accessory organs.

Integumentary System Structure

The integumentary system includes the skin and the accessory organs: hair, nails, and skin glands. The skin is a membrane. There are two types of membranes: epithelial and connective-tissue membranes. Epithelial membranes are composed of a layer of epithelial tissue and an underlying layer of connective tissue.

Epithelial membranes

There are three types of epithelial membranes: cutaneous, serous, and mucous.

Cutaneous membrane

The **cutaneous membrane** is better known as the skin.

Serous membranes

Serous membranes line body cavities and cover the organs within those cavities. The parietal portion of the membrane lines the walls of the body cavity; the visceral portion covers the organs. For example, the parietal peritoneum lines the walls of the abdominal cavity, and the visceral peritoneum covers the organs within the abdominal cavity. Serous membranes secrete serous fluid that lubricates and reduces friction between surfaces.

Mucous membranes

Mucous membranes line the surfaces that open to the external environment. Mucous membranes line the respiratory tract, digestive tract, urinary tract, and reproductive tract. This membrane secretes mucus to keep the tracts moist.

Connective-tissue membranes

Connective-tissue membranes do not contain epithelial tissue. One example of a connective-tissue membrane is the synovial membrane that lines the joints. Synovial membranes secrete synovial fluid. Both the synovial membrane and synovial fluid help to lubricate and reduce friction between joint surfaces.

Skin

Skin is generally 16 percent of a person's body weight. The skin has three layers: the epidermis, the dermis, and the hypodermis.

Epidermis

The epidermis is the uppermost layer of skin and is composed of stratified squamous epithelium. The epidermis is divided into two layers, the stratum germinativum (deep) and the stratum corneum (superficial). The cells of the stratum germinativum undergo mitosis and produce millions of cells daily. These cells progress though the middle layers (or strata) of cells and as they near the stratum corneum, their cytoplasm is replaced by the protein keratin. Keratin is a durable, waterproof protein that helps to protect the skin. Humans lose thousands of dead skin cells each day. This continual reproduction of skin cells gives human skin a natural healing quality. The innermost layer, the stratum germinativum, also contains the skin pigment (melanin) and the melanocytes that produce melanin.

Dermis

The dermis is the middle layer of skin. The dermis is thicker than the epidermis and is composed of connective tissue. It also contains two layers, the papillary and the reticular. The papillary layer contains rows of small bumps called dermal papillae. The dermal papillae form part of the dermal-epidermal junction and also make up fingerprints. The reticular layer contains collagen to provide strength and elastic fibers to allow for stretch. The number of elastic fibers decreases as a person ages, resulting in wrinkles. The dermis also contains sensory nerves, hair follicles, skin glands, blood vessels, and muscle fibers.

Hypodermis

The hypodermis is the innermost layer of skin and is composed of loose connective tissue and fat. The hypodermis is also called the subcutaneous layer. It insulates, cushions, and protects the body from injury, and stores potential energy in the form of fat.

Skin Accessory Structures

Hair

Each individual hair grows in a hair follicle. The root is the part of the hair that is hidden within the follicle, and the shaft is the part of the hair that is visible to the naked eye. Each hair is nourished by a blood vessel. Arrector pili muscles surround each hair follicle and contract involuntarily in cases of fright or cold temperatures.

Sensory receptors

Sensory receptors in the skin receive information regarding touch, pressure, temperature, vibration, and pain. Chapter 5, Nervous System, provides a detailed discussion of these receptors.

Nails

The nail body is the visible part of the nail. The nail root is the area that is beneath the cuticle. The cuticle is the folded-back portion of skin at the base of the nail. Beneath the nail body is the nail bed, which contains many blood vessels and normally appears pink. The nail bed can appear blue with decreased blood oxygen levels.

Skin glands

There are two types of skin glands: sudoriferous (sweat) glands and sebaceous glands.

Sudoriferous glands

Sudoriferous glands are the most common skin gland and are divided into two kinds, eccrine and apocrine. **Eccrine glands** are smaller and more abundant. They produce perspiration (sweat), and they function to rid the body of wastes such as ammonia and uric acid. Pores are the outlets of eccrine glands. **Apocrine glands** are found mostly in the axilla and the pigmented area of the genitals. Apocrine glands secrete a substance that is thicker than that secreted by the eccrine glands.

Sebaceous glands

Sebaceous glands function to secrete an oil called sebum to lubricate the hair and skin. These glands are found mostly in the areas of hair growth.

Skin Functions

- **Protection:** The skin serves to protect the body from bacteria, microbes, chemicals, physical tears, fluid loss, and ultraviolet rays.
- **Thermoregulation:** Evaporation of sweat and loss of heat by radiation from increased blood flow are examples of the skin's role in thermoregulation. Constriction of skin blood vessels and shunting of blood away from the skin helps to conserve heat. Increased blood flow to the skin can cause flushing, and decreased blood flow can cause a cyanotic (bluish or purplish) appearance of the skin.
- **Sensation:** The skin contains many sensory organs that identify touch, pressure, temperature, vibration, and pain.

Responses to Exercise

There is a continuous loss of water through the skin, called insensible perspiration. Skin also loses water through sweat loss. As sweat evaporates, the body temperature cools. Normally, sweat loss is between 500 and 700 mL per day. During maximal exercise in hot conditions, the skin can produce sweat at a rate of up to 1 L per hour. There is a risk of dehydration with excessive sweat or fluid loss. People who are exercising should be careful to drink adequate fluids to replace those lost during exercise.

The skin also dissipates the heat produced by the exercising muscles. Blood flow is shunted away from visceral organs to the skin, where heat can be released.

Pharmacology

Many prescription drugs that are taken for other diseases or conditions can affect the skin. Medical personnel should remember that corticosteroids hinder epidermal regeneration and collagen synthesis. Also, be aware of photosensitivities related to drugs, especially with the elderly. (Specific wound treatment materials are listed later in this chapter.) Drugs that affect the skin include antibacterials, antihypertensives, analgesics, tricyclic antidepressants, antihistamines, antineoplastic agents, and antipsychotics. Diuretics, hypoglycemics, sunscreens, oral contraceptives, hormones, steroids, and NSAIDs also have effects on the skin. Allergic reactions to drugs can manifest as skin rashes or irritations.

EVALUATION

During the evaluation process, it is important for the examiner to make decisions on what tests and measures are appropriate to establish a problem list in order to treat the patient's impairment. Again, during the examination process the patient must be viewed as a whole, whether the examination takes place in a hospital room, a home setting, an outpatient setting, or a long- or short-term care facility. In all cases each part of the examination process must be considered, although it is known that some portions of the examination are more appropriate for a certain setting or problem. Wound measurements and staging are important in the evaluation of wounds; pain, circulation, and vital signs are other important components.

Examination of the Integumentary System

- Patient/caregiver interview
- Systems review
- Past medical history
- Appearance of skin at bony prominences
- Skin quality: color, hydration, thickness
- Presence of wounds or incisions
- Incontinence
- Edema
- Previous skin breakdown
- Muscle atrophy
- Body weight
- Postural exam
- ROM
- Strength
- Sensation
- Cognition (related to ability to change position)
- Evaluation of scar: height, texture, pliability, measurement

Wound Measurement

If a wound is present, it should be measured and its depth, width, and length should be recorded. The presence of tunneling and undermining should be noted. Even the volume of the wound can be measured. Along with measurements, a description of the wound is needed that includes the presence, quality, and amount of exudate; smell; color; and presence and location of eschar.

Wound Staging

Stage	Description
Stage I	Discoloration, change of warmth, sensation, no open areas
Stage II	Superficial, loss of epidermis or dermis
Stage III	Full-thickness loss of tissue with damage to the underlying subcutaneous tissue that extends to the fascia
Stage IV	Full-thickness with extensive destruction; damage extends to deep tissues of bone, muscle, and tendon; tissue necrosis is present

Wound Assessment

When treating a patient for a wound, the physical therapist should make a detailed assessment of the wound. The therapist should identify the cause of the wound. The location, measurement, and stage of the wound should be examined. The therapist should examine the wound bed and edges, the presence of undermining, and the presence of any odor. The amount and quality of exudate should be assessed. An examination of the peri-wound skin is necessary. Finally, the patient should be evaluated for any pain or lack of protective pain. Any diagnosed or suspected infection, including signs or symptoms of infection, should be documented.

Pressure Measurement

Pressure measurement can be accomplished through handheld devices or large computerized mapping systems. These pressure measurements can be used for wheelchair positioning and prescription of pressure-relieving surfaces.

Classification of Burns

First-degree burns

First-degree burns damage the epidermis only.

Second-degree burns

Second-degree burns damage the epidermis and part of the dermis. First- and second-degree burns are also called partial-thickness burns.

Third-degree burns

Third-degree burns completely destroy the epidermis and dermis and are the least painful burns because the nerve endings are destroyed. Third-degree burns are also called full-thickness burns.

Fourth-degree burns

Fourth-degree burns are often from electrical burns. Fourth-degree burns extend to the subdermal tissue and involve muscle and even bone and often can result in serious medical issues and amputation.

Rule of Nines

The rule of nines is used to estimate the surface area of skin that has been burned. The body is divided into 11 areas of 9 percent each, with the genitals accounting for the remaining 1 percent.

- Head: 9 percent
- Front of torso: 18 percent
- Back of torso: 18 percent
- Arms: 9 percent each
- Front of each leg: 9 percent
- Back of each leg: 9 percent
- Genitals: 1 percent

Movement Analysis

Skin assessment is based on the propensity of skin to break down under pressure. Skin is more apt to break down if it is dry, aged, insensate, prone to excessive perspiration, or exposed to incontinence, friction, or shear. Therapeutic positioning of the patient who is prone to skin breakdown is paramount in preventing skin impairments. The major goal of positioning is to avoid weight-bearing over bony prominences. This can include equalizing weight-bearing (distribution of forces) or providing complete non-weight-bearing over bony prominences. Evaluation of friction and shear forces should be included in the assessment. Posture in sitting (particularly in a wheelchair) and shear forces during wheelchair propulsion should be noted. Reddened areas on the weight-bearing surfaces indicate friction and shear forces. Wheelchair cushioning, proper positioning, and education and training in avoidance of friction forces are essential components in the primary prevention of skin breakdown. Friction, shear forces, pressure, and scar tissue should be included in the movement analysis of a patient with skin impairments.

Friction

Friction is created when the surface of one object rubs against the surface of another object. Friction damages the epidermal layers, which makes the skin more apt to break down under pressure. Friction works with gravity to create shear forces.

Shear

Shear forces are the forces that act in parallel against the skin. Shear forces can cause ischemia in tissues by displacing blood vessels laterally. Shear forces stretch and twist tissues and blood vessels. These shear forces can often cause pressure ulcers that are larger than the bony prominence itself.

Pressure

Pressure is a force that acts perpendicularly against skin and tissues and causes ischemia. Immobility, inactivity, and impaired sensation contribute to pressure. With immobility, the patient is unable to reposition himself in order to avoid pressure buildup. With inactivity, the patient's movements are minimal and can lead to increased pressure along bony prominences. If a patient's sensation is impaired, he is unable to feel the pressure and thus does not recognize the need to reposition.

Scar tissue

The formation of scar tissue during wound healing can be disfiguring and functionally limiting. Scarring that occurs over joint surfaces can restrict joint motion. Scarring of the face can impair feeding and speech. Scars can also be a source of pain, paresthesias, and itching. Scars are at increased risk for sunburn. Medical treatment for troublesome scars includes surgical management, pressure therapy, and pharmaceuticals. There are three types of scar: normotrophic, hypertrophic, and keloid.

Normotrophic scar
A normotrophic scar is a visible scar that is of the same height as the surrounding skin.

Hypertrophic scar
A hypertrophic scar is a raised scar that does not extend beyond the wound boundaries.

Keloid scar
A keloid scar is a raised scar that extends beyond the original wound boundaries.

DIFFERENTIAL DIAGNOSIS AND PATHOLOGY

Based on the findings obtained during the evaluation of the skin, a list of differential diagnoses can be made. The type of wound and irritating factors can be identified. Each type of wound or condition of the integumentary system is unique and will dictate the medical management and treatment intervention choices made by the physical therapist. Skin impairments are multifactorial and vary in location and severity. By identifying the cause and mitigating factors of wound development, the physical therapist can then choose appropriate treatment interventions. Pathologies and conditions of the integumentary system are described below.

Pleurisy and Peritonitis

Since pleurisy is an inflammation of the pleural membranes, and peritonitis is inflammation of the peritoneal membranes, technically these are conditions of the integumentary system.

Burns

The severity of burns varies widely. Possible complications of more severe burns are increased risk of infection, extreme fluid loss, and the need for skin grafts. The medical management of burns includes protection against infection, rehydration, and skin grafts. There are several types of skin grafts, including allograft, autograft, and heterograft.

Types of skin grafts

- **Allograft:** skin graft from a donor
- **Autograft:** skin graft from the patient's body
- **Heterograft**: skin graft from another species

Skin Cancer

Squamous cell carcinoma is a slow-growing malignancy of the epidermis that looks like tough, raised nodules. Eventually, squamous cell carcinoma will metastasize to other organs if not treated.

Basal cell carcinoma is the most common type of skin cancer and is commonly seen on the face. This type of cancer appears as a small, elevated, bleeding crater. Basal cell carcinoma is unlikely to metastasize.

Malignant melanoma begins as a benign mole and changes to a cancerous lesion. Malignant melanoma is the most serious form of skin cancer. The ABCD rule applies to screening for malignant melanoma.

ABCD rule

Asymmetry: Malignant lesions are asymmetrical.
Border: Malignant lesions have an irregular shape or border.
Color: Malignant lesions have differing shades of color within the same lesion.
Diameter: Malignant lesions are generally larger than 0.25 inch.

Wounds

Wounds are the major pathology of the integumentary system that physical therapists treat. This section discusses the terms used in evaluating and describing wounds.

Slough

Slough is the yellow, thin, stringy necrotic material that can be found in a wound.

Eschar

Eschar is the brown or black, soft or hard necrotic tissue that signals full-thickness tissue destruction. Necrotic tissue slows wound healing, as it is a medium for bacterial growth and a barrier to granulation. Increased amounts of necrotic tissue represent more severe injury and prolonged healing times.

Exudate

Exudate is wound drainage. Exudate contains enzymes and growth factors that contribute to wound healing. This wound drainage may also contain infection.

Granulation tissue

Granulation tissue is the vascular connective tissue that forms grainy capillary loops in the wound bed. Granulation tissue is usually pink or red and signifies healing.

Fistula

A fistula is an abnormal passage between two structures or spaces.

Undermining/tunneling

Undermining, or tunneling, is the caving under of the wound edges that can tunnel into the underlying fascia.

Wound-healing factors

- Age
- Nutrition
- Smoking
- Circulation and perfusion
- Infection
- Gangrene
- Medications
- Diabetes

Types of wounds

There are several types of wounds and special considerations related to the healing of wounds. This section describes the different types of wounds, including the general medical treatment related to that specific type of wound.

Pressure ulcers

Pressure ulcers are areas of localized necrosis that develop after the compression of soft tissue between a bony prominence and another surface for a prolonged time. Prevention is the key factor in managing pressure ulcers. Assessment tests include the **Braden** and the **Norton** and the **Braden Q** for the pediatric population. The Braden and Braden Q identify the amount of risk for pressure ulcers. Pressure-reduction techniques include pressure-relief mattresses and cushions, position changes every two hours, heel elevation, and mobilization.

Risk factors for pressure ulcers

- Immobility
- Poor activity level
- Impaired sensation
- Moisture, friction, and shear forces
- Impaired nutrition
- Increased age
- Edema
- Smoking

Arterial ulcers

Arterial ulcers are a result of occlusion of an artery that decreases blood flow to tissue and results in ischemia. Typically, an extremity that is prone to arterial ulcers is shiny, dry, and hairless. Arterial ulcers are located distally, especially on the feet, and have well-defined borders, minimal exudate, and dry necrotic eschar. Physical therapy intervention includes exercise to increase blood flow. Compression should not be used for edema control.

Risk factors for arterial ulcers

- Diabetes
- Family history
- Hyperlipidemia
- Hypertension
- Smoking

Venous ulcers

Venous ulcers form as a result of impaired venous blood flow and congestion of blood in the veins that then spills over into the tissue. Chronic venous insufficiency often results in dark brown staining of the skin. The edges of venous ulcers are irregular and their bases are ruddy. There is moderate to large amounts of exudate. Crusting is seen around the ulcer. Pain is described as aching and worsening throughout the day and is relieved by elevating the affected area. Edema can be controlled by elevation, ankle-calf pumps, compression wraps, and/or medication. Surgical interventions include skin grafts and venous repairs.

Risk factors for venous ulcers

- History of ulcers
- Family history
- Deep vein thrombosis or thrombophlebitis
- Trauma

- CHF
- Increased age
- Obesity
- Immobility
- Malnutrition
- Pregnancy

Autoimmune wounds
Autoimmune wounds are related to chronic inflammation caused by an autoimmune response such as systemic lupus erythematosus. Medical treatment is treatment of the underlying disease and inflammation.

Neoplastic wounds
Neoplastic wounds are from malignancies on the skin or underlying tissue that extend to the skin. Treatment of the malignancy is of foremost concern, followed by treatment of the wound.

Allergic wounds
Allergic wounds are caused by allergic reactions to a topical or systemic substance. Medical treatment for allergic wounds consists of identifying the allergen and treating the systemic symptoms.

Infectious wounds
Infectious wounds are caused by differing types of infectious agents. Examples of infectious agents are staphylococcal, impetigo, candidiasis, herpes zoster, and necrotizing fasciitis. Medical treatment is pharmaceutical elimination of the infectious agent.

Traumatic wounds
Traumatic wounds include abrasions, lacerations, and skin tears.

Neuropathic wounds
Neuropathic wounds are a complication of neuropathy and are often related to diabetes. Neuropathic wounds are typically found on the sole of the foot. Wound borders are well defined, with a punched-out appearance. Infection and gangrene are common complications. Amputation is a common end result. Neuropathic wounds are non- or minimally painful due to the absence of sensation. Primary prevention of neuropathic wounds is an important component of the treatment of patients with neuropathy.

Medical Treatment and Management

There are several treatments, techniques, and interventions that can be performed by the medical team in the treatment of wounds. The medical management of vascular deficiencies is closely related to the integumentary system because impairments of the vasculature often result in arterial or vascular wounds. Some of the more common types of tools for assessing the vasculature are ones that visualize and inspect blood flow and ones that compare blood pressures.

Continuous-wave Doppler is used to assess blood flow within a vessel. **Arterial and venous duplex** can be used to diagnose thrombosis and chronic venous insufficiency. **Skin perfusion pressures** are determined via laser Doppler to predict limb ischemia. **Magnetic resonance angiography** is used to visualize the stenoses of vessels.

The **ankle-brachial index (ABI)** is used to compare the blood pressure of the ankle with that of the arm. **Segmental and digital plethysmography** compare the pressure of segments of the leg (segmental) or the pressure of the toes (digital) with the arm pressure.

Laboratory tests often performed for a patient with a wound include a complete blood count and a wound culture.

Surgical intervention for the debridement or closure of a wound is common for large, slowly healing, or infected wounds. Amputation of an extremity due to gangrene or severe peripheral vasculature disease can be a last option in the treatment of wounds.

General medical treatment for wounds

- Infection prevention
- Protection from further mechanical, chemical, or thermal trauma
- Pain control
- Improve nutrition and hydration
- Smoking cessation
- Edema control
- Medication to address underlying causes
- Weight control
- Topical treatments
- Debridement of necrotic tissue

TREATMENT INTERVENTIONS

Once the evaluation is completed, it is necessary to choose the proper interventions to treat the patient's impairments. Primary prevention of integumentary pathology is important. The integumentary system is unique in its treatment interventions, as most relate to the management of wounds. Thus, treatment interventions of the integumentary system focus on the healing of wounds.

Methods of Wound Closure

Primary closure

Normally, a wound quickly heals by first intention. An example is a normally healing surgical incision. This is primary wound closure.

Secondary closure

Secondary closure of wounds refers to large, open wounds that are slow to heal.

Tertiary closure

Tertiary closure refers to an open wound that heals via secondary intention initially but then is surgically closed.

Phases of Wound Healing

Inflammatory phase

The inflammatory phase usually lasts from the first to the third day and is the body's initial response to injury. This phase includes clot formation and destruction of bacteria by white blood cells. Erythema, pain, edema, exudate, and increased temperature are present during the inflammatory phase.

Proliferative phase

During the proliferative phase, granulation tissue is formed. The wound begins to contract, and epithelization takes place. Collagen is synthesized, and angiogenesis takes place.

Maturation phase

During the maturation phase, collagen matures and scar tissue is formed. Tensile strength is significantly less in a healed wound, so risk of subsequent breakdown at the site is increased.

Phases of Chronic Wound Healing

- **Inflammatory phase:** Inflammation
- **Epithelialization phase:** Generation of epithelial cells and resurfacing of the wound
- **Proliferative phase:** Chronic wound fluid interfering with proliferation
- **Remodeling phase:** Scar formation and tensile strength increasing

General Wound-Healing Principles

- Débride necrotic tissue
- Infection treatment
- Pack empty spaces
- Absorb exudate
- Maintain moist wound environment
- Open wound edges
- Protection
- Insulation

Wound-Healing Considerations

- If the wound is minimally exudative, maintain a moist environment.
- If the wound is moderately exudative, maintain a moist environment but absorb excess exudate.
- If the wound is shallow, protect and insulate it.
- If the wound is deep, eliminate dead space and protect it.

Specific Wound-Management Techniques

Antiseptics

Antiseptics are used to decrease bacterial counts. Examples are Betadine, Dakin's, acetic acid, and hydrogen peroxide.

Alginates

Alginates are used to absorb exudate in wet wounds. Alginates are nonadherent and biodegradable. They help to stop bleeding and are not for use in dry wounds. Examples are seaweed dressings, Sorbsan, and AlgiSite.

Antimicrobials

Antimicrobials are used to treat bacteria, yeast, MRSA, and VRE. Antimicrobials can be systemic or topical. Examples are Silvadene, mupirocin, and Polysporin.

Silver antimicrobial dressings

Silver antimicrobial dressings are used to control yeast, mold, bacteria, MRSA, and VRE. Examples are Granufoam AG, Acticoat, Silvadene, and $AgNO_3$.

Hydrocolloids

Hydrocolloids are used for wounds with slight to moderate amounts of exudate. Hydrocolloids protect wounds and promote autolysis. An example of a hydrocolloid is DuoDERM.

Hydrogels

Hydrogels are used for dry wounds to promote a moist wound environment. One complication of hydrogels is skin maceration. Examples are SoloSite, Flexigel, and Vigilon.

Transparent dressings

Transparent dressings are used in superficial, non-exudative wounds to protect from friction. Transparent dressings also promote autolysis. Examples are Tegaderm and OpSite.

Foams

Foams are used for light to moderately exudative wounds. Foams can absorb ten times their body weight. Foams are easily removed and are changed only weekly or as needed based on saturation. An example is Mepilex.

Nonadherent dressings

Nonadherent dressings do not stick to skin and are changed every two or three days. Nonadherent dressings are generally used for skin tears and superficial wounds. Examples are Telpha and Release.

Vaseline dressings

Vaseline dressings are used to promote a moist wound bed. Examples are Vaseline gauze, Xeroflo, and Adaptic.

Skin barriers

Skin barriers form protective barriers and are used before taping or dressing is applied.

Gauze

Gauze is used for wound packing and absorbing exudate.

Wound VAC (vacuum-assisted closure)

A wound VAC uses special equipment to remove exudate and to assist in wound healing. Vacuum pressure is applied to a sponge on the wound and exudate is eliminated.

Hyperbaric oxygen

Hyperbaric oxygen helps to increase oxygenation of plasma and vascularization. Hyperbaric oxygen tends to be used for more serious wounds such as fasciitis, gangrene, crush injuries, and chronic nonhealing ulcers.

Debridement

Debridement is the removal of necrotic tissue (slough and eschar). Once the areas of necrosis have been eliminated, the debridement should cease. Debridement can be classified as selective or nonselective.

Selective debridement

Selective debridement refers to debridement with tools such as a high-pressure water jet; by sharp debridement via tweezers, scissors, or scalpel; and with topical enzymatic and autolytic materials. In selective debridement, only the areas of necrosis are removed. However, this type of debridement tends to cause the patient more pain than nonselective debridement.

- **Enzymatic/chemical debridement:** Chemical debridement uses a special enzyme that is applied to the wound. The enzyme chemically degrades the necrosed tissue. This form of selective debridement may take 3 to 30 days to clean a wound.
- **Sharp debridement:** Sharp debridement is the removal of necrosed tissue with a sharp instrument. This is the fastest way of debridement, but this technique may cause increased pain to the patient.
- **Autolytic debridement:** Autolytic debridement refers to using the body's own mechanisms in the removal of necrotic tissue. This technique includes maintenance of a moist wound environment to allow rehydration of necrotic tissue. Also, the body's natural enzymes assist in cleaning the wound.

Nonselective debridement

Nonselective debridement refers to debridement that removes areas of necrosis but also may remove areas of viable tissue. **Mechanical debridement** is nonselective. Mechanical debridement refers to outside forces assisting in the removal of necrotic tissue. Examples are **wet-to-dry dressings**, **wound irrigation**, and **whirlpools**. A complication of mechanical debridement is the possibility of removing viable tissue.

Therapeutic modalities

Therapeutic modalities can also be used in the treatment of wounds. Electrical stimulation in many forms can increase blood flow, decrease edema, and encourage wound contraction. Pulsed electromagnetic fields (diathermy), ultraviolet light, ultrasound, whirlpool, and pulsative lavage with suction can also be used. For specifics on therapeutic modalities, please refer to chapter 8, Equipment and Devices, and Therapeutic Modalities.

Positioning

Bed and wheelchair positioning are of utmost importance in the prevention and treatment of wounds. Skin is more apt to break down with friction, shear, and pressure over bony prominences, and this should be avoided. A patient who is immobile or inactive has lost the ability to perform adequate weight shifts to redistribute forces adequately. Frequent turning and repositioning by caregivers is necessary to prevent skin breakdown. Patient, family, and caregiver education in positioning—including positions to avoid and positions to assume—may be needed. Use of appropriate wheelchairs, cushions, and mattresses can help to reduce risk of skin breakdown. Also, devices that "float" the heels or keep blankets and sheets from resting on the patient's toes can help to prevent pressure on the feet.

Exercise

Therapeutic exercise is useful in the treatment of wounds. A goal of exercise can be increased strength and functional mobility so the patient can perform position changes to avoid pressure buildup. Simple ankle pumps can assist in edema control and encourage venous return to prevent venous ulcers. Care should be taken to avoid friction and shear forces in the performance of exercises, as these can be detrimental to the prevention of wounds.

Scar Management

- Range of motion
- Exercise
- Splinting
- Positioning
- Massage
- Thermal modalities
- Scar mobilization
- Patient education

A FINAL WORD

To adequately evaluate and treat a patient or client, the physical therapist must have a strong knowledge of the foundational sciences and background, evaluation, differential diagnoses, and treatment interventions of the integumentary system. This chapter, which highlights each of these areas, along with your experience in lab practicals and clinical affiliations, will help prepare you to identify and treat impairments of these systems.

The following pages offer an end-of-chapter practice quiz to test your knowledge of some of the fundamentals of the integumentary system. It is not necessary to time this, as it is a chapter review quiz.

INTEGUMENTARY SYSTEM CHAPTER QUIZ

1. A physical therapist notices a wound on a hospitalized patient. The wound is on the distal lower extremity. Its edges are well defined. The wound appears dry and the area around the wound is shiny and hairless. Based on this appearance, what type of wound is this *MOST* likely to be?

   (A) Pressure ulcer
   (B) Arterial ulcer
   (C) Venous ulcer
   (D) Trauma wound

2. A physical therapist in an outpatient clinic is treating a patient who has a pressure ulcer of the right heel. At initial evaluation, the patient is afebrile, the wound has minimal exudate, and the patient denies pain. Two weeks later, the patient presents to the clinic and complains of chills and severe pain in the foot. The wound has purulent, malodorous drainage. The right leg also appears to have increased edema. What should the physical therapist do?

   (A) Call the patient's physician and have the patient seen by the physician
   (B) Continue with treatment per the treatment plan
   (C) Add transparent film to the treatment plan
   (D) Hold treatment and have the patient return when he is feeling better

3. A resident of a nursing home is referred to physical therapy for wheelchair positioning. The patient, who spends the majority of her day sitting in a wheelchair, starts to complain of pain on the left buttock. The nursing staff notices a reddened area on the left buttock. The physical therapist knows that prevention is key to managing pressure ulcers. The patient is continent of bowel and bladder. Besides pressure, what other risk factors does this resident have for developing a pressure ulcer?

   (A) Increased age and impaired mobility
   (B) Intact sensation and impaired mobility
   (C) Presence of moisture and impaired sensation
   (D) Impaired sensation and high activity level

4. An electrician experiences a third-degree burn from an explosion. His entire right arm and his head and neck are burned. What percentage of his skin is burned?

   (A) 9 percent
   (B) 18 percent
   (C) 22.5 percent
   (D) 27 percent

5. A physical therapist evaluates a patient's wound that has moderate amounts of exudate. The physical therapist should document what characteristics of the exudate?

   (A) Color, consistency, and amount
   (B) Location
   (C) Color only
   (D) Amount only

6. A patient is referred to physical therapy due to a third-degree burn of the right elbow. The physical therapist knows that a third-degree burn affects what layers of skin?

   (A) Damages the epidermis only

   (B) Damages the epidermis and part of the dermis

   (C) Completely destroys the epidermis and dermis

   (D) Extends to bone and muscle

7. A person with chronic obstructive pulmonary disease has nail beds that appear blue. What is the reason for this color change?

   (A) Increased tissue perfusion

   (B) Decreased tissue perfusion

   (C) Increased blood oxygen levels

   (D) Decreased blood oxygen levels

8. A patient has a stage III pressure ulcer on her coccyx. The wound appears red and has a purulent exudate. The patient is complaining of increasing pain. The ulcer is small, measuring 2 cm wide by 1.5 cm high. The surrounding tissue is pale and remains intact. The physical therapist is aware that this wound is most likely infected. The physical therapist may ask the physician to consider what treatment?

   (A) Skin cleaner

   (B) Antiseptics

   (C) Topical antibiotic

   (D) Systemic antibiotic

9. A patient sees her physician complaining of pain in the chest with deep breathing. The physician diagnoses the patient with pleurisy. What structure is *MOST* affected with this condition?

   (A) Lungs

   (B) Pleural membrane

   (C) Peritoneal membrane

   (D) Heart

10. A dependent adult living at home presents to the hospital with a stage IV pressure ulcer on the right heel. Bone and muscle can be visualized. What condition is the person *MOST* at risk for developing?

    (A) Arthritis

    (B) Hammer toe

    (C) Bleeding

    (D) Osteomyelitis

11. A physical therapist is treating a patient with diabetes. What risk factors put this patient at increased risk for a neuropathic foot ulcer?

    (A) Impaired sensation of the feet and good glycemic control

    (B) New onset of diabetes and nonsmoker

    (C) Impaired sensation of the feet and poor glycemic control

    (D) Daily inspection of the feet by the spouse and no history of ulceration

12. A hospitalized patient has signs and symptoms of wet gangrene of the right foot. What should a physical therapist do to *BEST* treat this area?

    (A) Sharp debridement

    (B) Wet-to-dry dressing changes

    (C) No debridement; refer the patient to a physician

    (D) Autolytic debridement

13. A patient has burns on 36 percent of the surface of his body, mainly on the lower extremities. The physical therapist is concerned about the patient's ability to regulate his body temperature. Which skin structure is *MOST* involved in thermoregulation?

    (A) Nails

    (B) Melanocytes

    (C) Skin blood vessels

    (D) Lymphatic vessels

14. A physical therapist uses the Braden Scale for Predicting Pressure Sore Risk for a patient in a nursing home. Two difficulties that this patient exhibits are sliding down in the bed and needing maximum assistance to reposition. The patient has knee flexion contractures and spasticity that make independent mobility impossible. The patient is continent of bowel and bladder and eats well. The physical therapist recognizes that the patient is at risk for pressure ulcer development due to:

    (A) poor nutritional status.

    (B) moisture.

    (C) cardiopulmonary compromise.

    (D) friction and shear.

15. A patient is referred to physical therapy for treatment of a venous ulcer. The physical therapist establishes a treatment plan that includes patient education about the care of venous ulcers. What is the *MOST* appropriate advice to give this patient?

    (A) Sit with the legs dependent for two hours every day.

    (B) Small skin tears do not require treatment.

    (C) Increase salt intake.

    (D) Elevate the legs as much as possible throughout the day.

ANSWERS

1. **B.**

   Arterial ulcers usually have distinct borders. The surrounding skin is shiny, dry, and hairless. These ulcers are typically located distally and have minimal exudate.
   (Baranoski, page 288)

2. **A.**

   The patient did not have signs of infection upon initial evaluation but has definite signs of infection two weeks later. The treatment plan should be modified and the patient should be referred to the physician. Transparent film should not be used for infected wounds.
   (Sussman, page 220)

3. **A.**

   Increasing age, impaired mobility, the presence of moisture, and poor activity level are risk factors for the development of pressure ulcers.
   (Baranoski, page 245)

4. **B.**

   According to the Rule of Nines, the entire arm accounts for 9 percent and the head and neck account for 9 percent. The total surface area is 18 percent.
   (Hanumadass, page 8)

5. **A.**

   The color, amount, and consistency of exudate should be documented for a wound.
   (Baranoski, page 87)

6. **C.**

   A third-degree burn completely destroys the epidermis and dermis.
   (Hanumadass, page 12)

7. **D.**

   The nails of a person with decreased blood oxygen levels often appear blue. Normally, the nail bed is pink.
   (Thibodeau, page 108)

8. **C.**

   Topical antibiotics are useful for reducing the bacterial burden in localized areas. Systemic antibiotics are effective in controlling advanced infection. Skin cleaners are too toxic to be used on open wounds. Antiseptics are toxic to all cells and therefore should not be used in treating wounds.
   (Baranoski, page 110)

9. **B.**

   Pleurisy is the inflammation of the pleural membrane.
   (Thibodeau, page 100)

10. **D.**

    Osteomyelitis is an infection of the bone and can be life-threatening.
    (Sussman, page 422)

11. **C.**

    Risk factors for development of neuropathic foot ulcers include impaired sensation, poor glycemic control, smoking, history of ulceration, lack of inspection of the feet, and diabetes of 15 years or longer.
    (Brown, page 183)

12. **C.**

    A patient with wet gangrene most likely has infection. Do not debride a gangrenous area. Refer the patient to a surgeon immediately.
    (Sussman, page 406)

13. C.

Thermoregulation is accomplished by dilatation and constriction of skin blood vessels.
(Baranoski, page 52)

14. D.

Friction and shear are problems for a patient who slides in bed and needs maximum assistance to reposition. Also, contractures and spasticity increase the risk for pressure.
(Brown, page 104)

15. D.

Patients with venous insufficiency should use elevation of the legs as much as possible. Small skin tears can become large ulcers quickly, so protection from skin tears and trauma is important. Limiting salt intake to limit fluid retention is important.
(Baranoski, page 304)

Other Systems: Metabolic and Endocrine, Gastrointestinal, Genitourinary, and Multisystem Pathologies

7

During physical therapy evaluation and treatment interventions, consideration must always be given to any signs or symptoms that may indicate underlying impairments that originate from other systems. Pathologies and conditions in the metabolic or endocrine system, the gastrointestinal system, and the genitourinary system can present as a musculoskeletal or neuromuscular system differential diagnosis. Any differential diagnosis that does not respond to treatment interventions appropriately and within a reasonable amount of time should be closely examined for other underlying pathologies. For this reason, you will need to be familiar with the other systems that may present themselves in physical therapy.

METABOLIC AND ENDOCRINE SYSTEMS

As a graduating physical therapy student, you should be familiar with the basic anatomy and physiology of the endocrine system. The endocrine system is composed of the glands in the body and the hormones they produce to regulate body function. The endocrine system is the slow communication pathway of the body, whereas the nervous system is the faster communication network. The endocrine system is crucial in development, growth, reproduction, and maintaining homeostasis. Hormone imbalance, either too much or not enough, can have detrimental effects on the growth and repair of musculoskeletal tissue. This section discusses the function of the endocrine system, how it affects other systems, and how it may present in your physical therapy practice.

Foundational Science and Background

A strong understanding of the basic background and fundamental science of the metabolic and endocrine systems is necessary before evaluation, interpretation, and intervention can take place. It is necessary to understand the major glands and their functions as well as their interactions with other systems. **Metabolism** is the process that uses food to provide energy and rebuild tissues as a part of constant homeostasis. The glands of the endocrine system and the hormones they secrete control metabolism. Some of the major glands and their functions in the endocrine system are discussed below

Pituitary gland

The pituitary gland is vital in regulating the function of other glands in the system. It is responsible for the synthesis of protein, and it releases endorphins.

Thyroid gland

The thyroid gland regulates the body's metabolism and protein synthesis. Disorders of the thyroid gland are hypo- or hyperthyroidism and cause secondary glandular problems throughout the body.

Parathyroid gland

The parathyroid gland is responsible for hormone secretion and regulates calcium and phosphorus metabolism.

Adrenal glands

The adrenal glands maintain electrolyte balance within the body, control the body's response to stress, control the inflammatory response, stimulate the heart to beat faster, and cause vasoconstriction.

Pancreas

The pancreas secretes glucagon and insulin to control blood glucose.

Gonads

The gonads are responsible for the maturation of sex characteristics, for sexual function, and for hormone regulation during pregnancy.

Pharmacology

The effects of medication or drug therapy must always be considered in the evaluation and treatment of metabolic or endocrine system disorders. Different drugs can have adverse or valuable effects on the rehabilitation process, depending on how and when they are used. Below is a list of common drugs prescribed for metabolic and endocrine system impairments.

Hormone replacement therapy

Hormone replacement therapy (HRT) consists of synthetic thyroid hormone (thyroxine); in addition to its other uses, it is administered to patients who have a hypo-functioning thyroid. HRT can have cardiac complications and is monitored closely when given to patients who have preexisting cardiac concerns.

Vasopressin

Vasopressin (ADH) is used in hormone replacement in diabetes insipidus to stimulate smooth-muscle contraction. Patients taking vasopressin may have increased blood pressure, diarrhea, or angina as a result of taking this medication.

Radioactive iodine

Radioactive iodine is used to treat hyperthyroidism. Iodine-131 can be given to patients, generally adolescents and older, to help regulate the thyroid. Coincident with this drug therapy is resultant hypothyroidism which, if it develops, can be treated with HRT.

Insulin

Insulin is used to regulate blood glucose in type 1 diabetics. Insulin is given intravenously as needed, or through an insulin pump if constant regulation is necessary.

Oral hypoglycemic drugs

Oral hypoglycemic drugs (OHDs) are used to regulate blood sugar in type 2 diabetes. Different types of OHDs can stimulate insulin secretion or improve a tissue's reception of insulin as needed by the patient.

Nonsteroidal anti-inflammatories

Nonsteroidal anti-inflammatory drugs (NSAIDs) are commonly used for pain relief of musculoskeletal injuries and also have anti-inflammatory benefits. Physical dependence is not an issue with these non-opioid analgesics. They are COX inhibitors, working to prevent the formation and release of prostaglandin, a hormone that is responsible for the pain and inflammation that often accompany injury. Long-term use of NSAIDs can cause gastrointestinal (GI) upset, drowsiness, dizziness, and possible fluid retention.

Bisphosphonates and estrogen

Bisphosphonates and **estrogen** are options for prevention and treatment of osteoporosis. Bisphosphonates such as alendronate, ibandronate, and risedronate work to prevent bone resorption by osteoclasts. These are the preferred treatments of choice for prevention of osteoporosis. **Estrogen** is also used to decrease osteoclastic activity. If used in conjunction with progesterone as hormone replacement therapy, there is increased risk of several life-threatening conditions, including CVA, heart attack, and pulmonary embolism. Parathyroid hormone (teriparatide) boosts the formation of new bone by osteoblasts but is less commonly used.

Calcitonin

Calcitonin prevents osteoclast activity and stimulates the increase of bone mass. It also has some pain-relieving effects related to bony injury or disease.

Disease-modifying antirheumatic drugs

Disease-modifying antirheumatic drugs (DMARDs) are used to retard the progression of rheumatic disease. They are thought to decrease the action of the T and B lymphocytes and monocytes that together cause inflammation and tissue destruction. Chloroquine and hydroxychloroquine are the safest DMARDs but still can cause retinal damage, headache, and GI distress. Other generic DMARDs include cycloserine (Necral) and etanercept (Enbrel). A more toxic yet more aggressive DMARD is azathioprine (Imuran), but it can cause fever, chills, vomiting, and fatigue. Another DMARD is gold sodium thiomalate, "gold therapy." Side effects from its use include GI distress and skin rash.

Responses to Exercise and Inactivity

Exercise and food intake can affect the rate of metabolism. Fluid and electrolyte balance directly affect the functions of the metabolic and endocrine systems. During exercise, dehydration can occur, especially in patients who are taking diuretics or other electrolyte supplements for other conditions.

Environmental influences

Exercise at higher altitudes can increase the rate of fluid loss and the risk of dehydration. In a cold ambient environment, epinephrine and norepinephrine are two hormones that are secreted to increase heat production. In a hot environment, the antidiuretic hormone is secreted during heat stress to conserve fluid, and aldosterone (a hormone) is increased to conserve sodium. There is also increased risk of dehydration from excess fluid loss.

Complications of exercise in hot environments can ultimately result in heat illness. The major forms of heat illness are heat cramps, heat exhaustion, and heat stroke.

Fluid imbalance

Any fluid imbalance can cause problems, whether it involves too much or too little fluid. If the body is unable to get rid of extra water or fluid, edema can occur. Distal pitting edema and, in some cases, pulmonary edema and congestive heart failure are associated with retention of water.

On the other hand, if the body eliminates too much water or does not receive enough water input, dehydration can occur. Symptoms of dizziness, lethargy, fatigue, cramping, or palpitations can occur with dehydration. Caffeine, alcohol, and diuretic medication can increase the risk of dehydration. Warm air or water temperatures, or high humidity, can also increase sweating, which in turn can cause fluid and electrolyte loss.

Electrolyte imbalance

Electrolyte imbalance is often associated with fluid imbalance, as one often directly affects the other. Electrolytes include sodium, potassium, calcium, magnesium, chloride, bicarbonate, and phosphate. These charged ions have a direct effect on the cells within the body as well as on the processes in proper functioning of the muscles (including the heart) and circulation.

Evaluation

During the evaluation process, it is important for the examiner to make decisions on what tests and measures are appropriate in order to establish a good list of differential diagnoses to treat the injury or disability. During the evaluation the patient must be viewed as a whole. The evaluation may take place in a hospital room, a home setting, an outpatient setting, or a long- or short-term care facility. In all cases each part of the examination process must be considered, although it is known that some portions of the examination are more appropriate for certain settings.

Signs and symptoms of metabolic or endocrine system involvement

Many of the signs and symptoms of endocrine system impairments are similar to musculoskeletal impairments. Connective tissues particularly are affected by either excessive or insufficient hormone production. It is important to learn of any endocrine or metabolic disorders in the patient's history. Undiagnosed endocrine or metabolic disorders can also surface during physical therapy, as some of the chief complaints are impairments that may be appropriate for treatment intervention. They can include, but are not limited to, the following:

- Fatigue
- Localized pain
- Muscle weakness (typically proximally)
- Stiffness

These symptoms may respond to treatment, as they should if the endocrine dysfunction is being addressed medically. But if the underlying cause has not yet been diagnosed, these signs and symptoms may not respond to treatment as would be expected.

Lab values and diagnostic imaging

Although the diagnosis of endocrine system and metabolic disorders is made through blood work, labs, and radiologic testing, the following table lists some important base values to be aware of when you are working with patients who have underlying endocrine system or metabolic disorders.

Base Lab Values

Blood glucose levels	• Normal: 100–120 mg/dL • Critically low: <50 mg/dL • Exercise is contraindicated if symptoms are present and blood glucose is 70–100 mg/dL or >250 mg/dL
Bone density testing (T-score)	• Normal: –1.0 or higher • Osteoporotic: –2.5 or lower

Differential Diagnosis and Pathology

A list of differential diagnoses is developed on the basis of the findings during your evaluation of the patient. Differential diagnoses represent all of the possible conditions or pathologies that could be causing the impairments found during the evaluation. Each condition or pathology is unique and will dictate what medical management is necessary and what physical therapy intervention is most effective. Comorbidities of conditions of other systems may play a role in the decision-making process when developing interventions, as well as affect the rate or success of tissue healing. In general, carpal tunnel syndrome, rheumatoid arthritis, and adhesive capsulitis are common musculoskeletal and neuromuscular diagnoses that can be related to endocrine system dysfunction. The following are some conditions that are specific to the metabolic and endocrine systems.

Hyperthyroidism

Hyperthyroidism is an overactive thyroid causing increased secretion of thyroid hormone and increased metabolism; Graves' disease is one type of hyperthyroidism. Clinical manifestations are proximal muscle weakness, spinal muscle pain, goiter, uncontrolled weight loss, nervousness/restlessness, and palpitations, among other symptoms. Medical management includes drug therapy and, in some cases, surgery to remove part or all of the thyroid. Physical therapy management may include treatment for the proximal muscle weakness and pain; with exercise, special consideration must be given to the fact that the patient's exercise tolerance is probably greatly diminished compared to a patient with a well-functioning thyroid gland.

Hypothyroidism

Hypothyroidism is an underfunctioning thyroid that does not produce an adequate amount of thyroid hormone, thus slowing the metabolism. Clinical manifestations include proximal muscle weakness, muscle pain, stiffness, fatigue, and sometimes paresthesias. There may also be some connection between fibromyalgia and hypothyroidism. Skin breakdown may be a concern with an individual who has hypothroidism. Drug therapy of hormone replacement is the typical medical treatment. Physical therapy intervention should include a controlled exercise program to gradually increase activity tolerance, if needed, and to improve the patient's cardiovascular function and profile.

Hyperparathyroidism

Hyperparathyroidism is an overactive parathyroid. Clinical manifestations may include increased bone loss causing increased fractures, proximal muscle weakness in the extremities, atrophy, muscle and joint pain, depression, fatigue, and damage to the kidneys. Medical management is surgical removal of the thyroid. Physical therapy management includes low-intensity core and proximal muscle strengthening, range of motion, and pain management.

Also appropriate are fall prevention measures for home safety and the use of an assistive device, if necessary, to prevent fractures. Use caution with any manual joint activity, as there is increased fracture risk.

Hypoparathyroidism

Hypoparathyroidism is an underactive parathyroid. Clinical presentations are neuromuscular, with tingling and muscle spasm from tetany (one-sided). Medical management may include intravenously administered calcium to decrease tetany in acute conditions, and drug therapy in more chronic presentations. Physical therapy intervention primarily includes fall prevention measures.

Addison's disease

Addison's disease is an autoimmune, insufficiently functioning adrenal gland. Clinical manifestations include weakness, fatigue, weight loss, and decreased tolerance for stress. Medical management includes steroid drug therapy. Physical therapy intervention may include low-level exercise and education in stress reduction/relaxation techniques.

In general, carpal tunnel syndrome, rheumatoid arthritis, and adhesive capsulitis are common musculoskeletal and neuromuscular diagnoses that can be related to endocrine system dysfunction. There may also be some connection between fibromyalgia and hypothyroidism. Tendonitis conditions can present from parathyroid impairments such as Addison's disease.

Diabetes mellitus

Diabetes mellitus is an endocrine system dysfunction that has systemic complications from an excess of blood glucose. There is dysfunction in the production and/or action of insulin and its interaction with blood glucose. There are two types of diabetes: type 1 (insulin-dependent) and type 2 (non-insulin dependent).

Diabetes Mellitus

Type 1 (insulin-dependent)	• Juvenile onset (age <20 years) • Nonproduction or diminished secretion of insulin • Direct genetic correlation
Type 2 (non-insulin dependent)	• Adult onset • Resistance to the action of insulin • Can sometimes be controlled with diet and exercise • Risk factors include family history, obesity, high blood pressure, and elevated HDL cholesterol levels

Clinical presentations of diabetes are varied but can include abnormal blood glucose levels, increased thirst, frequent urination, weight change, and fatigue. As diabetes progresses, it can cause such secondary problems as osteoporosis, congestive heart failure, vision impairment/loss, comprised cardiovascular system, peripheral vascular changes, and peripheral neuropathy. Medical management of diabetes is to control the blood glucose with exercise, diet, and if necessary, insulin. If kidney failure occurs, transplant or dialysis is necessary to maintain life.

Physical therapy intervention may include low-intensity exercise prescription, low-resistance strength training, and education for prevention and control of type 2 diabetes. Wound care and treatment of other secondary complications of diabetes may also be appropriate (i.e., management of adhesive capsulitis, assistive device training, pulmonary physical therapy, cardiac physical therapy, footwear evaluation). The feet of diabetic patients require special attention to monitor sensation, skin integrity, joint support, and sometimes orthotics or casting. In the case of amputation, prosthetic training is necessary. These patients generally do not respond well to the stresses of too-intensive exercise (i.e., dehydration, low blood pressure, myocardial infarction). Morning exercise may be preferred to avoid fluctuations in blood glucose caused by growth hormone. Exercise programs should be regular (same time, same duration each day). Exercise may be best one hour after eating a meal; by then the patient should have adequate blood glucose levels. Patients must also be closely monitored for signs and symptoms of hypoglycemia during exercise or treatment.

Diabetic response to exercise

Signs of **hypoglycemia** may include increased irritability or difficulty focusing, decreased coordination, headache, weakness, and decreasing responsiveness. Orange juice or glucose tablets can be used to increase blood glucose quickly. **Hyperglycemia** can occur if a patient is in need of insulin to decrease blood sugar levels either before, during, or after exercise. Patients needing insulin should be taught to always carry insulin with them to therapy but if possible, should not use insulin within one hour before exercise. In severe cases of either hypoglycemia or hyperglycemia, diabetic coma can occur.

Osteoporosis

Osteoporosis is a decrease in bone density that can put the individual at greater risk of multiple fractures. It is most common in women, and there is greater risk if the patient is inactive or immobilized, has had long-term corticosteroid use, is postmenopausal, or has a calcium and/or magnesium deficiency. Bone mass is controlled by the regulation of osteoblasts and osteoclasts, and in osteoporosis there is an imbalance with osteoclasts predominating. Patients with osteoporosis present with low back pain and often thoracic kyphosis. They have an increased risk of fracture, especially in the spine. Prevention may include hormone replacement, calcium supplement, weight-bearing exercise (the National Osteoporosis Foundation recommends exercising 45–60 minutes 4 times/week), calcium- and magnesium-rich foods, vitamin D (sunshine), and avoidance of alcohol and tobacco. Medical management includes diagnostic imaging using dual-energy X-ray absorptiometry (DXA) to measure total body bone density. Physical therapy intervention includes education in posture, body mechanics, and fall prevention; a balance retraining program; and weight-bearing or controlled-resistance exercise, particularly of muscles attached to affected bone. These patients should avoid spinal flexion, side-bending, or rotation during activity. Treatment may also include pain management and range of motion for restrictions resulting from the osteoporosis. Caution must be taken with any mobilization techniques, especially in the thoracic spine.

Osteomalacia

Osteomalacia is a softening of the bony mass of the skeletal system due to a calcium or phosphate deficiency. Inadequate exposure to sunlight (vitamin D deficiency) can also contribute to the development of osteomalacia. Long-term use of some anticonvulsants or antacids can also increase the risk of osteomalacia. Osteomalacia most commonly occurs in patients who are shut-ins or in long-term care settings. Clinical presentations include general achiness, proximal muscle weakness, neuropathy, postural abnormalities, and decreased functional mobility. Medical management is dietary and drug therapy supplements. Physical therapy intervention is the same as for osteoporosis.

Paget's disease

Paget's disease involves increased bone density but decreased bone strength. It is characterized by increased activity of the osteoclasts. Bone is absorbed at an abnormally fast rate, and the new bone that is made is much weaker than normal bone tissue. This patient population is generally <50 years in age, with equal prevalence in men and women. There does appear to be a genetic component to Paget's disease. Clinically, the typical presentation is bone pain, bone deformity, and increased thoracic kyphosis. The spine and pelvis are more affected than the extremities, causing secondary problems of stenosis and peripheral nerve syndromes. Hearing loss, headaches, and vertigo are also common symptoms. The progression of Paget's disease is very slow and varies greatly among patients. Some may even have the disease for quite some time before it is actually diagnosed. Treatment includes drug therapy to decrease osteoclast activity. Similar to osteoporosis, caution must be taken when using manual techniques on individuals with a known Paget's diagnosis. Physical therapy intervention should include education on posture, body mechanics, gentle range of motion, and low-intensity exercise. Assistive devices for safe mobility and orthotics to help maintain good positioning may be beneficial.

Treatment Interventions

Once the evaluation is completed and the differential diagnosis is listed, it is necessary to choose the proper interventions to treat the patient's impairments. Typically, the use of functional mobility, exercise, range of motion, mobilization, and modalities are combined to work toward the patient's physical therapy goals. Exercise prescription, the use of assistive devices, implementation of orthotics and prosthetics, and the application of modalities are covered in their own chapters. Specific recommendations for treatment interventions have been listed associated with each differential diagnosis.

Prevention as intervention

Although family history plays a large role in dictating the incidence of metabolic and endocrine system disease, physical therapy can aid in preventing—or at least slowing the progression of—some of the processes associated with these diseases. Patients at risk can be educated in the posture, body mechanics, general strengthening, and balance exercises that were described in chapter 4, Musculoskeletal System.

Metabolic and endocrine system response to intervention

The metabolic system is vital in total-body homeostasis and responds reactively when the fluid or electrolyte balance is not what it should be. Patients with metabolic or endocrine system dysfunction should be encouraged to drink plenty of water, eat regularly, and rest frequently before and during exercise. This is especially true when the patient is first beginning an exercise program. Since metabolic or endocrine system dysfunction may be a preexisting condition to another impairment that is being treated, patients should always be monitored for the abnormal responses to exercise. In the clinic, hospital, or home, any of these symptoms can put the patient at an increased risk for falls or injury.

Signs and symptoms of dehydration include the following:

- Fatigue
- Cramping
- Palpitations
- Dizziness and dysequilibrium

- Dry mouth and/or dry skin
- Lethargy or confusion
- Irritability

GASTROINTESTINAL SYSTEM

As a graduating physical therapy student, you should be familiar with the basic anatomy and physiology of the gastrointestinal (GI) system. The GI system is responsible for the movement of food and water through the body, absorption of fluid and nutrients, and the processing of waste for removal from the body. This section discusses the function of the GI system, how it affects other systems, and how it may present in your physical therapy practice.

Foundational Science and Background

A strong understanding of the basic background and fundamental science of the GI system is necessary before evaluation, interpretation, and intervention can take place. This section examines the function of the GI system and how it relates to evaluation and treatment intervention in physical therapy. The GI system is made up of the upper and lower GI tracts.

The upper GI tract

- Organs: Mouth, esophagus, stomach, duodenum
- Function: Receives and digests food and liquid

The lower GI tract

- Organs: Small and large intestines
- Function: Digestion and absorption of nutrients, electrolytes, and water; and storage until disposal

Exercise and the GI system

Problems with ingestion and digestion of food and water can have a direct effect on electrolyte balance and an indirect effect on the musculoskeletal system. Low levels of potassium prevent adequate muscle contraction and can contribute to muscle weakness, muscle pain, and possible injury. Inadequate calcium absorption can lead to bone loss, increasing the risk for fractures. Underlying GI system dysfunctions can lead a person to physical therapy and/or can complicate the success of physical therapy treatment.

Differential Diagnosis and Pathology

Based on the findings during the evaluation of the patient, a list of differential diagnoses is developed. Differential diagnoses represent all of the possible conditions or pathologies that could be causing the impairments found during the evaluation. Each condition or pathology is unique and will dictate what medical management is necessary and what physical therapy intervention is most effective. Comorbidities of conditions of other systems may play a role in the decision-making process when developing interventions and may affect the rate or success of tissue healing.

Common signs and symptoms of GI dysfunction

- Nausea/vomiting
- Diarrhea/constipation/fecal incontinence

- Anorexia/diminished appetite
- Heartburn
- Dysphagia
- Abdominal pain
- GI bleeding

Pain Referral Patterns for GI Pathology

Thoracic pain	• Stomach pathology • Liver pathology • Pancreas pathology
T4-T6	• Ulcer
T6-T10	• Duodenal perforation
Low back pain	• GI bleed • Pancreatic tumor
Shoulder pain Left shoulder pain (Kehr's sign) Right shoulder pain	• GI bleed • Blood in abdomen (ruptured spleen, ulcer; diverticulitis) • Blood in the peritoneal cavity
Right scapula	• Gallbladder pathology
Low back/sacral pain	• Constipation
Right lower abdomen	• Lung pathology
Abdominal pain	• Spinal nerve root irritation
Lower right quadrant pain	• Intestinal (ileum) pathology
Umbilicus	• Appendix/pancreas pathology
Left pectoral region	• Spleen pathology

Any of the pain complaints listed in the table above, most commonly low back and hip pain, coupled with GI symptoms could indicate an underlying GI pathology. Look for intestinal symptoms, pain relief after bowel or bladder elimination, or any changes in content of bowel or bladder (i.e., discoloration, etc.).

Gastroesophageal reflux disease

Gastroesophageal reflux disease (GERD), or reflux, presents as pain or burning in the chest that sometimes radiates into the back or neck. It usually starts during or after a meal or in a supine position. GERD can limit a patient's ability to tolerate supine positioning with exercise. Positioning in an elevated supine or left side-lying direction can decrease symptoms during exercise or sleep. Pulmonary physical therapy intervention may be indicated postsurgically. Proper breathing techniques coincident with exercise or lifting should be taught to avoid increasing abdominal pressures by Valsalva.

Gastritis

Gastritis is an inflammation of the stomach lining that presents as chest pain and abdominal fullness. This is a common side effect with prolonged use of anti-inflammatory medications, particularly NSAIDs. Taking anti-inflammatory medication with milk or antacids can decrease the incidence of gastritis. If gastritis progresses to a bleed, the patient should follow up with her physician.

Peptic ulcer

Peptic ulcer (stomach or duodenal ulcer) is a breakdown of the lining of the stomach, allowing digestive juices to move into the abdominal cavity. Ulcers present as burning pain and cramping that is intermittent and can last for minutes at a time. As with GI bleeds, weakness and sweating may also be present.

Malabsorption syndrome

Malabsorption syndrome is decreased absorption of the nutrients in the intestines. It presents as general weakness and fatigue, loss of appetite, cramping, and diarrhea. The loss of adequate nutrition can affect muscle strength and increase fall risks due to poor proprioceptive reactions. In the long term, there is increased risk for fractures and postural abnormalities. Paresthesias can occur due to the nervous system receiving poor nutrition.

Inflammatory bowel disease

Inflammatory bowel disease (IBD), or **Crohn's disease**, is the inflammation of any portion of the intestines and is usually sporadic in nature (good spots, bad spots, good days, bad days). It can typically present along with rheumatoid arthritis. IBD causes joint pain and joint inflammation (enteropathic arthritis). It is more pronounced in the lower extremity, particularly in the PIP joints of the toes. The arthritis resolves as the IBD is successfully treated.

Irritable bowel syndrome

Irritable bowel syndrome (IBS) is the most common GI pathology. It is a chronic, non-inflammatory intestinal bowel disruption in the intestines. IBS presents as constant or intermittent abdominal pain that is lessened with a bowel movement. Clinically, symptoms must exist for three months and must follow a specific group of symptoms to be diagnosed as IBS. Exercise in general assists with the regularity of bowel movements and decreases the associated pain.

Hernia

A **hernia** is the protrusion of part of an organ through any of the surrounding tissue in the abdominal cavity, most commonly in weakened abdominal muscle tissue. It presents as a bulge in the lower abdomen with accompanying pain. It can be caused by any kind of strain that elicits a Valsalva maneuver. Neuralgic pain may come from compression by surrounding tissues on the ilioinguinal nerve. Instruction in proper lifting mechanics and in correct breathing techniques with lifting and exercise is preventative and a corrective treatment intervention.

Treatment Interventions

Once the evaluation is completed and the differential diagnosis is listed, it is necessary to choose the proper interventions to treat the patient's impairments. Typically, functional mobility, exercise, range of motion, mobilization, and modalities are combined to work toward the patient's physical therapy goals. Exercise prescription, the use of assistive devices, implementation of orthotics and prosthetics, and the application of modalities are covered in their own chapters. Specific recommendations for treatment interventions have been listed associated with each differential diagnosis described above.

GI system implications for exercise

Pathologies of the GI system can directly affect a patient's tolerance of exercise and activity. There are some special considerations, however, that may be necessary in the patient's adapting to these pathologies. Positioning in an elevated supine or left side-lying direction can decrease symptoms of GERD during exercise or sleep. Avoidance of the Valsalva maneuver, or bearing down, during exercise must be emphasized to avoid, among other dangers, increased pressure on the GI tract.

Effects of exercise on the GI system

Regular activity or exercise can help to regulate bowel function and assist with movement through the GI tract. Exercise can decrease the incidence of GI bleeding as well. Strenuous exercise can cause GERD. With inappropriate breathing techniques, particularly with abdominal exercise, abdominal pain and constipation can occur. Inadequate fluid intake before or during exercise can lead to dehydration and an imbalance in fluid and electrolytes similar to that mentioned earlier.

GENITOURINARY SYSTEM

As a graduating physical therapy student, you should be familiar with the basic anatomy and physiology of the genitourinary (GU) system. The GU system is responsible for ridding the body of wastes in fluid form, as well as for reproduction and, in women, childbearing. This section discusses the function of the GU system, how it affects other systems, and how it may present in your physical therapy practice.

Foundational Science and Background

A strong understanding of the basic background and fundamental science of the GU system is necessary before evaluation, interpretation, and intervention can take place. In this section we will look a little deeper into the function of the GU system and how it relates to evaluation and treatment intervention in physical therapy.

The urinary tract

The **kidneys** play a large role in regulating metabolism by filtering waste and forming and excreting urine. The kidneys help to regulate electrolytes and the acid-base balance. They form red blood cells and control blood pressure. The ureters, bladder, and urethra form the exit route for the urine formed by the kidneys.

Gender-specific systems

There are also gender-specific reproductive system functions and impairments.

Females

The female reproductive system includes the ovaries, fallopian tubes, uterus, and vagina. The ovaries produce estrogen and progesterone, hormones that are specific to females and that work together to prepare women for childbearing and nursing.

Males

The male reproductive system includes the testes, epididymis, vas deferens, seminal vesicles, prostate, and penis. The male hormone testosterone is produced in the testes and influences male characteristics.

Motor learning and motor control

Motor control is the ability to perform quality and effective movements. Intrinsic feedback, generated from within the human body, involves how a particular movement feels and compares it to the reference of how that movement *should* feel. **Motor learning** is the process used to learn new motor skills. Motor learning requires feedback. Often, motor control can be impaired in the GU system, and motor learning activities are then needed to make changes to reduce impairments. The treatment intervention portion of this section explains some of the motor learning processes that can improve motor control of the GU system.

Differential Diagnosis and Pathology

Based on the findings during the evaluation of the patient, a list of differential diagnoses is developed. Differential diagnoses represent all of the possible conditions or pathologies that could be causing the impairments found during the evaluation. Each condition or pathology is unique and will dictate what medical management is necessary and what physical therapy intervention is most effective. Pathologies such as prostatitis, endometriosis, and ovarian cyst disease can present with low back, sacral, or pelvic pain. It is important for the therapist to recognize GU pathologies and to know when referral for medical management is needed.

Common signs and symptoms of genitourinary system pathology

- Low back or leg pain
- Ipsilateral shoulder pain
- Costovertebral palpation tenderness
- Fatigue
- Fever, chills, and general malaise
- Dysuria, proteinuria, hematuria, nocturia
- Change in frequency of urination
- Abnormal discharge
- Swelling or mass in the genital area

During the patient interview, general questions about pain or difficulty associated with urination and about changes in urinary habits may be appropriate to rule out GU involvement.

Urinary tract infections

Urinary tract infections (UTIs) are the most common pathology of the GU system. UTIs can afflict any age group but are more prevalent in women than men. The incidence of UTIs is greater in long-term care facilities. Causes of UTI include catheterization and instrumentation, general inactivity, bladder or kidney dysfunction, and sexual inactivity. The presence of a UTI can increase the chance of infection elsewhere in the body. This is an important consideration when treating patients with a recent surgical history or a healing wound. Indications of a UTI include increased frequency of urination, pain or burning during urination, fever, chills, and general malaise. In more advanced cases, pain in the low back, ipsilateral shoulder, and hip may be present. Medical management includes patient education on preventative measures: increased hydration, increased frequency of urination, hygiene, and nutritional considerations (decreased alcohol, tobacco, caffeine, chocolate, spicy foods). Bacterial counts and urine leukocyte counts are taken to diagnose UTI. Drug therapy with antibiotics is also necessary. Physical therapy intervention is not treatment for a UTI, but it is important to consider a UTI as a differential diagnosis. A UTI can also inhibit successful physical therapy intervention of other diagnoses if not treated appropriately or left untreated. The presence of UTI symptoms may limit a patient's activity tolerance. Recognition of referred pain to the shoulder, low back, or hip without mechanism of injury may indicate a need for referral.

Chronic renal failure

Chronic renal failure (CRF) is the permanent loss of nephrons in the kidney. This has implications in the filtering of waste and the elimination of urine from the system. These insufficiencies cause disruption in the body's electrolyte balance and systemic changes. Common comorbidities of CRF are lupus, diabetes, high blood pressure, osteoporosis, and long-term acetomenophin or NSAID use. The onset is gradual, and it presents in multiple systems, including blood, cardiovascular, GI, musculoskeletal, and neurologic. Common findings in the physical therapy examination may include decreased mental alertness, osteoporotic changes to bone, calcification of soft tissues, lower-extremity neuropathy, and musculoskeletal pain and deformity. Medical management of CRF is widely variable and can include surgical intervention to improve blood flow, medication to control blood pressure, and nutritional intervention for improved electrolyte balance. Creatinine and BUN levels are monitored during the course of the disease. In more advanced cases, dialysis or kidney transplant may be indicated. Physical therapy management of patients with CRF includes low-intensity exercise to improve muscle strength, functional mobility, and overall quality of life while avoiding fatigue. Exercise intensity should be adjusted using the rate of perceived exertion instead of the heart rate, as changes in maximum heart rate may be a secondary affect of CRF. To be most beneficial, physical therapy should be coordinated so that it takes place the day after dialysis.

Urinary incontinence

Urinary incontinence (UI) is the involuntary loss of urine when bladder pressure is greater than the strength of the sphincter muscle. It is more common in women than men, and incidence increases as age increases. UI is further defined as follows:

- **Stress incontinence:** Occurs during activity that increases intra-abdominal pressure (sneezing, lifting, running, etc.).
- **Urge incontinence:** The rapid loss of urine as soon as the urge to urinate is felt
- **Functional incontinence:** Functional incontinence is normal urinary control, but the patient cannot get to the toilet in time.
- **Overflow incontinence:** Continuous urinary leakage because the bladder cannot empty completely
- **Mixed incontinence:** Any combination of two or more of the above UI can result from pelvic floor muscle weakness that occurs as age increases, coincident with pregnancy and childbirth, and from surgical interventions. The use of medications such as sedatives can also promote UI. The bladder expands and contracts, depending on the amount of fluid it holds. When the bladder is full, it relays that message to the brain with the urge to urinate and the urine is voluntarily expelled. When the bladder shrinks from inadequate fluid intake, it senses a nearly constant fullness, sending the brain a constant message on the need to void. The result is increased urge and less-frequent complete emptying of the bladder. Medical management may include drug therapy to decrease urine output and improve sphincter muscle tone, or surgical intervention to correct the position of the bladder. Physical therapy intervention can be very successful and calls for bladder retraining and behavioral modifications that include pelvic floor strengthening, biofeedback therapy, and electrical stimulation of weakened muscles, thus improving the patient's overall quality of life. Soft-tissue mobilization, stretching of hypomobile areas, and resistive

strengthening of weakened muscles may also be necessary. Treatment considerations should also address arthritic and functional limitations that may impede the patient's ability to get to, and get on and off, the toilet. Difficulty and unsafe techniques in attempting to get to the bathroom can contribute to increased fall risk and fall-related injuries. The comorbidity of low blood pressure and associated lightheadedness can further increase the risk for falls.

Neurogenic bladder

Neurogenic bladder is urinary dysfunction caused by disruption of the normal innervation of the bladder. The disruption can occur at several neurologic levels and can cause a decrease in bladder volume, inability of the bladder to contract, dysfunction of the sphincter muscle, and decreased sensory perception of the bladder. A neurogenic bladder can be a secondary dysfunction from other diseases or conditions, including spinal cord injury, dementia, stroke, multiple sclerosis, and CNS tumors. Which bladder dysfunctions are present depends on the cause of the dysfunction. Patients with neurogenic bladder present with increased frequency and urgency, incontinence, and/or urinary retention. The latter largely contributes to the increased incidence of UTIs in these patients. Early identification of a UTI can prevent the spread of infection to other systems. Medical management includes catheterization and drug therapy to restore normal muscle tone. Surgical intervention may be necessary to restore sphincter function. Physical therapy intervention includes a bladder training program and pelvic floor muscle strengthening, if appropriate.

Pelvic floor dysfunction

Pelvic floor dysfunction covers a broad category of pelvic floor inadequacies and pain. Although it can affect both men and women, it is more commonly seen in women. Pelvic pain lasting longer than six months can contribute to pelvic floor dysfunction. Low back pain, pain with intercourse, and incontinence may also be present. Medical management may include diagnostic testing with ultrasound and drug therapy for hormonal effects. Physical therapy management includes biofeedback, pelvic floor strengthening, and bladder training techniques, if necessary. Modalities, soft-tissue mobilization, and postural training may be used for pain management.

Treatment Interventions

Once the evaluation is completed and the differential diagnosis is listed, it is necessary to choose the proper interventions to treat the patient's impairments. Typically, functional mobility, exercise, range of motion, mobilization, and modalities are combined to work toward the patient's physical therapy goals. Exercise prescription, the use of assistive devices, implementation of orthotics and prosthetics, and the application of modalities are covered in their own chapters. Specific recommendations for treatment interventions have been listed associated with each differential diagnosis above.

Bladder programs

Bladder training involves education on proper fluid intake, dietary considerations to limit fluid retention, and a regular voiding schedule to train the bladder to function properly. Intervals between voiding can be increased gradually as function improves.

Pelvic floor strengthening

Pelvic floor muscle (pubococcygeal muscles) strengthening uses Kegel exercises as an isometric resistance program. Emphasis is on isolated pelvic floor contractions without co-contraction of the gluteals or abdominals. Additionally, it is beneficial to strengthen the abdominals, hip adductors, and hip external rotators separate from the pelvic floor to improve resting muscle tension. Motor control and motor learning are important concepts in retraining the pelvic floor musculature; often, it is the patient's lack of awareness of these muscles that makes them dysfunctional. Coordination of pelvic floor muscle contraction with diaphragmatic breathing is necessary to further isolate function.

Diaphragmatic breathing

Diaphragmatic breathing involves educating the patient in using the normal movement of the diaphragm superiorly and inferiorly to expand and contract the lungs while breathing during exercise. The use of this technique helps the patient to avoid the bearing down, or Valsalva maneuver, that can increase pressure on the pelvic floor.

Relaxation techniques

Relaxation techniques or physiologic quieting exercise can be used to help decrease muscle tension and pressure on the pelvic floor, thus decreasing the usually associated urinary incontinence. Relaxation techniques include closing the eyes; darkening the room; slow, deep breathing; mental imagery; music and meditation.

Biofeedback

Biofeedback uses electromyography (EMG) to differentiate between contracting the isolated pelvic floor and contraction of surrounding muscle. EMG provides visual and auditory feedback on contraction of the pelvic floor musculature and can be done with vaginal or surface electrodes. Biofeedback is an effective method of feedback to allow successful motor learning for improved motor control.

Effects of exercise on the GU system

Benefits of increasing the strength of the pelvic floor and surrounding musculature include:

- Improved blood flow to the GU organs
- Improved fertility
- Improved mental well-being

Negative effects of exercise include:

- Amenorrhea
- Compromised bone density when coupled with inadequate nutrition

Surgical interventions

Complications of surgical interventions for GU pathologies can include infection and urinary incontinence. Surgical interventions, including prostatectomies, cesarean section births, and abdominal emergencies, can cause abdominal and pelvic floor weakness. Identification of signs and symptoms of infection related to any of these surgeries necessitates a physician referral for antibiotic treatment. Physical therapy intervention may be necessary for pelvic floor and abdominal strengthening.

MULTISYSTEM CONDITIONS

As a graduating physical therapy student, you should be familiar with the basic anatomy and physiology of the entire body. This section discusses the special conditions that have systemic effects and how these conditions may present in your physical therapy practice.

Foundational Science and Background

In addition to the individual systems already discussed in this book, there are many diseases and conditions that can affect more than one system. These systemic pathologies can also have an impact on the evaluation and treatment of a physical therapy patient. Systemic pathologies primarily affect homeostasis within the body. Many systemic diseases also predispose patients to developing secondary impairments such that patients may seek physical therapy intervention. Certain impairments and what seem to be localized injuries can also produce changes in systems other than just the musculoskeletal or just the cardiovascular, etc. Although physical therapy itself is not going to cure systemic disease, various treatment interventions can greatly improve the patient's quality of life and the function of the affected systems, and can improve outcomes. Some physical therapy interventions that are used in multisystem pathologies are as follows:

- Pulmonary function activities
- Positioning, gait training, and functional mobility
- Soft-tissue mobilization
- Exercise
- Pain management techniques
- Edema management techniques

In many cases the physical therapist may have the most frequent health-care interactions with these patients; the therapist must keep a close eye on any decline in status or change in the patients' presentation.

Pharmacology

The effects of medication or drug therapy must always be considered in the evaluation and treatment of multisystem disorders. Different drugs can have adverse or valuable effects on the rehabilitation process, depending on how and when they are used. The following are some drugs commonly prescribed for multisystem impairments.

Antipsychotics

Antipsychotics are used to help normalize thought disturbances. It is thought that they work by blocking dopamine receptors. Haloperidol (Haldol) is an older antipsychotic (traditional) medicine but can cause significant motor side effects, including dystonia, dyskinesia, movement disorders, restlessness, and anxiety. Long-term use of antipsychotics can cause worsened involuntary muscle movements. Newer, atypical antipsychotics such as risperidone, clozapine, and olanzapine cause fewer motor problems. These drugs' side effects can include dry mouth, sedation, vision blurring, constipation, urinary retention, and orthostatic hypotension.

Antidepressants

Antidepressants are used to improve the patient's mood and lessen the associated symptoms of depression. They can be further divided into tricyclic antidepressants (TCAs), selective serotonin reuptake inhibitors (SSRIs), and monamine inhibitors (MAOIs).

TCAs work by increasing norepinephrine and serotonin levels. Side effects that must be taken into consideration during physical therapy interventions are increased heart rate, palpitations, low blood pressure, drowsiness, and sometimes tremor. Examples of TCAs are amitriptyline, amoxapine, desipramine, doxepin, and imipramine.

SSRIs block removal of serotonin so that it remains present in the neural cleft. Important side effects include GI distress, headaches, and sleep disruption. Some common brand-name SSRIs are Prozac (fluoxetine), Zoloft (sertraline), and Paxil (paroxetine).

MAOIs do just what their name indicates, leaving serotonin and norepinephrine in circulation. Side effects may include headaches, muscle weakness, hyperreflexia, GI distress, and sleep disruption. Examples of MAOIs are phenelzine, tranylcypromine, and selegiline.

Disease-modifying antirheumatic drugs

Disease-modifying antirheumatic drugs (DMARDs) work to prevent the progression of rheumatoid arthritis (RA). They are typically used with NSAIDs and corticosteroids to treat RA. GI upset is the most common side effect. Methotrexate, azathioprine, and hydroxychloroquine are examples of DMARDs.

Differential Diagnosis and Pathology

Based on the findings during the patient's evaluation, a list of differential diagnoses is developed. These conditions have systemic effects and most definitely play a role in the decision-making process when you are developing interventions; they also affect the rate or success of tissue healing. Some of the conditions discussed in this section are not pathological but rather something that affects the body system as a whole. Each condition or pathology is unique and will dictate what medical management is necessary and what physical therapy intervention is most effective.

Aging

Although not a pathology, age has a systemic effect on the body. As advances are continuously being made in health-care treatment and prevention, the population continues to age. Aging causes change in all organ systems in the body; and that change, in turn, has an impact on treatment outcomes. Generally, as age increases most organ system function deteriorates at variable rates. Specific changes are discussed below:

- **Cardiovascular system:** As age increases, there is decreased elasticity of the aorta and vessels and degeneration of the heart valves.
- **Integumentary system:** As age increases, there is increased pigmentation and degeneration of collagen and elastin, making the skin more fragile and less elastic.
- **Eye:** As age increases, there is degeneration of the oculomotor muscles and loss of elasticity in the lens.
- **Ears, nose, and throat:** As age increases, there is impaired elasticity of the membranes of the ear, increased earwax, atrophic changes in mucous linings, and atrophy of laryngeal muscles.
- **Nervous system:** As age increases, there is cerebral atrophy, increased plaques, meningeal thickening, and a reduced number of neurons.
- **Musculoskeletal system:** As age increases, there is general skeletal muscle atrophy, osteoporosis, and decreased tensile strength of ligaments and cartilage.
- **GI system:** As age increases, there is a decrease in digestive enzymes.
- **Respiratory system:** As age increases, there is sclerosis of the bronchi, decreased elasticity of the cartilage, and weakness of the accessory muscles of breathing.
- **GU system:** As age increases, there is atrophy of the prostate and generalized system degeneration.

These changes are important to consider when you are choosing treatment intervention techniques and assessing the success of those interventions. It may take longer to see benefits of treatment in a 70-year-old patient than in a 20-year-old patient. As functional mobility declines with aging, it is also necessary to educate the patient in safety and exercise to prevent or minimize the risk for falls and injuries due to falls.

Bariatrics (obesity)

In all areas of physical therapy, it is not uncommon to see patients that are overweight. They present with back pain, joint pain, decreased functional mobility, and general deconditioning. Obesity is defined as a weight greater than 20 percent over that individual's optimal weight. The term obesity is dependent on body composition, gender, and height. It is thought that obesity is a combination of environmental, psychological, and biochemical factors. Obesity is generally the result of an imbalance between caloric intake and caloric expenditure. The distribution of fat over the waist indicates an overall greater health risk than does fat distributed elsewhere. A person with a body mass index (BMI) over 30 is considered obese. Systemic changes that occur with obesity include the following:

- Increased insulin resistance
- Increased blood pressure
- Decreased action of the sodium-potassium (ATPase) pump
- Increased number of adipose cells
- Shortness of breath with or without exertion
- Increased risk of development of type 2 diabetes, cardiovascular disease, cerebrovascular disease, cancer (breast, cervical, liver, prostate, colon, and rectal), menstrual disorders, infectious disease, sleep apnea, and pregnancy complications

Medical management of obesity is primarily education on nutrition and activity level, with a goal of weight loss. Drug therapy may be used for appetite suppression. Newer surgical intervention techniques are being used to physically change the GI system, but *physical therapy intervention begins with prevention!* Education on healthy lifestyle choices, diet, and general exercise can prevent many of the complications associated with obesity. In treating the obese patient, instruction in posture, body mechanics, resistive and aerobic exercise, and functional mobility are all necessary. Special considerations for the obese patient include the following:

- Use of appropriate equipment that is safe for the increased weight
- More gradual progression into an exercise program, to avoid injury
- Aerobic exercise at least four to five times per week for 30 minutes each for weight loss
- Caution must be used when exercise is coupled with obesity, due to the previously mentioned systemic effects of obesity. During exercise, the obese patient is at greater risk for heart attack, stroke, loss of balance, and dehydration/overheating.

Pregnancy and postpartum considerations

A full-term pregnancy is considered 38 to 42 weeks in length. Often the pregnant woman seeks physical therapy for impairments either related or completely unrelated to pregnancy. In either case special considerations must be made when treating the pregnant woman due to hormone-related systemic changes. Pregnancy and the related hormonal changes have profound effects on all of the body systems.

Reproductive system

The size of the uterus increases as the fetus grows. This also changes the spacing and orientation of some of the organs in the abdominal cavity and puts added physical pressure on many of those organs.

Cardiopulmonary system

In pregnancy, the diaphragm is displaced upward. The depth of respiration increases with slight hyperventilation to increase the oxygen exchange necessary for pregnancy. The overall blood volume increases (plasma especially), lower-extremity venous pressure increases, and the heart rate increases 10–20 bpm. In healthy pregnancies, blood pressure decreases. Venous-pressure and blood-pressure changes are due to increased stretching of venous walls.

Musculoskeletal system

Ligaments become more lax in preparation for childbirth. This causes hypermobility of the joints. The pelvic floor and abdominal muscles become stretched. The pregnant woman's postural changes move toward a forward head and rounded shoulders due to the change in the center of gravity (upward and forward). Other postural changes include shoulder protraction, lumbar lordosis, and knee hyperextension.

Conditions and pathology specific to pregnancy

The systemic changes generated by hormones and pregnancy put the pregnant woman at greater risk for several pathologies or conditions that are musculoskeletal in nature and may benefit from physical therapy intervention.

- **Low back or sacroiliac pain:** This is due to increased weight anteriorly, requiring greater opposition by lumbosacral paraspinal muscles for upright postures. Depending on the position of the fetus, especially in the third trimester, the sciatic nerve can become irritable from direct compression by the fetus.
- **Pelvic floor muscle dysfunction:** This can progressively worsen as gestation increases, due to direct pressure and weight on the pelvic floor. It can cause urinary incontinence. Surgical episiotomy can also disrupt pelvic floor muscle function.
- **Diastasis recti:** This is a >2 cm separation of the rectus abdominis muscle. This separation puts the muscle at a less efficient position for activation, thus causing weakness. Abdominal weakness can lead to low back pain and postural changes.

In healthy progressing pregnancies, exercise can help the woman maintain good posture, promote healthy weight gain, and prevent pregnancy-associated muscle pain and dysfunction. Due to all of the organ system changes, you must take special consideration when you are treating a pregnant woman. Some of the considerations for exercise during healthy pregnancy are as follows:

- The obstetrician or family practitioner should always approve exercise before starting treatment.
- Avoid the supine position after the first trimester to avoid occluding the vena cava.
- Modalities such as diathermy, ultrasound, heat, electric stimulation, and iontophoresis are contraindicated over the low back and abdomen and must be used cautiously and with obstetrician approval over other areas.
- Dyspnea can occur with even low-intensity exercise.
- Avoid dehydration and overheating during exercise (avoid increasing core body temperature).
- Use caution with stretching due to increased ligamentous laxity. Avoid aggressive joint mobilization for this same reason.
- The heart rate should not increase to >140 bpm during exercise.
- Cardiac output is greatest in left side-lying, so this may be a good position for exercise.
- Watch for signs and symptoms of UTI, as the incidence is increased with pregnancy.

- Discontinue exercise if any pain, abdominal cramping, or bleeding occurs.
- With exercise, there is an increase in heart rate, hematocrit level, caloric expenditure, core body temperature, blood insulin levels, and norepinephrine/epinephrine levels.
- General postural strengthening and lumbosacral stabilization exercises are beneficial to the pregnant patient. Low-intensity aerobic exercise (walking, aquatic activity) is also recommended. Specific exercises for pelvic floor muscle strengthening, such as Kegels, are also good.
- For the patient on bed rest, exercise is clearly contraindicated. Physical therapy intervention for these patients may include positioning (left side-lying and changing position frequently) and ROM or stretching, if allowed by the physician. Sometimes these patients are allowed a brief upright time during the day.

Postpartum considerations
Postpartum aerobic exercise can be started soon after an uncomplicated delivery, with physician approval. Pelvic floor and abdominal muscle strengthening can begin almost immediately if there is no tear or episiotomy. In the case of a cesarean delivery, exercise and lifting are usually contraindicated for six to eight weeks while the abdominal and uterine wall are healing.

Rheumatoid arthritis

Rheumatoid arthritis (RA) is a chronic, progressive inflammatory condition that primarily affects synovial fluid and the surfaces and surrounding tissues of articulating joints. Along with the obvious negative effects on the joints, RA also affects the cardiovascular, pulmonary, and GI systems. Initial diagnosis of RA is between the ages of 25 and 50, and women tend to be more commonly afflicted than men. Musculoskeletal presentation is joint swelling, pain, and limited motion. Symptoms are usually symmetrical, whereas osteoarthritis is often unilateral. Classically advanced RA presents with "swan neck" deformity, ulnar deviation at the wrist, and boutonnière deformity of the fingers. In addition to the joint dysfunctions, there may be skin rash, depression, fatigue, weight loss, fever, anemia, osteopenia, and general weakness. Patients with RA can also be predisposed to other autoimmune disorders. As RA progresses, there can be weakening of the transverse ligament supporting the atlantoaxial joint, leading to cervical instability and vertebrobasilar symptoms. Effects can also be seen in the lymphatics, the spleen, and the eyes.

Medical management of RA includes early detection to slow the damage caused by the disease. Analysis of synovial fluid will identify a high white-blood-cell count. Treatment is with drug therapy, using antirheumatic drugs to slow disease progression and manage symptoms. Other drug therapy may include NSAIDs and immunosuppressants. Physical therapy intervention for those patients already diagnosed with RA follows with medical management in controlling edema and with modifying activity and educating the patient in the use of assistive devices or orthoses, if needed. Physical therapy for maintenance of range of motion, improved functional mobility, education on posture and body mechanics, and pain management is also necessary. Modalities may be beneficial. Caution must be taken with aggressive joint or soft-tissue mobilization over inflamed areas. Frequent rest breaks may be necessary during an individual treatment session. Low- to moderate-intensity exercise may help to improve cardiovascular function, maintain joint motion, and strengthen atrophied muscles.

Juvenile rheumatoid arthritis

Juvenile RA (JRA) refers to arthritis specifically diagnosed in childhood. JRA is further divided into three types of arthritis, varying in the number of joints affected and the probability of systemic signs and symptoms. JRA affects both sexes, and onset can be as early as two to three years of age. Medical management is similar to that of RA, including early diagnosis and drug therapy to lessen the severity of damage and to control symptoms. Physical therapy intervention in children is, again, pain and edema control and also evaluation and intervention using adaptive equipment or assistive devices to allow the child to be more functional. ROM, stretching, and exercise may also be necessary.

Systemic lupus erythematosus

Systemic lupus erythematosus (SLE) is a chronic inflammatory disease of connective tissues affecting multiple systems in the body. There is a strong genetic link with this diagnosis. SLE is much more common in women than men, with onset at ages 15–40 years. SLE presents with symptoms including, but not limited to, joint and muscle pain, skin rash (classic butterfly presentation), fatigue, shortness of breath, and decreased medical alertness. Signs and symptoms come and go, with periods of exacerbation and remission. Medical management includes control of exacerbations, generally with drug therapy to control pain, inflammation, skin rashes, and cardiovascular dysfunction. Physical therapy intervention is important for the impairments related to joint changes, skin changes, and general fatigue. Patient education for a balance between rest, daily activity, and low-intensity exercise is imperative.

Multiple organ dysfunction syndrome

Multiple organ dysfunction syndrome (MODS) is the progressive deterioration of two or more organs and their function in critically ill or critically injured patients. Many patients who have MODS also have signs/symptoms of systemic inflammatory response syndrome (SIRS). SIRS is a metabolic response to illness or injury and includes tachycardia, fever, declining mental alertness, and increased respiratory rate. The pattern of MODS development is as follows:

- Lung dysfunction
- Liver/kidney failure
- GI/immune system failure
- Cardiac failure

Once it has started, MODS cannot be stopped. It is fatal, usually around three to four weeks after onset. Physical therapists will not see MODS in the clinic but may encounter the patient with MODS in the intensive care unit. Physical therapy intervention is usually for ROM and/or positioning only.

Acquired immune deficiency syndrome

Acquired immune deficiency syndrome (AIDS) is an infection of the immune system that eventually leads to suppression of the system altogether. Patients with AIDS are more likely than a healthy individual to acquire infections and cancers. The HIV-positive patient can progress from having no symptoms to having full-blown AIDS, with symptoms of muscle and joint pain and dysfunction, peripheral neuropathy, skin lesions, and neuromuscular dysfunction. Medical management is to attempt to treat the secondary complications, as there is yet no cure for AIDS. Although not seen frequently in the physical therapy realm, patients with HIV/AIDS may need treatment for some of the secondary complications named here. Physical therapy intervention can include pain management techniques, including ROM, stretching, and low-level exercise. Mobility training and activity modification as the patient's conditions worsen may also be necessary.

Cancer

There are many situations in which physical therapists treat patients who have had or are currently receiving cancer treatment. The incidence of primary cancer of the musculoskeletal system is rare. However, many primary cancers can metastasize to the bone as a secondary cancer. The lumbar vertebra is the most common bone for metastasis. The most common primary cancers to metastasize to the bone are breast, prostate, lung, kidney, and thyroid. Since some primary cancers are thought to move through the blood, it makes sense that the common sites of metastasis are in the bone marrow.

Identifying cancer

As physical therapists we may be the first to recognize an abnormal response to treatment or a combination of signs and symptoms that indicates something outside of our scope of practice. Risk factors can be first identified in the patient interview: age, family history, ethnicity, contributing environmental factors (tobacco use, exposure to radiation or UVA rays, or exposure to certain industrial chemicals). The American Cancer Society lists seven early warning signs of cancer, with the mnemonic CAUTION:

- **C**hanges in bowel or bladder habits
- **A** sore that does not heal in six weeks
- **U**nusual bleeding or discharge
- **T**hickening or lump in the breast or elsewhere
- **I**ndigestion or difficulty swallowing
- **O**bvious change in a wart or mole
- **N**agging cough or hoarseness

The patient with cancer may present with fatigue, unexplained weight loss, and anemia. Symptoms of cancer that may be found during physical therapy evaluation could include severe pain that is unchanged by activity or rest, or pain that is worse at night. Clinical assessment by the physical therapist may identify unexplained proximal muscle weakness and increased deep tendon reflexes without other contributing pathology.

Treatment interventions with cancer patients

Medical management includes thorough diagnostics to identify the cancer. Medical treatment by an oncologist may include chemotherapy, radiation, and/or surgical intervention to remove the neoplasm.

Physical therapy intervention for a patient with the diagnosis of active cancer may include lung function testing and education in breathing techniques. Improving functional mobility through ROM and exercise, along with pain management, are also goals of physical therapy. Low-intensity exercise can help to lessen fatigue and improve mental health. In the case of breast cancer with mastectomy, lymphedema treatment and soft-tissue mobilization may be appropriate. In all cases of primary or metastatic cancer, some joint mobilization techniques and therapeutic modalities are contraindicated.

For those patients who have had **radiation as a cancer treatment**, another list of side effects presents itself. Impairments caused by radiation that may be significant during physical therapy evaluation and intervention include the following:

- General malaise
- Skin toxicity
- Fibrosis of connective tissue (hypomobility, decreased function)

- Reduced lung function, reduced endocrine function
- GI distress
- Scarring of tissue in the heart and lungs
- Permanent damage to nerve tissue, particularly to the brachial plexus or lumbosacral plexus

Low- to moderate-intensity exercise is allowed during active radiation treatment. Exercise is not recommended within two hours of radiation or chemotherapy treatment. Monitoring of vitals and the Rate of Perceived Exertion (RPE) is recommended to avoid overworking the patient. Caution should be used in contact with radiated skin, as it may be tender, painful, and fragile. Caution should also be used with stretching and mobilization techniques due to the presence of fibrosis.

Fibromyalgia

Fibromyalgia is a syndrome characterized by the presence of pain in at least 11 of 18 specific locations in the body. Along with the tender points, there are sleep disturbances and abnormal stress responses. Fibromyalgia is much more prevalent in women and has been seen through all age groups. A solid cause for fibromyalgia is not yet known. Patients present with general fatigue and diffuse muscular pain that is easily flared. Medical management of fibromyalgia is primarily educating the patient on coping mechanisms, stress management, and nutrition. Physical therapy intervention is primarily for pain management and patient education. Instruction in a low- to moderate-intensity exercise program may also help to lessen the physical and emotional symptoms of fibromyalgia. The use of modalities, stretching, and soft-tissue mobilization may reduce pain and improve the patient's quality of life.

Depression

Depression is a feeling of excessive sadness or dejection different from normal response to loss. It can influence the onset, change, and treatment of pain. Depression can be a disorder in and of itself or a part of another mood disorder. Psychosocial, biological, and genetic factors can all contribute to the presence of depression. Patients suffering from depression present with general lack of interest, decreased energy, and poor concentration.

Physical therapy intervention: Exercise is known to improve mood and mental health and to decrease pain through the release of endorphins. Exercise can also improve reception of the neurotransmitter serotonin. Untreated depression can inhibit treatment success, so it is important to address this and provide treatment options for the patient.

Dementia

Dementia most profoundly affects a patient's ability to learn new information and the recall memory. Patients may have some confusion and may feel that they know the answers to questions or situations when in reality they do not. Special considerations for patients with dementia are necessary for their safety, as they may not be aware of balance deficits, weaknesses, or impairments of functional mobility and daily activity. Use of consistent, one-step instructions in a simple, repetitious routine may provide the patient with the ability to remember key information. If the patient has a support system, it is important to educate these people about instructions for home programs and recommendations. Patients with dementia will have trouble following weight-bearing restrictions or learning how to use new assistive devices, such as may be necessary following a hip fracture. In this case, it may be necessary to speak to the physician about giving the patient either a non-weight-bearing or full-weight-bearing status. Rather than teaching the patient how to use a new device, it may be better to wait until he is safe for either no device or a familiar device before putting emphasis on gait training.

Schizophrenia

Schizophrenia is a psychological disorder that is characterized by disturbed thought processes, delusions, hallucinations, decreased social function, and flattened affect, all of greater than six months' duration. Although the exact cause of schizophrenia is unknown, it is attributed to overactive dopamine pathways in the brain. The overactivity can be from oversynthesis, decreased breakdown, or increased sensitivity of receptors. The disorder cannot be cured, but it can be normalized.

A FINAL WORD

Any of the conditions and pathologies discussed in this chapter can affect patient management as coexisting conditions. In all cases, it is important that a patient with any of these conditions or pathologies is under a physician's care and that no recent change in the status of that condition has occurred. In physical therapy the patient is treated as a whole, which means that factors other than purely musculoskeletal or neuromuscular or cardiopulmonary issues come into play. It is necessary to continuously reassess each patient's condition to know if there is systemic involvement. If treatment intervention does not progress as would be expected, referral to the primary physician may be necessary to rule out other contributing pathology.

The following pages offer an end-of-chapter practice quiz to test your knowledge of some of the information covered in this chapter. It is not necessary to time this, as it is a chapter review quiz.

METABOLIC AND ENDOCRINE, GASTROINTESTINAL, GENITOURINARY, AND MULTISYSTEM PATHOLOGIES CHAPTER QUIZ

1. A patient is referred to physical therapy with pain and stiffness in her knee. Which one of the following treatment interventions may be contraindicated in a patient with an acutely inflamed flare-up of rheumatoid arthritis?

   (A) Low-intensity exercise
   (B) Moist hot packs
   (C) Passive stretching
   (D) Grade III tibial mobilizations

2. In designing a bladder program for a patient with urinary incontinence, "quick-flick" exercises are *MOST* appropriate for which type of incontinence?

   (A) Stress incontinence
   (B) Urge incontinence
   (C) Overflow incontinence
   (D) Functional incontinence

3. Which of the following medications would be *MOST* likely to have negative side effects on the GI system with prolonged use?

   (A) Immunosuppressants
   (B) Corticosteroids
   (C) Nonsteroidal anti-inflammatories
   (D) Disease-modifying antirheumatic drugs

4. Which of the following is one correct way of differentiating between osteoarthritis and rheumatoid arthritis?

   (A) Osteoarthritis is typically diagnosed before age 40.
   (B) Rheumatoid arthritis typically presents unilaterally.
   (C) Rheumatoid arthritis typically presents with joint pain, fatigue, and general malaise.
   (D) Osteoarthritis most commonly affects the fingers.

5. A patient returns for his third physical therapy treatment session for low back pain. Today he complains of fever, chills, and increased frequency of urination. A possible explanation for the new symptoms could be which of the following?

   (A) Urinary tract infection
   (B) Influenza
   (C) Irritable bowel syndrome
   (D) Chronic renal failure

6. Which of the following would be the *MOST* likely bone to develop metastatic breast cancer lesions?

   (A) The calcaneus
   (B) The sternum
   (C) The radius
   (D) The femur

7. Which gland is responsible for the secretion of epinephrine and norepinephrine?
   (A) The pancreas
   (B) The pituitary gland
   (C) The thalamus
   (D) The adrenal medulla

8. A 40-year-old patient is being seen in the hospital for gait training following a total knee arthroplasty. He also has type 2 diabetes mellitus. His most recent labs, just taken, show his blood glucose level at 140 mg/dL. What would be the *MOST* appropriate treatment plan?
   (A) Bed exercise only
   (B) No activity
   (C) Gait training as planned
   (D) Transfer training only

9. A patient who has type 2 diabetes would benefit from a regular exercise program but needs some direction on what to do. Which one of the following recommendations is *MOST* appropriate for setting up a home program?
   (A) Exercise should be done before bedtime.
   (B) Exercise should be done just before lunchtime.
   (C) Exercise should be done midmorning.
   (D) Exercise should be done in the late afternoon.

10. A physical therapist is treating a woman for low back pain who is also 28 weeks pregnant. Which exercise is *NOT* appropriate for this woman to do at home?
   (A) Quadruped "fire hydrant"
   (B) Standing wall push-ups
   (C) Side-lying pelvic floor isometrics
   (D) Side-lying posterior pelvic tilts

11. A physical therapist is treating a woman for knee pain who is also 14 weeks pregnant. She is riding a stationary bicycle for a ten-minute warm-up prior to exercise. Three minutes into the ride, her heart rate is 110 bpm, and seven minutes into the ride, it is 120 bpm and she has no physical complaints. What is the appropriate treatment?
   (A) Decrease the intensity on the bicycle.
   (B) Stop the bicycle and end the treatment.
   (C) Continue at the current intensity.
   (D) Increase the intensity on the bicycle.

12. A physical therapist is reviewing a patient's lab values and tests, taken at a recent physical examination. Which one of the following would the therapist need to look at to *BEST* evaluate the patient's bone density?
   (A) The hematocrit
   (B) The blood glucose level
   (C) The dual-energy X-ray absorptiometry (DXA)
   (D) The magnetic resonance imaging (MRI)

13. A 78-year-old woman is being seen for insidious onset of pain in her midback after rising from a chair. The pain is worse with bending forward. She has a long, intermittent history of NSAID use for patellofemoral pain. Which of the following information from her past medical history would *BEST* guide the physical therapist as to the reason for the injury?
   (A) Osteoporosis
   (B) Type 2 diabetes mellitus
   (C) Total knee arthroplasty two years ago
   (D) Osteoarthritis of the knees

14. A physical therapist is reviewing a patient's current medication list and notices she is taking Haldol. She is being seen today for chronic shoulder pain. For which of the following conditions is this woman *MOST* likely using this medication?
    (A) Depression
    (B) Schizophrenia
    (C) Anorexia
    (D) Diabetes mellitus

15. In considering risk factors for cardiac complications, and if all other contributing factors are equal, which bariatric patient is at *GREATEST* risk?
    (A) The patient with adipose tissue distribution over the thighs and hips
    (B) The patient with adipose tissue distribution over the waist and abdomen
    (C) The patient with adipose tissue distributed evenly over the body
    (D) The patient with adipose tissue distributed through the chest and arms

Answers

1. **D.**

   In an inflamed rheumatic joint, aggressive mobilization techniques are not recommended. Gentle stretching, low-intensity exercise, and heating modalities are usually the preferred treatment for flare-ups.
   (Goodman/Pathology, page 953)

2. **A.**

   "Quick-flick" exercises involve short-duration, frequent contractions of the pelvic floor muscles to improve the strength of the appropriate fast-twitch muscles. These are the muscles most necessary for preventing stress incontinence, such as from a sneeze or cough.
   (Goodman/Pathology, page 727)

3. **C.**

   Prolonged or repetitive use of nonsteroidal anti-inflammatory drugs (NSAIDs) frequently causes GI distress and possible GI bleeds.
   (Goodman/Pathology, page 90)

4. **C.**

   Rheumatoid arthritis typically presents with joint pain, fatigue, and general malaise. Symptoms of osteoarthritis are generally localized to the painful joint and do not have systemic influences.
   (Goodman, page 947)

5. **A.**

   The presence of symptoms such as fever and chills indicates there is something systemic going on. The change in bowel or bladder function points in the direction of a GU system dysfunction. Low back pain is also a symptom associated with a UTI if the infection is untreated and moves further up the tract.
   (Boissonault, page 706)

6. **D.**

   Breast cancer most likely metastasizes to the pelvis, ribs, vertebrae, or femur.
   (Boissonault, page 924)

7. **D.**

   The adrenal medulla secretes epinephrine and norepinephrine.
   (Thibodeau, page 266)

8. **C.**

   Safe blood glucose levels are between 100 and 250 mg/dL. Exercise should be avoided if blood glucose levels are greater than 250 mg/dL. This patient's labs indicate he is at a safe level to continue activity.
   (Boissonault, page 356)

9. **C.**

   Exercise done midmorning avoids the increased risk of hypoglycemia associated with changes in other hormones that occur in the afternoon hours. By midmorning, the blood glucose levels should be normal after eating breakfast.
   (Boissonault, page 357)

10. **A.**

    For a pregnant woman, any exercise that puts the pelvis above the level of the head can increase the risk of placenta previa.
    (Kisner, page 567)

11. **C.**

    The rise in this patient's heart rate is less than 10 percent, which is safe for a woman who is pregnant. Pregnant women should always be educated to stop exercising if there are any abnormal responses such as pain, shortness of breath, vaginal bleeding, or cramping.
    (Kisner, page 560)

12. **C.**

    The dual-energy X-ray absorptiometry measures total-body bone density. The DXA can specifically measure bone loss at the hip and spine, which are common areas of fracture in patients with osteoporosis.
    (Boisonnault, page 877)

13. **A.**

By themselves, diabetes mellitus, knee replacement, and osteoarthritis would not drive the differential diagnosis. A current medical history of osteoporosis coupled with insidious onset of pain in the midback that is worse with flexion can point toward a spinal fracture. There is increased risk of fracture with osteoporosis.
(Boisonnault, page 881)

14. **B.**

Haldol is an antipsychotic drug and is used for treatment of conditions such as schizophrenia and bipolar disorder.
(Ciccone, page 180)

15. **A.**

The higher the patient's waist-to-hip ratio, the greater the risk of cardiac pathology along with other complications. Visceral fat around the abdomen puts the patient at greatest risk for other disease.
(Boisonnault, page 32)

Equipment and Devices, and Therapeutic Modalities

8

The preceding chapters have discussed the basic knowledge—including foundational sciences, evaluation, differential diagnoses, and treatment interventions—that an entry-level physical therapist should possess. Not only does a physical therapist need to be able to evaluate the patient, identify impairments, and create treatment interventions, a good physical therapist must be able to identify the need for equipment and devices to maximize a patient's function and quality of life. This chapter reviews some of the most commonly issued equipment and devices in physical therapy. It also covers the therapeutic modalities used as adjuncts to other treatment intervention techniques.

EQUIPMENT AND DEVICES

In some situations it is necessary to issue equipment or assess the patient's safety and independence with assistive and prosthetic devices. Equipment and assistive devices allow the patient greater functional mobility and maximize safety with that mobility. Treatment intervention of gait training, balance training, exercise, and patient education should be used when issuing, and when assessing a patient in using, equipment and assistive devices.

Assistive Devices

Assistive devices are given to patients to allow them to control the amount of weight or weight-bearing allowed on a joint or to improve balance by increasing the base of support below the center of gravity. An assistive device can allow weight to be shifted from the painful or affected lower extremity to the upper extremities. In addition to allowing weight-bearing adjustments and less pain with mobility, assistive devices provide another point of contact with the ground to aid in balance. The additional tips or points of contact further widen the patient's base of support, allowing greater area for the center of gravity to cover for safe mobility. The following assistive devices are listed in the order of most to least support given.

Standing frame

A **standing frame** is used for static standing only and provides the greatest support to the patient. It can be adjusted to allow the patient to add upper-extremity activity while standing, for more functional gains and improvement in standing tolerance.

Parallel bars

Parallel bars provide support that does not move, and allow the patient to ambulate or exercise while holding onto a stationary assistive device.

Walker

Walkers can provide varying levels of support, as they can be front-wheeled, four-wheeled, or standard in design. Some walkers have brakes that engage with hand controls or weight-bearing.

Axillary and forearm crutches

Axillary crutches can be used as a pair or singly, depending on the amount of assistance needed or the amount of weight-bearing allowed. **Forearm (Lofstrand) crutches** do not support at the axilla but rather via a band around the forearm, with weight-bearing through the forearms and wrists.

Canes

Canes can also provide varying amounts of support, depending on the design. Hemi-walker, quad (four-pointed), and standard single-point are examples of the different canes available. Among all assistive devices, canes provide the least amount of support.

Gait Patterns Using Assistive Devices

With each assistive device there are several gait patterns that can be taught to the patient, depending on the patient's weight-bearing status and physical abilities.

Three-point pattern

This gait is used with a walker, crutches, or cane. Instructions: Advance the assistive device first, followed by the weak or painful leg, and then the strong leg. This is typically used post-operatively, following weight-bearing precautions given by the surgeon.

Swing-to pattern

This is used with a walker or crutches. Instructions: Advance the assistive device, and then swing both legs forward to the assistive device. This gait can be used for patients with lower-extremity impairments who have good trunk stability and can stabilize with the hips and trunk, or if there are weight-bearing restrictions bilaterally.

Two-point pattern

This gait is used with crutches or cane(s). Instructions: Advance one assistive device and the opposite leg at the same time, and then advance the other device and the opposite leg together in a walking motion. This is typically used as a graduation from lesser weight-bearing to full weight-bearing, with the expected progression to no device if/when the patient is able.

Four-point pattern

This is used with crutches or cane(s). Instructions: Advance one assistive device first, then the opposite leg, then the other assistive device, and finally the other leg (i.e., right crutch, then left leg, then left crutch, then right leg). This gait can be used by patients who have cerebral palsy and use Lofstrand crutches for balance during mobility, or by those who need extra assistance with gait due to pain or balance.

Amputations and Prosthetic Devices

Amputations can result from damage to vessels, soft tissue, or bony tissue caused by peripheral vascular disease, diabetes, infections, or tumors. Amputation can also be traumatic in nature and in those cases does not always leave the limb at an ideal length for prosthesis. In the case of surgical amputations, consideration is taken to make the residual limb a size and length that is conducive to fitting with a prosthesis to improve function. A **prosthesis** (**prosthetic device**) is a synthetic device made to compensate for the loss of part of a limb or an entire limb. Prosthetic devices can be for upper or lower extremities and can assist in function and cosmetics after amputation. Prostheses are also appropriate for congenital limb deficiencies.

Stages of prosthetic devices

Changes in the residual limb occur following amputation. This is particularly true in lower-extremity amputations and is the reason for the development of different stages of prosthetic wear.

Immediate postoperative prosthesis (IPOP)

This is the prosthesis that is applied in the operating room or in the first few days postop. It utilizes a socket, suspension belt, pylon, and foot. This allows for immediate weight-bearing on the affected limb and also protects the residual limb.

Temporary (preparatory) prosthesis

This includes the socket, suspension belt, pylon, and foot. It allows for fitting and adjusting of the prosthetic components while the patient is able to ambulate with the prosthesis. The volume changes can be large in the residual limb in the first six months after amputation, and this change can be accommodated with the temporary prosthesis.

Definitive prosthesis

This is the final prosthesis. It typically consists of a custom-made socket, pylon, and foot. Some patients will also need an additional suspension component.

Partial Foot Amputations

These patients are often able to ambulate without the use of a prosthesis, but a prosthesis can provide protection for the residual foot.

- **Single- or multiple-ray resection:** Removal of one or more toes of the foot
- **Chopart disarticulation:** Disarticulation of the talonavicular and calcaneocuboid joints
- **Lisfranc disarticulation:** Disarticulation of the tarsometatarsal joint
- **Syme amputation:** Ankle disarticulation with preservation of the heel fat pad and removal of distal projections of the tibia and fibula
- **Transmetatarsal amputation:** Amputation that dissects the metatarsals

Prosthetics for partial foot amputations include a neuropathic walker (custom-molded ankle-foot orthosis with a rocker bottom), toe fillers, custom-molded shoes, a socket fitted to the foot, a prosthetic foot, or a solid ankle-cushioned heel (SACH) foot.

Transtibial Amputations

A transtibial, or below-knee, amputation is just what the name implies: amputation through the middle of the tibia. If possible, the length of the residual limb is left to best fit into the appropriate prosthesis. Although the components of any prosthetic device are similar, there are a multitude of adjustments and materials that can be used to allow greater mobility or provide greater stability to the patient. Components are also different based on the location of the amputation. The following are the components of a prosthetic device for a transtibial amputee.

Sockets

This is the component that fits against the residual limb.

Total contact sockets

Total contact sockets are important for patients with impaired sensation and vascular compromise. These sockets can provide maximal sensory feedback and can give a massaging effect to assist with vascular return.

Supracondylar/suprapatellar sockets

Supracondylar/suprapatellar sockets are used for amputees with short residual limbs and can allow for self-suspension.

Silicone suction socket

A silicone suction socket is a silicone liner that minimizes shear forces on the skin and allows for suction suspension.

Patellar tendon-bearing sockets

Patellar tendon-bearing (PTB) sockets use the patellar tendon as the main weight-bearing area.

Suspensions

The following all secure the prosthesis to the residual limb.

Elastic sleeves

Elastic sleeves are rolled on, provide full contact, and seal the socket.

Valve suspension

Valve suspension allows excess air to be released through a valve.

Gel liners

Gel liners provide cushioning and suspension.

Pin lock or lanyard system

These use a locking device such as a pin or lanyard system to maintain suspension.

Vacuum-assisted suspension system

The vacuum-assisted suspension system (VASS) uses a vacuum pump that helps to maintain volume levels of the limb.

Pylon

This is the component of the prosthesis that is between the socket and the foot. It can help with torque absorption and propulsion.

Foot and ankle components

These components simulate the motion of the foot and ankle and are variable based on the amount of movement or control desired.

Solid ankle-cushioned heel
The SACH foot is the standard foot that provides shock absorption at heel strike.

Single-axis
This allows for limited plantar flexion and dorsiflexion.

Multiple-axis
This allows for plantar flexion, dorsiflexion, eversion, and inversion.

Dynamic response
This allows for the storage of energy. It can be coupled with multiple-axis to allow for plantar flexion, dorsiflexion, eversion, inversion, and storage of energy.

Prosthetic sock

This is worn between the socket and residual limb. Prosthetic socks are measured in plies (thickness), from one-ply to six-ply. The patient needs to change to different-ply prosthetic socks throughout the day to allow for volume changes of the residual limb.

Transfemoral Amputations

Transfemoral, or above-knee, amputations are through the femur. In addition to the socket, suspension, pylon, and foot components, a transfemoral prosthesis also requires a prosthetic knee, which can be single-axis (hinged) or polycentric (changing center of rotation). The prosthetic knee uses different types of friction mechanisms. Mechanical friction is unvarying. Pneumatic friction and hydraulic friction are speed-dependent, offering minimal resistance at low speeds (initial swing) and increased friction at higher speeds (terminal swing). For weak or uncoordinated patients, a braking mechanism can be added to the knee that helps to lock the knee during stance.

Sockets

This is the component that fits against the residual limb.

Quadrilateral socket
This socket contains four walls. The posterior wall allows for weight-bearing on the ischial tuberosity and the gluteal muscles. This is the preferred socket for a longer residual limb.

Ischial containment socket
This has a wider anteroposterior dimension with a more narrow mediolateral dimension than the quadrilateral socket. It allows for containment of the ischial tuberosity and the pubic ramus and distributes the forces along the shaft of the femur. This is the preferred socket for a shorter residual limb and for active patients.

Suspensions

The following suspensions all secure the prosthesis to the residual limb.

Suction
The following utilizes surface tension, negative pressure, and muscular contraction.

Hypobaric
This is a fabric/silicone ring positioned 5 cm below the ischial tuberosity. It fits into the socket, then air is pushed out through a valve in the distal socket.

Soft belt

This is a belt that encompasses the pelvis on the patient's sound side. Common examples are the total elastic suspension (TES) and the Silesian bandage. A soft belt can be used in addition to other suspension components.

Pelvic belt

This is a belt that encompasses the pelvis for suspension.

Knee Disarticulation

This is complete separation of the femur and tibia with disarticulation of the knee. The procedure is used infrequently in adults due to prosthetic concerns and cosmesis.

Transpelvic Amputation

A hemipelvectomy is a hindquarter or complete hip amputation. Sockets encase the abdominal cavity and protect the abdominal contents so this area can accept weight-bearing. Weight-bearing is shifted to the ischial tuberosity and buttock of the sound leg.

Hip Disarticulation

This is complete thigh amputation and is done through the trochanter, femoral neck, or hip joint. Sockets are made to bear weight on the ischial tuberosity and the gluteal musculature and also to encase the opposite pelvis.

Upper-Limb Amputations

The functional goals of using an upper-extremity prosthetic device are much different than those of using lower-extremity prosthetics. Fine motor skills and functional use become more important than weight-bearing and mobility.

Levels of amputation

The following are some of the common surgical upper-limb amputations:

- **Wrist disarticulation:** Separates the carpal bones from the radius and ulna
- **Transradial amputation:** Through the radius and ulna
- **Elbow disarticulation:** Separates the radius and ulna from the humerus
- **Transhumeral amputation:** Through the humerus
- **Shoulder disarticulation:** Surgical separation of the shoulder at the glenohumeral joint

Terminal device

A **terminal device (TD)** is a component that is used in place of a hand. Prosthetic hands or hooks are terminal devices and can be active or passive. Active TDs can be opened and closed through a harness system. Passive devices can be adjusted by using the sound hand to change the position of the TD. Active TDs can be voluntarily opened or closed through use of the harness system. With an active, voluntary-opening TD, the fingers are closed at rest and opened with tension to the harness. With an active, voluntary-closed TD, the fingers are usually opened at rest and closed with tension to the harness.

Wrist component

This allows for supination and pronation of the TD, which can be maintained by friction or a lock. The wrist component may have a quick-disconnect feature to allow the patient to change TDs for different activities.

Elbow component

This allows for flexion and extension and can be locked at a desired angle.

Transradial sockets

These are situated around the radius of the forearm; usually proximally, if possible.

Self-suspending transradial socket
This includes the epicondyles of the humerus and the olecranon process. This socket must be a tight fit to allow for maximum elbow range of motion.

Silicone suction socket
This is a silicone liner that is locked to the socket.

Transhumeral sockets
Transhumeral sockets can be open or closed. Closed shoulder sockets encase the shoulder and are used most commonly when there is a short residual limb.

Power for Upper-Extremity Prosthetic Use

Harness
This allows for suspension and control of a body-powered upper-extremity prosthesis. It fits around the torso, with a strap under the opposite axilla. A figure-eight configuration is most common.

Body-powered control
This uses the force of proximal muscular contractions within a harness to control distal components such as the elbow, wrist, and terminal device.

Externally powered control
This is a battery-powered control system for the active upper-limb prosthesis.

Physical Therapy Management of Amputees and Prosthetic Devices

The standard examination should include patient history, environmental barriers, and an overall systems review. Specific objective measures prior to prosthetic-device training should include the following:

- Aerobic capacity
- Edema measurements, stable or unstable
- Cognition
- Circulation
- Sensation
- Skin integrity
- Strength
- Pain
- Posture
- Range of motion

Physical therapy interventions

Immediately after surgery, intervention may include wrapping of the residual limb, positioning to avoid contractures, and range of motion and strengthening exercises for the nonaffected surrounding joints. Special consideration is needed to maintain full knee and hip extension for success with prosthetic training. Treatment should also include cardiovascular exercise for whole-body fitness. Early ambulation training with the appropriate assistive device and assistance to the prosthetist for prosthetic prescription are also necessary. Prosthetic training includes donning and doffing the prosthesis, prosthetic care, and application of proper prosthetic socks. The residual limb may need daily skin inspection and desensitization.

Gait deviations and possible causes

Remember that any gait deviation can be caused by habit or fear.

Gait Deviations

Lateral whip (lateral heel movement at toe-off)	• Excessive internal rotation of the knee
Medial whip (medial heel movement at toe-off)	• Excessive external rotation of the knee • Poor prosthetic positioning with donning
Lateral trunk bending	• Prosthesis is too short • Excessive abduction of the socket • Weakness of the gluteus medius • Poorly aligned prosthesis • Pain along the medial wall
Abducted gait (wide-based gait)	• Prosthesis is too long • Pain along the medial pubic ramus • Small socket
Circumduction (wide lateral swing of the prosthesis during swing phase)	• Prosthesis is too long • Poor knee flexion • Muscle weakness • Fear of flexing or inability to flex the knee
Vaulting (rising on the toe of the sound leg to swing the prosthetic leg through)	• Prosthesis is too long • Excessive knee friction • Fear of flexing or inability to flex knee
Rotation of the forefoot at heel strike	• Heel cushion plantar flexion bumper is too stiff • Muscular uncoordination or weakness

Amputation-associated patient symptoms

There are several common symptoms associated with amputations, both traumatic and surgical.

Nonpainful phantom limb sensations
This is a sensation of numbness, pressure, itch, temperature, or pins-and-needles feeling in the amputated limb.

Residual limb pain
This is a feeling of pain in the residual limb associated with the trauma or surgery.

Phantom limb pain
This is a sensation of pain in the amputated limb despite the fact that the limb is no longer attached to the body. The pain can be burning, cramping, or shooting. Medical management may include pharmacologic interventions using tricyclic antidepressants, antiseizure medication, narcotic and non-narcotic analgesics, or local analgesic or steroid injections. Surgical intervention may be appropriate for patients with other pathology of the residual limb such as bone spur, neuroma, or heterotopic bone formation. Physical therapy interventions include early rehab in a multidisciplinary approach, stretching to prevent contractures, strengthening, and early ambulation.

Orthotic Devices

Orthotic devices are used to control or resist unwanted motion. They can assist with performance of motion to perform a function. Orthotic devices transfer force from one area to another. They also protect from injury and inhibit tone.

Orthotic considerations

- Maximal area that the orthosis covers results in increased comfort
- Duration of use, both in hours per day and days/weeks/ months
- Cognitive abilities for wearing schedule, skin inspection, donning/doffing, care of orthosis
- Skin integrity
- Stable or unstable edema
- Muscular weakness
- Presence of, and reason for, contracture

Foot orthosis

A **foot orthosis** is a shoe insert or an external orthosis. Shoes can be considered foot orthoses. They can help control the position of the foot, support deformities, add support for leg-length discrepancy, or help to decrease pain. They can be standard-size or custom-molded.

Ankle-foot orthosis

An **ankle-foot orthosis (AFO)** supports the foot, the ankle, and part of the lower leg. It controls the foot and ankle and may affect the knee, hip, and pelvis as well. A custom-molded AFO is usually molded with the patient in subtalar neutral position. A posterior leaf spring is used for patients with weak dorsiflexion to prevent toe drag and foot slap. A posterior leaf spring has no ankle articulation, as the ankle motion is through recoil of a plastic orthosis. Ankle motion can be controlled by inclusion of the malleolus in the orthosis, which allows for the control of dorsiflexion/plantar flexion as well as eversion/inversion. An ankle articulation can be added into the AFO that can allow full motion or limited dorsiflexion or plantar flexion. Solid ankle AFOs can prevent knee hyperextension. Tone-reducing or tone-inhibiting AFOs are used in the neurologic population to prevent hypertonicity and prevent an extensor synergy.

Knee-ankle foot orthosis

A **knee-ankle-foot orthosis** (**KAFO**) supports the foot, ankle, knee, and distal thigh. The knee joint can be single-axis or polycentric. Active patients tend to favor the polycentric knee, which can be more stable but is bulkier. Knee joints often contain a lock such as a drop lock, which requires full passive knee extension. These are most often used for patients with knee extensor weakness or paralysis.

Knee immobilizer

A **knee immobilizer** immobilizes the knee in extension. It is used after surgery to immobilize and stabilize the knee joint.

Knee orthosis

A **knee orthosis** (**KO**) is a fracture or hinged orthosis that allows immobilization or limited range of motion and the inspection of the limb. A functional KO supports the weakened or lax knee. A rehabilitative KO is a temporary orthosis used after knee surgery. A prophylactic KO is used to prevent knee injury. A contracture-reducing KO is used to increase range of motion. A supportive KO such as a neoprene sleeve is used to support patellar tracking.

Hip-knee-ankle-foot orthosis

A **hip-knee-ankle-foot orthosis** (**HKAFO**) supports the pelvis, hip, knee, ankle, and foot and incorporates both lower extremities. This orthosis is useful for patients with paraplegia. It controls hip abduction, adduction, and rotation and can limit flexion and extension.

Trunk-hip-knee-ankle-foot orthosis

A **trunk-hip-knee-ankle-foot orthosis** (**THKAFO**) supports the torso, both thighs, and the legs down to the feet. It is used for limited ambulation by patients with paraplegia. It is often cumbersome and of limited use due to high energy expenditure and difficulty with donning. The patient must use an assistive device for ambulation with a THKAFO.

Standing frame

This is a frame that provides four-point support for the patient in standing, allowing for use of the upper extremities. Physiological benefits of standing include prevention of osteoporosis via weight-bearing on the skeleton; improved digestion, respiration, and urinary system function; position change to maintain skin integrity; and psychological benefits. Standing frames are particularly useful for children with neurologic disorders and adults with spinal cord injuries.

Parapodium

This is an articulated standing frame.

Reciprocating gait orthosis

This is an articulated THKAFO that is used to allow a patient with paraplegia to walk using an assistive device. It limits the step length and provides for hip stability during swing and stance.

Hip orthosis for hip dislocations

This is for infants with congenital hip dislocation who may benefit from an orthosis that maintains the femoral head in the acetabulum.

Trunk orthoses

A trunk orthosis may be a sacroiliac corset used to prevent pubic symphysis separation and sacroiliac diastasis, or a lumbosacral corset that helps to support the spinal extensors and prevent spinal hyperextension. Other lumbosacral orthoses are used to prevent motion as needed: trunk flexion, extension, lateral flexion, and rotation. Thoracolumbosacral orthoses (TLSOs) are also prescribed to prevent motions of the trunk, including flexion, extension, lateral flexion, and rotation. These are often used after a vertebral fracture or spinal surgery. Special scoliosis and kyphosis orthoses are made for children. These orthoses are designed for long-term use (until spinal maturity) and long-day use (16 to 23 hours per day).

Cervical orthoses

These include soft collars, cervical-post orthoses, and halos. Soft collars serve as motion-restriction reminders. Cervical-post orthoses are rigid and more restrictive and, depending on the design, restrict flexion, extension, rotation, and lateral flexion. A halo is used for immobilization of the cervical spine in cases of vertebral fracture.

Upper-limb orthoses

Upper-limb orthoses can be classified according to their function:

- **Assistive:** These are used for patients with neuromuscular weakness to place a limb in a functional position.
- **Substitutive:** These are used for patients with paralysis and augment prehension with more proximal joint movements.
- **Protective:** These are used to prevent contractures or to protect from painful movement. They include a shoulder sling to prevent subluxation, a forearm cuff to treat lateral epicondylitis, or a wrist-hand orthosis to treat carpal tunnel syndrome.
- **Corrective:** These are used to increase range of motion.

Devices Used for Special Considerations

These devices are not necessary for each patient but rather are specific to the needs of certain patient populations. Patients at risk for development of wounds need protective and supportive equipment. Patients who are not able to perform functional mobility training on conventional equipment may benefit from gravity-assisted devices. Bariatric patients need special equipment for support and function that will support their weight.

Protective and supportive devices

These include pressure-reducing mattresses, used to reduce pressure on bony prominences. They are made from materials such as foam, air, dynamic air, gel, and water. Pressure-relieving mattresses completely eliminate pressure on bony prominences. Seat cushions are also considered protective and supportive.

Gravity-assisted devices

Gravity-assisted devices are used as physical therapy aids and include aquatic therapy, which may be gravity-assisted or gravity-resisted; gravity-assisted treadmill devices; and gravity-assisted exercise devices.

Bariatric devices

This group of equipment is specially made for patients who weigh more than 350 lb. Bariatric devices can include beds, wheelchairs, commodes, walkers, and mechanical lifts. Bariatric beds can have optional bed scales, foot exits, or cardiac chair conversion mechanisms.

Wheelchairs

Wheelchair evaluations can be performed by several health-care professionals, including physical therapists. Wheelchairs allow patients who may otherwise be nonmobile the ability to move about their environment with assistance or independently. Options for additions and specialized wheelchairs are constantly developing to provide patients with the best quality of life and function.

Wheelchair positioning principles

There are principles for positioning that are in place to prevent injury and promote good postural alignment. Back height, seat depth, seat width, and footrest length should be measured for each patient.

Pelvic control
The pelvis should be maintained in a neutral spine position, avoiding anterior or posterior tilt. The backrest should support the normal curvatures of the spine.

Thigh control
The thighs should be horizontal to the floor, and the hips and knees should be horizontally aligned.

Seat depth
The seat should extend to between one and a half and two inches from the popliteal fossa.

Footrest
The footrest maintains proper leg position and should keep the thighs parallel to the floor.

Wheelchair options

- Manual or power mobility
- Hemi-height to allow for propulsion via foot
- Sport or lightweight to allow easier mobility for the athlete and energy conservation for the frail person
- Rigid, nonfolding frame for lower maintenance
- Reclining back to allow for a multitude of seat-to-back angles
- Wheelchair cushions to reduce pressure, shear, and friction forces; to resist moisture and heat; and to assist in postural control

The use of equipment and devices allows patients to be more functional despite their impairments. Sometimes the goal of physical therapy is not to treat the impairments but rather to maximize the nonimpaired function. This section has reviewed some of the most common equipment and devices used in physical therapy. Once you are familiar with the section on therapeutic modalities, you will be ready to test your knowledge with the end-of-chapter review quiz.

PAIN AND THE INFLAMMATORY RESPONSE

Before making the decision of which modalities to use, if needed, you must first have a better understanding of pain and the inflammatory response to injury.

Pain

Pain can be categorized as either acute or chronic in nature. **Acute pain** is that which occurs as a result of recent injury, surgical intervention, infection, or disease. It can be characterized by localized swelling and redness and usually has a specific point of irritability. **Chronic pain**, on the other hand, is less specific. It can be vague, diffuse, and long-lasting in nature. In some cases pain may even be referred from another point of injury or dysfunction. Either type of pain can cause limitations in function, including weakness, range of motion deficits, muscle spasm, and general immobility.

Pain pathways

There are two types of nerve fibers that carry the pain stimulus: A-delta and C fibers. A-delta fibers relay quick pain messages and sensory stimulation from the skin. C fibers carry a slower, deep, dull pain message. The route of the pathway begins when a noxious stimulus is perceived by the A-delta or C fibers. The signal is transmitted to the dorsal horn of the spinal cord; and from the dorsal horn, connections are made to various tracks of the lamina. Lamina V carries the message to the lateral spinothalamic tract of the spinal cord. In the lateral spinothalamic tract, the signal crosses over to the other side of the cord, where it then enters the brain stem to be perceived as pain. Mechanoreceptors that sense pain from tissue injury relay the impulse to A-beta and A-gamma fibers. The A-beta and A-gamma fibers transmit signals to the dorsal horn, laminae, and substantia gelatinosa.

Methods of measuring pain

Measurement of pain is difficult because it is a subjective measure. Pain measurements can be useful when comparing changes in pain before, during, or after treatment interventions, or with certain activities. One of the most common measurement methods is the numeric pain scale that asks patients to rate their pain from 1 to 10. The visual analog scale uses an individual line along which the patient can mark the intensity of the pain. A more in-depth measure of pain may be the McGill Pain Questionnaire, which asks specific questions about the location, strength, type, and characteristics of the pain. Whichever method is chosen should be used throughout treatment for comparison and consistency.

Inflammatory Response

The **inflammatory response** occurs as a response to tissue injury. Signs of inflammation are as follows:

- Pain caused by edema and activation of pain receptors within the nervous system
- Edema caused by vasodilation of vessels to allow fluid entry to the affected area that is needed for tissue healing
- Redness (erythema), also as a result of the vasodilation of vessels and increased blood flow to the area
- Increased tissue temperature, again as a result of the vasodilation and increased blood flow to the area
- Decreased functional use and limited range of motion due to all of the four previous points

THERAPEUTIC MODALITIES

Therapeutic modalities are used to treat the signs and symptoms associated with the differential diagnoses and pathologies that have been discussed in the previous chapters. Use of heat and cold, ultrasound, electrotherapy, hydrotherapy, and traction are some of the most commonly used modalities. Generally, modalities help to control pain and inflammation and may promote improved conditions for healing to occur. This section discusses some of the common therapeutic modalities and the indications for their use.

Thermal Agents

Both heat and cold can be used as superficial methods of controlling pain and edema. There are five methods of transfer of temperature modalities:

- Conduction (hot packs, cold packs)
- Convection (fluidotherapy)
- Conversion (ultrasound)
- Evaporation (perspiration, vasocoolant sprays)
- Radiation

Superficial **heat** can cause increased blood flow both to the local treatment area and to the periphery. Heat provides an increase in the metabolic rate that translates to an increase in tissue healing and tissue viability, and it can also be successful in pain relief as a mechanism for the gate control theory discussed later in this chapter. Muscle spasm is controlled with heat by decreasing the firing of type II muscle fibers and increasing the firing of the Golgi tendon organs. The use of heat on a tightened area of soft tissue is said to increase tissue extensibil. A temperature ranging from 40–45°C (113°F) along with static tissue elongation can maximize this stretch.

Effects of thermal agents

One effect of heat is the local increase in the metabolic rate and local vasodilation, causing local increase in blood flow. These local changes can allow for delivery of increased amounts of oxygen and leukocytes, as well as the removal of metabolites. The benefits of the local vasodilation can also spread to surrounding tissues when the heat intensity remains high for a sustained period of time. This can be helpful if there are multiple injured sites or if the primary site of injury does not allow for local heating methods. Heat also provides a perception of pain reduction, thereby acting as an analgesic. It can also decrease muscle guarding and increase tissue extensibility. It is understood that the use of heat prior to exercise may actually decrease the muscle's ability to gain strength.

Methods of Applying Superficial Heat

Superficial heat can be applied in a number of ways, mostly depending on the desired area of use and the availability of the modality in the physical therapy setting. The following are some of the common methods of applying superficial heat.

Hydrocollator packs

Hydrocollator packs provide superficial moist heat as one of the most basic methods of conduction in therapeutic treatment. Hot packs are stored in hydrocollators at a temperature range of 71–79°C (approximately 170°F). To prevent tissue injury, six layers (roughly one inch) of padding are placed between the hot pack and the patient's skin. Skin temperature changes within ten minutes. Treatment time is usually from 15 to 20 minutes, depending on patient comfort. If there is a history or comorbidity that would indicate a compromised response to heat, the skin should be checked after five minutes of treatment. For home use there are hot-water bottles, electric heating pads, and microwaveable heating items.

Paraffin baths

Paraffin baths allow a greater degree of heat to the injured area since they contain paraffin wax and mineral oil. This combination has a lower melting point than water, allowing the patient to tolerate a much higher temperature. Paraffin baths are typically used for extremities, particularly the hands and feet. Paraffin is stored for treatment use at 47–54°C (approximately 126°F). Typical treatment time is 15–20 minutes.

Dip and wrap method

The dip and wrap method involves dipping the area to be treated into the paraffin seven or eight times, forming a paraffin "glove" or "sock," then wrapping that area in a plastic bag and covering it with a towel to hold in the heat.

Dip and submerge method

The dip and submerge method involves dipping the area to be treated into the paraffin seven or eight times, and then leaving the area submerged in the paraffin bath for the treatment duration. This method allows the greatest amount of tissue heating but also has the greatest risk for burns.

Paraffin precautions

Prior to starting any paraffin treatment, the patient should remove all jewelry from the hand or foot, and the skin should be inspected for any open wounds or cuts. When the treatment is completed, the paraffin can be peeled off and should be discarded to avoid contamination (unless the paraffin bath is being used by only one patient).

Fluidotherapy

Fluidotherapy can allow the combination of convection heat, manual techniques, and skin desensitization all in one treatment. The fluidotherapy machines contain small particles of solid, natural cellulose being driven by warm air to float in a contained tank. Temperature can be adjusted as needed but usually ranges from 43 to 53°C (110–125°F). Fluidotherapy is intended for use on the distal extremities. The movement of the particles against the skin can desensitize the skin and healed incisions and decrease edema. Because the method of transfer is convection vs. conduction, the patient tolerates higher temperatures. Treatment time is typically 15–20 minutes. Since the patient can freely move the involved limb within the unit, manual techniques by the therapist or exercise by the patient can be coupled with this thermal treatment.

Short-wave diathermy

Short-wave diathermy can be used for slightly deeper heat penetration than the previously discussed superficial thermal agents. This uses electromagnetic energy to pass waves through the body, causing an increase in tissue temperature. The technique is a conversion from electromagnetic energy to mechanical energy within the tissues. Short-wave diathermy uses a frequency of 27.12 MHz. The greatest heating effects are superficial, near the electrodes. Plates or electrodes should be one to three inches from the patient's skin. Treatment duration is 20–30 minutes.

Hydrotherapy

Hydrotherapy is the use of water to achieve the goal of treatment. This section covers hydrotherapy as a modality; aquatic therapy is covered in chapter 4, Musculoskeletal System, as part of exercise intervention. Warm whirlpools are generally used for musculoskeletal disorders or wound care. Whirlpools can have a therapeutic effect on managing pain and decreasing muscle spasm to allow greater ROM. A warm whirlpool is thought to oxygenate tissues, soften necrotic tissues for later debridement, and stimulate the formation of granulation tissue over the wound bed (see chapter 6, Integumentary System, for more on debridement). Hydrotherapy used as wound care should be done at temperatures around 33.5–35.58°C (92–96°F). Special considerations and techniques should be employed when cleaning whirlpools to prevent the spread of infection between patient uses.

Contraindications to hydrotherapy

Contraindications to warm whirlpool therapy include the following:

- Edema
- Cardiovascular or pulmonary complications
- Being febrile
- In wound care, dry gangrene or maceration

Effects of Cryotherapy

Cold modalities are known to cause a decrease in tissue temperature and local vasoconstriction, allowing a decrease in blood flow to the treated area. There is also a reflex vasoconstriction and an increase in the patient's pain threshold that occurs as the cold stimulates free nerve endings. These effects decrease metabolism in the area and prevent extra fluid from accumulating there in the case of acute injuries to the musculoskeletal system. Cold is also well known as an analgesic and is thought to actually slow nerve conduction velocities and modulate pain via the gate control theory. It is suspected that after 30 minutes of cold treatment, vasodilation takes place for a short time (4–6 minutes), followed again by vasoconstriction for 15–30 minutes, and then again by vasodilation. This is the **Hunting response** and is actually the body's way of preventing tissue injury/death from extended cold exposure. Cold modalities are thought to penetrate deeper than heat modalities, up to 4 cm in depth. In acute injuries, cold modalities are preferred for the first 48–72 hours. For maximum benefit in acute injuries, ice should be applied within 20 minutes after injury or after completion of athletic event. With all cold modalities, care must be taken to avoid frostbite of the skin or nerve palsy, which can occur in individuals with low body fat or in cases of treatment times that are too long.

Methods of Superficial Cryotherapy

Superficial cold can be applied in a number of ways, mostly depending on the desired area of use and the availability of the modality in the physical therapy setting. The following are some common methods of applying superficial cold.

Cold packs

Cold packs are most commonly used as cold modalities. They come in various shapes and sizes and are stored in a freezer at –5°C (8°F). A towel is placed between the cold pack and the skin to prevent frostbite. Treatment time varies, depending on the size of the patient, but is typically 15–20 minutes. The use of a moist towel may help facilitate the cold conduction. If the patient has a history or comorbidity that would indicate a compromised response to cold, the skin should be checked after five minutes of treatment.

Ice massage

Ice massage is a method of decreasing temperature at a more rapid rate than the cold pack. Ice is applied directly to the skin in a constant massage motion. Application is usually over a small area. The patient will experience cold, burning, and aching before the desired numbness from the ice massage occurs. Treatment time varies based on the location of the application and the size (body fat) of the patient, but typically ranges from 5 to 15 minutes.

Ice bath or whirlpool

An **ice bath or whirlpool** allows the desired body part to be submerged in a mixture of cold water and ice for more direct contact with the surface area. Cold baths are typically kept at

13–18°C (55°F). Treatment time ranges from 5 to 15 minutes. As with the warm whirlpool, the agitator should be plugged into a ground fault interrupter switch to avoid injury from electrical shock.

Vapocoolant sprays

Vapocoolant sprays such as fluoromethane can be used for quick cooling or spray-and-stretch techniques in the clinic. Typically, this is used for trigger-point stretching to increase ROM.

Cold compression units

The use of compression may be combined with cryotherapy in a fitted compression sleeve in which cold water circulates for the duration of the treatment. These do not cool as efficiently as ice packs but can be used for longer durations and are common postsurgical modalities.

Therapeutic Ultrasound

Ultrasound is a form of sound-wave energy that can be transmitted through soft tissue for both thermal and nonthermal effects. Sound waves transmit vibration, causing a transfer of energy. This energy transfer is initiated by voltage passing through the crystal in the sound head of the ultrasound, causing alternating compression and expansion of the crystal. This is known as the piezoelectric and reverse piezoelectric effect.

Effects of ultrasound

The **effects of ultrasound** can be thermal or nonthermal. Ultrasound is considered a deep-heating modality and therefore has the same thermal effects—decreasing muscle guarding, increasing blood flow, reducing pain, and improving tissue extensibility—as superficial heat, but at a greater tissue depth. Adjustment of treatment time, frequency, and intensity can help determine the depth of penetration of the ultrasound (see below). The mechanical effects of ultrasound can be seen with cavitation causing a greater ability for ions to permeate back and forth across the cell membrane. This allows a greater ability to repair tissue and increase blood flow.

Ultrasound parameters

Ultrasound parameters can be adjusted to best treat the condition of the patient. Most typically, the frequency, mode, intensity, and duration of treatment can be adjusted as follows.

Frequency

Frequency can be set at either 1 or 3 MHz. The 3 MHz frequency penetrates to 1–2 cm, and the 1 MHz frequency is thought to penetrate 2–4 cm.

Mode

Mode of treatment can be either continuous or pulsed. The pulsed mode is variable based on the duty cycle and is written as a percentage determined by the duration of the pulse divided by the pulse period. Generally, continuous mode is used to achieve thermal effects, and pulsed mode is used for nonthermal effects on tissues.

Intensity

Intensity can be adjusted based on the desired strength of the ultrasound, measured in watts per square centimeter (W/cm^2). Intensities of 0.5 to 1.0 W/cm^2 are typically used for thermal effects and chronic conditions. To achieve nonthermal effects, or for acute injuries, intensities less than 0.5 W/cm^2 are used.

Duration
Duration can be determined on the basis of the size of the area to be treated, the desired depth of penetration of the ultrasound, and the desired heating effects. Treatment time should be approximately five minutes for every treatment area that is five times the size of the ultrasound head. For example, if the sound head is 5 cm diameter and the area to be treated is 50 square cm, the duration would be ten minutes (50 cm/5=10).

Ultrasound precautions
Keep in mind that it is a combination of all of the parameters that determines the desired effects of the ultrasound. A lower intensity at a continuous frequency can have the same energy output as a higher intensity at a pulsed frequency. Likewise, for changes in muscle tissue temperature, a 3 MHz mode for 2.5 minutes at 2.0 W/cm^2 can cause the same temperature change in superficial tissues as a setting of 1 MHz at 2.0 W/cm^2 for ten minutes can cause in deeper tissues. The area that is receiving the ultrasound should not be more than four to five times the size of the sound head to be used.

Indications for ultrasound

Indications for the use of ultrasound include, but are not limited to, the following:

- To improve soft-tissue tightness or ROM by increasing tissue elasticity (parameters: 1.0–2.5 W/cm^2, continuous)
- For pain reduction (parameters: 0.5–1.0 W/cm^2, continuous, daily if needed)
- To decrease muscle guarding
- To increase circulation, thus increasing the release of macrophages to decrease inflammation (parameters: 0.5–1.0 W/cm^2, pulsed, daily if needed)
- To promote tissue healing by increasing collagen secretion (parameters: 0.5 W/cm^2, pulsed, 1 MHz)

Contraindications to ultrasound use

Contraindications to the use of ultrasound include the following:

- Treatment area is over the eyes or genitals.
- Treatment area is over the pelvic, lumbar, or abdominal areas in a pregnant woman.
- During periods of active cancer
- Treatment area is over growth plates in children and adolescents.
- Treatment area is over an unprotected spinal cord (such as in laminectomy).
- Use of thermal ultrasound settings over an area of acute injury or infection
- Treatment area is in the vicinity of a cardiac pacemaker.
- Treatment area is over the carotid sinus or cervical ganglia.

As with any thermal modality, care should be taken when using ultrasound on a patient who has compromised sensation or circulation or decreased ability to communicate, as the patient may be at risk of tissue injury from a burn.

Phonophoresis

Phonophoresis is the use of ultrasound waves to noninvasively administer medication to a desired treatment area. Typically, either the NSAID dexamethasone or cortisone is used to control inflammation. Some clinicians use lidocaine for pain control. It is unclear whether continuous or pulsed frequency is most efficient for delivery. There is not yet strong support for the use of phonophoresis as a treatment modality.

Electrotherapeutic Modalities

An electric current is the movement of charged particles such as electrons or ions from one place to another. Electrodes can be either positive (cathode) or negative (anion) and will repel like charges and attract opposite charges. This allows the flow of ions to be either toward or away from the appropriate electrode. Both a positive and a negative electrode are needed for a complete circuit. The type of current produced during electrical stimulation can be either alternating (AC) or direct (DC). Direct current flows in just one direction, from the cathode to the anode or vice versa, as indicated on the machine. This can allow an accumulation of ions under the electrode, which can be beneficial for certain treatments discussed below. Alternating current moves in two directions, changing each second. With AC there is no buildup of charged particles under the electrodes because they are constantly changing polarity throughout the treatment. Pulsatile current (PC) can be either AC or DC but is characterized by brief periods of no current at all. This is the most typical current used in treatment, for patient comfort. There is minimal ion or charge buildup because of the pulsed current and depending on whether it is AC or DC.

Effects of electrotherapy

The effects of electrotherapy are quite variable based on adjustments of parameters that are discussed below. Chemical changes can take place since there is an accumulation of ions under an electrode, such as in the use of a DC stimulator. Chemical changes in the skin and soft tissues cause increased blood flow to the area beneath the electrodes. Another cause of the increased blood flow can be the vibration from the current movement through the tissues resulting in mechanical heating. The electrokinetic effect of electrotherapy is what allows for the depolarization of peripheral nerves for the therapeutic effects of sensory stimulation or muscle contraction.

Theories of pain control with electrotherapy

There are several theories that attempt to define how electrotherapy influences pain control in the body. Each theory carries its own particular method of electrotherapy, with parameters, indications, and contraindications discussed later in this section.

Gate control theory

The **gate control theory** suggests that electrical stimulation can work as a pain control modality by blocking, or "gating," the ascending pain pathway. Some pre- or postsynaptic transmission inhibition may take place. This method of pain control works best during the actual stimulation, with short-lasting effects once treatment is complete.

Endogenous opioid release mechanism

The **endogenous opioid release mechanism** suggests that a stronger stimulation producing a motor response can actually encourage the release of some of the body's natural painkillers—endorphins and enkephalins. This mechanism has longer-lasting effects since it is an actual release of hormones that is controlling the pain.

Descending inhibition

The **descending inhibition** theory uses yet a stronger stimulation to produce a noxious sensation that stops the pain perception at the spinal cord. In this case, the smaller pain fibers are activated with the strong stimulation and relay a message to the periaqueductal gray in the midbrain. A descending pathway is then activated that inhibits pain perception in the spinal cord. This pathway also provides longer-lasting pain relief; but to reach it, the electrotherapy parameters that are necessary create a current that may be uncomfortable for the patient during treatment.

Parameters of electrotherapy

Parameters of electrotherapy can be adjusted for both the individual pulse and the pulse train based on treatment goals and the desired tissue response. Variables of the individual pulse include the following.

Waveform

The **waveform** of the individual pulse can be monophasic, biphasic, or polyphasic. This describes the shape of the pulse and how many phases it contains. A monophasic pulse has a cathode and anode and is unidirectional, with similar but lessened effects to the DC. A biphasic pulse moves similar to the AC, in two directions, with similar effects. The biphasic pulse can be further divided into symmetrical or asymmetrical. The asymmetrical biphasic pulse creates a small buildup of charge since the waveforms do not cancel each other out. The symmetrical biphasic waveform is typically most comfortable for the patient. A polyphasic waveform consists of more than two phases.

Pulse duration

Pulse duration (measured in microseconds) is the time interval between the beginning and the end of one complete waveform cycle. In biphasic or polyphasic waveforms this also includes the period of time between the end of one phase and the beginning of the next phase of the pulse (also known as the intrapulse interval). Shorter pulse duration is needed at a higher pulse frequency. The cycle can be further broken down to **phase duration**, which is the time between the start and the end of one phase of the pulse.

Amplitude

Amplitude (measured in milliamperes or volts) is the peak current in one phase of a pulse. This determines the strength of the current and the depth of penetration (higher amplitude = greater depth). As the duration of treatment increases, the amplitude may need to be adjusted as the patient accommodates to the stimulation. Amplitude can result in subsensory, sensory, motor, or noxious effects.

Duty cycle

Duty cycle (measured as a percentage) modulates the on/off time relative to the total time of a pulse train (on time/total time). This is important in muscle fatigue because the longer the stimulus is on, the greater the fatigue.

Frequency

Frequency is the number of pulses per second of stimulation (measured as pps). The higher the frequency, the greater the muscle fatigue. An increase in pulse frequency can achieve tetany for a sustained muscle contraction.

Ramp time

Ramp time (measured in seconds) is the time it takes to reach the maximum amplitude of the pulse train. It can be either from baseline to max or from max to baseline. This allows the clinician to make the transition from on/off more comfortable for the patient. This time should be added to the time of muscle contraction when determining the on time of a duty cycle.

Treatment time

Treatment time is variable based on the desired results or can be adjusted to coordinate with completion of an exercise or activity.

Electrodes/electrode placement

Placement of at least two leads is needed to complete the electrical circuit. If the treatment is using two channels or is quadrapolar, four electrodes and fours leads are needed. Electrodes are carbon, adhesive, or suction.

Modulation

Modulation allows the delivery of the electrical stimulation to change throughout the treatment time for greater effect. Adaptation can occur if the current remains unchanged for the treatment duration. Modulation can be achieved by adjusting the delivery of the current as continuous or interrupted (see duty cycle, above, for on/off settings) or by adjusting ramp time, frequency, or amplitude.

Body tissues of skin and adipose tissue offer the greatest resistance to electrical current, whereas muscle and tendinous tissue offer the least resistance. This translates to the fact that a greater current is needed to penetrate a muscle that is beneath a layer of fatty tissue than to reach a muscle or tendon that may be more superficial. Because the skin offers greater impedance to the current, a stronger current is needed to penetrate the muscle underlying the fat—which may be uncomfortable for the patient. Possible ways to decrease skin impedance can be by warming the skin prior to treatment, by cleaning away oils and lotions in the area under the electrodes, and/or by shaving away excess hair.

The four levels of electric stimulation effect on the body are as follows:

- **Subsensory:** The patient cannot feel any stimulation (no nerve activation).
- **Sensory:** The patient feels a tingling sensation but it is not painful (activates the A-beta nerve fibers).
- **Motor:** The patient feels a strong tingling sensation and there is visible muscle contraction (activates the A-alpha nerve fibers).
- **Noxious:** The patient feels an uncomfortable or even painful sensation accompanied by a strong muscle contraction (activates the A-delta and C nerve fibers).

Indications for electrotherapy

Indications for the use of electrotherapy as a treatment modality include the following:

- For pain relief, it is thought that electrical stimulation works through the gate control theory. The electrical current inhibits the sensation of pain by blocking nociceptive impulses with afferent nerve impulses.
- For edema reduction through either the muscle-pump technique or the use of a polarized current to repel inflammation from the affected area
- For neuromuscular reeducation, electrical stimulation allows the clinician to activate denervated muscle for function and to actually strengthen weakened muscle tissues.
- To increase tissue healing/wound healing/fracture healing by increasing circulation (see chapter 6, Integumentary System)
- For delivery of medications noninvasively through the skin
- To decrease muscular spasm and allow greater ROM

Contraindications for electrotherapy

Contraindications for the use of electrotherapy include the following conditions:

- Pregnancy (unless used as pain relief during labor/delivery)
- Pacemaker or other electrical stimulators/defibrillators

- Cancer
- Treatment area is over the carotid sinus
- Treatment area is over an area of suspected thrombophlebitis or phlebothrombosis
- Epilepsy/seizure disorder
- Caution over areas of decreased sensation
- Caution over metal implants or fixators
- Caution in using with patients who are unable to communicate
- Treatment area is over areas of superficial metal (staples, pins, fixators)

Methods of Electrical Stimulation Application

There are a variety of methods of electrical stimulation application based on the desired goals of treatment intervention. Certain applications are more suitable for achieving pain control via the pathways mentioned previously. The following are some of the common methods of electrical stimulation application.

Transcutaneous electrical nerve stimulation

Transcutaneous electrical nerve stimulation (TENS) is a portable, battery-operated device that uses electrical stimulation across the skin barrier as a pain management technique. The theory behind the use of TENS is that it blocks the pain pathway via the gate control mechanism discussed previously. TENS can provide sensory analgesia either without muscle contraction or through the endogenous opioid theory with muscle contraction.

TENS parameters
TENS parameters are as follows:

- *Specific indications*: Acute/chronic pain, circulation
- *Frequency*: 75–200 pps (80 pps has greatest inhibitory effect on C fibers). Frequency should range from 40 to 80 pps for motor effects.
- *Phase duration*: 60–250 seconds
- *Amplitude/intensity*: Strong but comfortable sensory level only
- *Mode*: This is variable by device and controls the delivery of the pulse chains. Burst, amplitude-modulated, random, and continuous modes all seem to work equally well.
- *Treatment duration*: Variable; usually used for two hours before a 10-to-30-minute period of no stimulation. The TENS unit can be worn during work or activity; then the duration can be long enough to finish the activity.
- *Electrode placement*: Should be directly over or surrounding the area of pain. It can also be over the nerve trunk that communicates with the area of pain.

Interferential current

Interferential current (IFC) in the quad-polar (or four-electrode), two-channel technique uses two medium-frequency currents to pass through the skin comfortably; and then it mixes, or interferes, to generate a lower-frequency current needed for soft-tissue healing. The two frequencies mix to result in areas of large amplitudes where the waves are together and zero amplitude when the waves cancel each other out. Bipolar IFC modulates the amplitude, not the frequency (effects may be quicker).

IFC parameters
IFC parameters are as follows:

- *Specific indications*: Acute/chronic pain, Complex Regional Pain Syndrome
- *Frequency*: Usually preset at 4,000 pps
- *Beat frequency*: Endogenous opioid mechanism, 5–20 pps; gate control theory, 50–100 pps
- *Phase duration*: 125 μs
- *Amplitude/intensity*: Strong and comfortable (gate control) or to muscle contraction (endogenous opioid)
- Treatment duration: 20–30 minutes
- Electrode placement: Surrounding the area of pain
- Optional scan/sweep mode: Can be used to vary the position of treatment. If this option is chosen, longer treatment duration should be used.

Neuromuscular electrical stimulation
Neuromuscular electrical stimulation (NMES), also known as electrical muscle stimulation (EMS), is primarily used for muscle reeducation. It is said to work in a manner opposite to that of voluntary muscle strengthening, recruiting type II fibers first, and allowing greater fatigue. It is a biphasic, pulsatile, or burst-alternating current.

NMES parameters
NMES parameters are as follows:

- *Specific indications*: Muscle activation
- *Frequency*: 30–75 pps (>50 pps needed for smooth tetanic contraction)
- *Pulse duration*: 200–400 μs
- *Amplitude/intensity*: To patient comfort and desired muscular contraction
- *Treatment duration*: Ten minutes or until concurrent exercise is complete
- *Electrode placement*: Active electrode is as close as possible to the motor point. Smaller electrodes elicit a greater contraction than the large. Either one or two channels with either two or four electrodes may be used, depending on the goal of treatment. Two channels may be preferable if the desired outcome is co-contraction of antagonist muscles or production of two-joint movement.
- *On/off option (duty cycle)*: 10–15 sec on/15–20 sec off to avoid fatigue. The most optimal ratios are generally 1:3 or 1:5 for muscle activation and strengthening. As strength improves, the on time should be lengthened and the off time shortened accordingly.
- *Optional ramp time*: one to two seconds to allow gradual motor recruitment

The use of NMES can be coupled with active exercise such as straight leg raises or long-arc quadriceps sets to enhance strengthening. NMES has also been used for muscle retraining to treat urinary incontinence, as functional electrical stimulation (FES), or to inhibit muscle spasticity. In FES, the parameters remain the same except for on/off time, which is instead controlled by a foot or hand switch that can be triggered to maintain the contraction long enough to complete the task. An example would be FES placed over the tibialis anterior to assist with dorsiflexion during gait. The hand trigger holds the contraction to maintain the muscle activation through the heel strike and foot flat portions of gait (see the gait section in chapter 4, Musculoskeletal System). In the case of spasticity reduction, NMES again uses essentially the same waveform, pulse duration, and frequency as the other electrical stimulation systems discussed here. But the amplitude must be high enough to achieve at least a 3+ muscle contraction, and the duty cycle is altered to a 1:1 or 3:4 ratio to achieve muscle fatigue, thus decreasing spasticity.

NMES contraindications

Contraindications are the same as those for general electrotherapy but also include acute inflammation because edema may be exacerbated.

High-volt pulsed current

High-volt pulsed current (HVPC) is a monophasic stimulation that is very comfortable for the patient because of the short pulse duration and high amplitude. This level of stimulation can reach sensory, motor, and nociceptor fibers. HVPC can produce a polarized potential under the anode or cathode. An anode over the treatment area repels tissue fluids, thus decreasing edema. It is thought that injury polarity peaks positive at 48 hours and then peaks negative at nine days after injury. If HVPC is used for wound care, the current can be polarized negative over the wound for bacterial infection or positive over the wound to stimulate tissue healing and wound closure.

HVPC parameters

HVPC parameters are as follows:

- Specific indications: acute/chronic pain, edema, wound healing
- Frequency: 1–200 pps
- Pulse duration: 30–100 μs
- Amplitude/intensity: Sensory threshold only
- Treatment duration: 10–20 minutes

Iontophoresis

Iontophoresis uses direct-current electric stimulation to deliver medication through the skin to the area of pain or injury. Medications used for iontophoresis are ionized solutions. The "delivery" electrode is of the same polarity as the medication, to repel the ions and push the medicine through the skin. Some common medications and their polarities are:

- Dexamethasone (negative); anti-inflammatory
- Lidocaine (positive); local anesthetic
- Salicylates (negative); pain relief and anti-inflammatory

Iontophoresis parameters

Iontophoresis parameters are as follows:

- Specific indications: Inflammatory syndromes, trigger-point pain
- Amplitude/intensity: 1–4 mA, based on patient comfort
- Dosage: 40 mA min (up to 80 mA min)
- Treatment duration: Determined by amplitude and dosage
- Treatment frequency: Every other day, as the direct current can potentially harm the skin if used too often or too long

Mechanical Spinal Traction

Traction uses a mechanical force to lengthen soft tissues and separate vertebral joints, and it is typically used on the cervical or lumbar spine. Specific indications for traction include decreased sensation or radicular symptoms, acute/chronic back or neck pain, and decreased spinal mobility. Traction should be done in an open packed position (slight flexion) for both the lumbar and cervical spine. The patient is positioned supine with the appropriate halter secured tightly above and below the segment(s) to be treated. Pull can be up to 25 lb for the cervical spine. It should be at least one-quarter to one-half of the patient's body weight for the lumbar spine. Initial trials of traction should only be 5–10 minutes in length to assess patient tolerance. Total traction time can be increased to 20–30 minutes as needed. There is usually an option for continuous or intermittent pull. On/off time can range from 7–60 seconds on to 7–20 seconds off, depending on the treatment goal.

Contraindications to mechanical traction

Mechanical spinal traction of the lumbar or cervical spine is not appropriate for all patients with back or neck pain or radicular symptoms. Some contraindications to use of spinal traction are:

- Meningitis
- Cancer
- Cauda equina signs
- Osteoporosis
- Rheumatoid arthritis
- Caution with hypermobile conditions, including pregnancy
- Caution with cardiopulmonary comorbidities

Intermittent Compression

Intermittent compression can be used as a modality to control edema formation and encourage movement of fluid away from the site of injury. Intermittent compression sleeves are worn over the affected limb.

Intermittent compression parameters

Variable parameters that can be adjusted on the basis of patient need, as allowed by individual devices, include the following:

- On/off time: Ranges from 30 seconds to 5 minutes on and 30 seconds to 5 minutes off.
- Total treatment time: Ranges from 0 to 30 minutes or longer if needed.
- Sleeve pressure: Usually set at 30–60 mm Hg for the upper extremity and 40–80 mm Hg for the lower extremity. There is conflicting evidence on the maximum recommendation of pressure due to the concern about the danger of occlusion of lymphatic vessels.
- Concurrent cold therapy: See Cryotherapy section, above.

Other Methods of Compression

Other methods of compression can include, but are not limited to, distal-to-proximal bandaging and measured compression garments. Both of these help to maintain hydrostatic pressure and stimulate a muscle-pump method of edema reduction in the extremity.

In **distal-to-proximal bandaging**, variable amounts of stretch are available up to 140 percent stretch; these are identified as short, medium, and long stretch.

Compression garments can be measured to individual limb girth or purchased by general size once fluctuating edema has stabilized and reached a plateau. These garments provide a gradient pressure to the affected limb.

Contraindications to use of compression modalities include the comorbidity of congestive heart failure, pulmonary emboli, thrombophlebitis, and active infections.

Other factors to consider when using compression to control edema include caution with diminished sensation, arterial insufficiency, active cancer, and diabetes.

A FINAL WORD

The trend in physical therapy has definitely been toward limited use of modalities in treatment intervention. The fact remains, however, that certain impairments do benefit from the use of therapeutic modalities to supplement other treatment intervention techniques. With your educational background in modalities and the review presented in this chapter, you should have a better understanding of which modalities may be most appropriate when needed. You are now ready to move on to the end-of-chapter review quiz to test your knowledge of equipment and devices, including information about amputations and therapeutic modalities.

EQUIPMENT AND DEVICES, AND THERAPEUTIC MODALITIES CHAPTER QUIZ

1. A patient is referred to physical therapy following an acute ankle sprain. She has significant edema and would benefit from intermittent compression/cryotherapy intervention. What inflation pressure is *MOST* appropriate for this injury?

   (A) 20 mm Hg
   (B) 40 mm Hg
   (C) 90 mm Hg
   (D) 120 mm Hg

2. Which one of the following patients would be *MOST* appropriate for the use of functional electrical stimulation?

   (A) A patient with foot drop from a CVA
   (B) A patient with decreased ankle dorsiflexion due to an ankle sprain
   (C) A patient with shuffling gait from Parkinson's disease
   (D) A patient with diabetic neuropathy

3. A patient with diabetes and impaired sensation of bilateral feet presents with a Chopart disarticulation. Where is this disarticulation?

   (A) Between the talonavicular and calcaneocuboid joints
   (B) Between the tarsometatarsal joints
   (C) Between the distal tibia and fibula
   (D) Between the tarsal and metatarsal joint

4. An 83-year-old patient with a transfemoral amputation has a personal goal of household ambulation on level indoor surfaces. He does not plan to ambulate on uneven ground or participate in sports. He is also oxygen-dependent, with low activity tolerance. What type of prosthetic foot is *MOST* appropriate for this patient?

   (A) Multiple-axis foot
   (B) Dynamic-response foot
   (C) Single-axis foot
   (D) Solid ankle cushioned heel (SACH) foot

5. A physical therapist has chosen to use ultrasound to assist a patient in increasing tissue extensibility and reducing muscle guarding prior to passive stretching. Which of the following parameters should be adjusted on the basis of the depth of the tissues to be treated?

   (A) Duty cycle
   (B) Power/intensity
   (C) Frequency
   (D) Length of treatment

6. A 74-year-old patient is diagnosed with T8 compression fracture. The surgeon orders a rigid thoracolumbar orthosis. The physical therapist educates the patient on the purpose of the orthosis. The main purpose is to:

   (A) prevent spinal movement.
   (B) position the spine in flexion.
   (C) strengthen the paraspinal musculature.
   (D) protect the skin.

7. A physical therapist is seeing a patient with post-polio syndrome. The patient presents with bilateral weakness of dorsiflexors, quadriceps, and hip extensors. His left lower extremity tends to collapse with weight-bearing. First, the physical therapist performs gait training with a wheeled walker, but the patient still has difficulty with left leg collapse. What orthosis is appropriate for this patient?

   (A) Ankle-foot orthosis
   (B) Knee-ankle-foot orthosis
   (C) Hip-knee-ankle-foot orthosis
   (D) Knee immobilizer

8. A physical therapist is performing manual cervical traction on a patient with cervical pain, with the goal of temporarily increasing the patient's intervertebral joint space. What position of the neck is *BEST* to achieve this goal?

   (A) 5° flexion
   (B) 25° flexion
   (C) 45° flexion
   (D) Neutral

9. A patient is referred to physical therapy for preoperative gait training with crutches. The physical therapist measures the patient for the proper height of crutches. Ideally, the patient should have what position of the elbows when using the crutches?

   (A) Full elbow extension
   (B) 15 to 25° of elbow flexion
   (C) 45 to 55° of elbow flexion
   (D) Elbow hyperextension

10. A physical therapist is treating an athlete who has a diagnosis of turf toe due to hyperextension and valgus stress of the great toe. The physical therapist decides to use a taping technique in treating this patient. What is the purpose of taping in the treatment of turf toe?

   (A) Position the great toe in hyperextension and limit valgus stress
   (B) Limit great-toe terminal dorsiflexion and prevent valgus stress
   (C) Position the great toe in hyperextension and limit varus stress
   (D) Limit great-toe terminal dorsiflexion and prevent varus stress

11. Which one of the following pain control theories postulates that pain relief can come from stimulating the production and circulation of the body's natural painkillers: endorphins, enkephalins, serotonin, and dopamine?

   (A) Gate control theory
   (B) The hunting response
   (C) Endogenous opiate theory
   (D) Spinothalamic tract theory

12. Which one of the following types of electrical stimulation would be an example of a monophasic waveform?

   (A) Transcutaneous electrical nerve stimulation
   (B) Interferential current
   (C) Russian stimulation
   (D) Iontophoresis

13. A 27-year-old sustains a transtibial amputation due to a motorcycle accident. Immediately following the injury, the patient has severe edema of the residual limb. The physical therapist establishes a goal of independence with elastic bandage application to minimize edema. What method should be used to wrap the residual limb properly?

   (A) Circular wrapping
   (B) Proximal-to-distal wrapping
   (C) Light pressure throughout wrapping
   (D) Diagonal wrapping

14. A 45-year-old patient with a transfemoral amputation ambulates independently with a wide base of support and holds the affected lower extremity in abduction. What is the *MOST* likely prosthetic cause for this gait deviation?

    (A) Prosthesis is too short.

    (B) Prosthesis is too long.

    (C) Prosthesis is too big.

    (D) Prosthesis is too low at the medial wall.

15. Which one of the following types of electrical stimulation would be *MOST* appropriate to assist with pain and range of motion in a patient who has just had a CVA with resultant shoulder subluxation due to muscle dysfunction?

    (A) Transcutaneous electrical nerve stimulation

    (B) Interferential current

    (C) Neuromuscular electrical nerve stimulation

    (D) Russian stimulation

ANSWERS

1. **B.**

   The amount of pressure can range from 30 to 60 mm Hg for the upper extremities and 40 to 80 mm Hg for the lower extremities. Some recommendations include never exceeding the diastolic blood pressure due to possible occlusion.
   (Behrens, page 124)

2. **A.**

   Functional electrical stimulation can be used to assist with ankle dorsiflexion in an otherwise denervated tibialis anterior. It is most commonly used in patients with weakness due to a CVA.
   (Michlovitz, page 261)

3. **A.**

   A Chopart disarticulation disarticulates the talonavicular and calcaneocuboid joints.
   (Lusardi, page 579)

4. **D.**

   Solid ankle cushioned heel (SACH) foot is appropriate for persons at a household level of ambulation. SACH foot is inappropriate for those involved in high-level activity and those who plan to ambulate on uneven ground.
   (Lusardi, page 647)

5. **C.**

   The frequency of the ultrasound can be adjusted to 1 MHz or 3 MHz. For deeper tissues a frequency of 1 MHz is used, and for superficial tissues (1–3 cm) 3 MHz is recommended.
   (Behrens, page 60)

6. **A.**

   The purpose of the thoracolumbar orthosis prescribed for compression fracture management is to prevent spinal movement.
   (Lusardi, page 409)

7. **C.**

   A hip-knee-ankle-foot orthosis is appropriate for a patient with paraplegia.
   (Edelstein, page 82)

8. **B.**

   The optimal position for increasing intervertebral joint space is 25° of cervical flexion. Too much flexion can actually decrease joint space.
   (Behrens, page 105)

9. **B.**

   The handpiece height of the crutches should be positioned so that the elbows are flexed 15–25°.
   (Pierson, page 107)

10. **B.**

    In treatment of turf toe, taping is used to restrict terminal dorsiflexion and prevent valgus forces.
    (Nawoczenski, page 160)

11. **C.**

    The endogenous opiate theory indicates that endorphins, enkephalins, serotonin, and dopamine are naturally produced in the body and can provide pain-relieving effects that are both immediate and longer-lasting.
    (Behrens, page 13)

12. **D.**

    The monophasic waveform is unidirectional and carries a charge that is either from positive to negative or vice versa. There is no alternating current. Iontophoresis is the only such example listed as an answer choice.
    (Behrens, page 143)

13. **D.**

    The wrap should be on the diagonal, never circular, because circular wrapping tends to constrict. Wrapping should start distally and progress proximally and should have firm pressure distally, becoming less proximal.
    (Karacoloff, page 16)

14. **B.**

If the prosthesis is too long, the patient may abduct the leg to compensate.
(Karacoloff, page 169)

15. **C.**

Neuromuscular electrical nerve stimulation (NMES) can be used to strengthen the shoulder girdle and decrease the subluxation of the humeral head in the glenoid fossa. This, in turn, can decrease the associated pain and improve both range of motion and function.
(Michlovitz, page 260)

Safety Issues, Professional Responsibilities, Learning, and Research

9

The preceding chapters have discussed the basic knowledge that an entry-level physical therapist should possess, including foundational sciences, evaluation, differential diagnoses, and treatment interventions. This chapter integrates the physical therapist's role in ensuring the safety and protection of patients, other medical professionals, and the physical therapist him/herself. Physical therapists and other health-care professionals have legal and moral responsibilities that are important in every aspect of their practice. The patient's preferred style of learning and the therapist's best teaching methods to ensure maximal benefit of physical therapy are also discussed here. Finally, this chapter discusses the principles of research and evidence-based practice.

PROFESSIONAL RESPONSIBILITIES

Physical therapists practice according to the Code of Ethics set by the American Physical Therapy Association (APTA). As a physical therapist, you have obligations to the patient to do the following:

- Maintain proper education and licensure
- Adhere to local, state, and national rules and regulations
- Adhere to the American Physical Therapy Association Code of Ethics
- Maintain ethical compliance with rules of documentation and billing
- Maintain patient confidentiality and respect patient privacy at all times
- Avoid discrimination of any kind

MEDICAL PROFESSIONALS

Physical therapists work with a variety of health-care professionals. Included in this group are physical therapist assistants, occupational therapists, occupational therapy assistants, speech language pathologists, physicians, physician assistants, nurses, social workers, athletic trainers, exercise physiologists, and many others. Physical therapy aides and administrative staff also complement the work of physical therapists. It is important to know how these professionals contribute to the client's plan of care. Physical therapists work as part of an interdisciplinary health-care team to provide their clients with the highest quality of care.

Physical therapist assistants are capable of providing physical therapy to clients under the supervision and direction of a licensed physical therapist. The physical therapist should direct the assistant to perform specific procedural interventions that are within the assistant's scope of education, training, and experience. Physical therapy assistants are not qualified to perform evaluations, establish plans of care, or determine diagnoses of a client. Communication between the physical therapist and the assistant is key to maintaining proper and legal use of the assistant's talents and abilities. State regulations and licensure laws govern physical therapist assistants.

Physical therapy aides or technicians can also provide some ancillary services to the physical therapist. These positions are unlicensed; aides and technicians are typically provided with on-the-job training. Aides can provide support services such as cleaning of equipment, donning of orthoses and prostheses, patient preparation and transportation, setup of treatment modalities and assistive devices, and general clerical work.

Physicians, physician's assistants, and nurses work hand in hand with physical therapists throughout the continuum of care. These professionals are a source of referrals to physical therapy. To provide their clients with the highest quality of care, physical therapists must communicate reciprocally with all appropriate health-care professionals.

Direct access is a term meaning a client is able to access the services of a physical therapist without a referral from another health-care professional. Several U.S. states allow for direct access. Physical therapists should be aware of the direct-access requirements and regulations of the state in which they practice.

PROFESSIONAL LIABILITY

Physical therapists have professional liability and a legal responsibility to keep their patients safe. Even so, physical therapists have approximately a one in ten chance of being sued. The patient injuries that most frequently lead to litigation are:

- Fracture
- Hot pack burns
- Electrical/chemical burns
- Reinjury
- Soft-tissue injury
- Other injuries, not specified

At the time of injury, patients were involved in the following activities:

- Using heat/electrical modalities
- Exercise
- Manipulation
- Slips and falls

Physical therapists should be sure to monitor patients closely and to treat within their own scope of practice to avoid patient injury. Maintenance of equipment is important. Be sure to follow the physician's orders, and refer back to the physician as needed to avoid injuring the patient.

EMPLOYEE RIGHTS

Human resource offices provide employee assistance for legal issues such as sexual harassment and occupational safety and health.

Sexual Harassment

It is the right of any employee to be protected by its employer from sexual harassment. According to Title VII of the Civil Rights Act of 1964, the employee is protected against unwanted physical or verbal conduct of a sexual nature from another person of either sex that interferes with the work environment or the individual's ability to perform work-related tasks.

Occupational Safety and Health

The regulatory laws of the Occupational Safety and Health Act (OSHA) provide safety and health standards and regulations to protect the employee in the workplace. Some of the laws pertaining to health-care professionals include, but are not limited to, regulations on blood-borne pathogens; the use of personal protective equipment; and hazardous chemicals with regard to use, employee exposure, and storage.

PATIENT RIGHTS

Maintenance of patient autonomy or self-determination can be ensured in several ways. These include informed consent, the right to privacy, the Individuals with Disabilities Education Act (IDEA), the Americans with Disabilities Act (ADA), and mandatory reporting.

Informed Consent

In 1973, the American Hospital Association established the Patient's Bill of Rights. This states that the patient should be an active participant on the health-care team, as a part of his or her own treatment plan. Patients need to be informed about treatment and to provide consent to be treated. This is better known as informed consent. The APTA Standards of Practice for Physical Therapy state that the patient and/or family should be involved in establishing the treatment plan, in the treatment itself, and in any revision of the treatment plan. Patient input should be included during goal-setting, establishing a problem list, and modifying the treatment plan.

To obtain informed consent, the physical therapist should use plain language and explain the purpose(s), risks, and benefits of treatment or nontreatment; should offer alternative interventions; should discuss the patient's current health status; and should answer any questions the patient may have. Then informed consent should be documented. Often a signature of the patient or family member is obtained.

Right to Privacy

The privacy of patients and clients is protected by preventing disclosure of medical records or information without the consent of the individual. Enforcement of this rule began April 13, 2004, by the Office for Civil Rights of the Department of Health and Human Services.

Individuals with Disabilities Education Act (IDEA)

The Individuals with Disabilities Education Act (IDEA) governs services to children with disabilities that include early intervention and special education. Physical therapists provide early intervention and services in the schools to promote effective education of children with disabilities.

Americans with Disabilities Act (ADA)

The Americans with Disabilities Act (ADA) provides guidelines that were set by Congress in 1992 to require all new and renovated health-care facilities or buildings to provide handicapped accessibility for all patients. This access can include, but is not limited to, wheelchair-accessible restrooms and treatment rooms, larger parking spaces, ramps, and handrails, where necessary.

Mandatory Reporting

There is a legal and ethical obligation to report any suspicion of abuse or neglect of a child or dependent adult that the physical therapist may encounter. There may be different legal obligations in each U.S. state for mandatory reporting.

CLINICAL SAFETY AND INJURY PREVENTION

Hazard

A **hazard** is any situation for likely electrical injury. Physical therapy modalities and equipment should be inspected annually for safety, upkeep, and repair.

Line Voltage

Line voltage is any source of high electrical potential; for example, an electrical outlet. Normal leakage of an electrical device is referred to as **leakage current**.

Impedance

Impedance is the resistance to current flow. Excess current, as a safety mechanism, flows to a ground (literally, an electrical connection with the earth). The third prong on an electrical cord is usually the ground. Electrical shock occurs when electricity flows from a high source to a low source.

Ground Fault Circuit Interrupters

The electrical outlets in a clinic should be installed with **ground fault circuit interrupters (GFCIs)**. These compare the "hot" wire to the neutral wire to evaluate the amount of current that is flowing. These amounts should be equal. If they are more than 5 mA different, the GFCI shuts the outlet off to avoid electric shock and potential serious injury. The reset button is then used to turn the outlet back on.

Emergency Response to Electrical Shock

In an emergency, quick action by the physical therapist is key. If there is an electrical emergency, the response should be as follows:

1. Do not touch the person being electrocuted.
2. Disconnect the cord from the electrical outlet.
3. Use a piece of wood or other nonconducting material to push the person being electrocuted out of circuit.
4. Call EMS/911.
5. Initiate CPR.

Response to Fire

1. Rescue those in immediate danger; remove any other people from the area. If a person is on fire, use "stop, drop, and roll," or smother the flames with a blanket.
2. Alert EMS/911.

3. Contain the fire, if possible (i.e., remove nearby combustible materials, close the door to the room, etc.).
4. Extinguish the fire, if possible.

PATIENT POSITIONING, DRAPING, AND GENERAL SAFETY

It is important that you always respect a patient's privacy and maintain a safe environment during evaluation and treatment in any setting. This can be ensured by incorporating proper patient positioning, draping, and general safety techniques.

Patient Positioning

The patient should be positioned in a way that is comfortable for both the patient and the therapist or staff member. In side-lying, a pillow may be placed under the head and between the knees. In supine, a flattened pillow should be placed behind the head and under the knees for comfort. If it is necessary that the patient be prone, a pillow under the hips and under the feet maximizes comfort. Ideally, a facial cutout to maintain a neutral cervical position should be used while the patient is in prone. In all cases, if a high/low table or bed is available, it should be placed at a height that allows the physical therapist to work in a position with a neutral lumbar spine and with elbows in a slightly flexed position while avoiding knee hyperextension. To avoid the therapist being in potentially injurious positions of prolonged lumbar or thoracic flexion, the patient may move closer to one side of the bed temporarily. For patient safety, once treatment is completed he should return to the middle of the plinth or bed; the bed should then be lowered to its original setting to prevent the patient from falling off it from an elevated position.

Draping

Proper patient draping refers to the use of appropriate covering (clothing, sheets, towels, etc.) to shield the patient from cold, to prevent unexpected exposure to others, and to allow exposure of a specific body part for treatment.

General Safety

Other safety considerations during evaluation and intervention may include, but are not limited to, the use of a gait belt for fall prevention; the patient wearing shoes or nonslip socks; the use of support personnel for two-person assist transfers and gait training; and the proper monitoring of IV lines, catheters, feeding tubes, etc.

CARDIOPULMONARY RESUSCITATION

According to the American Heart Association, the most recent recommendations for cardiopulmonary resuscitation (CPR) by a health-care provider include the following.

- In the case of a sudden collapse, the health-care professional should first notify EMS/911, then retrieve an automatic external defibrillator (AED) and apply the AED as directed.
- Upon finding an unresponsive victim, the rescuer should provide two rescue breaths, then check for the pulse for ten seconds before beginning chest compressions.

- If there is a pulse, rescue breaths should be given at a ratio of 10–12 breaths per minute in the adult and 12–20 breaths per minute in the infant or child.
- In the case of a victim with an advanced airway, rescue breaths must be given at approximately 8–10 breaths per minute.
- A ratio of 30 compressions to two ventilations should be used for all single rescuers on all adult, child, and infant victims. A ratio of 15 compressions to two ventilations is recommended for all infant and child victims or in two-rescuer situations. If participating in two-person CPR, the rescuers should switch positions every two minutes, performing either compressions or ventilations.

BODY MECHANICS AND ERGONOMICS

For a physical therapist, utilization of proper mechanics with bending and lifting is essential to having a long and injury-free career.

- Stand with a wide base of support.
- Bend at the knees and hips, not the waist; bending at the waist increases lumbar or thoracic flexion.
- The therapist should keep his body close to the patient for a shorter lever arm, allowing less stress on the back. Keep equipment, therapist, and patient inside the base of support.
- Maintain a neutral lumbar spine.
- If movement is expected (i.e., transfers), stand with one foot slightly ahead of the other to stabilize and further widen the base of support.
- During movement, the therapist can position herself behind the object or subject to allow full view of the intended path and to maximize motor efficiency for lifting or pushing, as needed.
- Not only should therapy staff follow these guidelines, but these must also be shown to patients in all potentially injurious situations.
- In the sitting position (such as at a desk), the feet should be flat on the floor or on a footrest, with the individual's hips and knees bent to 90° each. At a computer workstation, the monitor should be set at a height that allows the individual to look directly at the screen with the head in a neutral position. The keyboard should be set at a position that allows the elbows to be flexed to 90° and the wrists to be in slight extension.

Adjustments to the body mechanics and ergonomics will have to be made depending on the task at hand. Maintaining the basic principles will prevent injury and maximize the body's efficiency.

INFECTION CONTROL PROCEDURES

Universal Precautions

Universal precautions are given by the Centers for Disease Control (CDC) to mandate how health-care workers should handle blood and bodily fluids with all patients and clients. The purpose is to protect against transmission of blood-borne disease.

All health-care workers are expected to wash their hands thoroughly with appropriate soap and water and dry the hands thoroughly before and after each patient interaction. Personal protective equipment (PPE) should be used as necessary and may include gloves, eye protection, gowns, hats, and/or shoe covers. Special care should be taken when using "sharps," equipment that could inadvertently puncture the skin.

Any open wound or lesion on the provider or patient needs to be covered properly to avoid contact and transmission of infection. Any equipment or material that comes into contact with blood or bodily fluid must be sterilized or disposed of properly in the appropriate hazardous material waste receptacle.

Standard Precautions

Standard precautions are in place to protect the health-care provider and the patient from any type of infectious transmission, whether blood-borne or otherwise (bodily fluid, air, droplet, etc.). These include all of the precautions listed above as universal precautions, plus the following:

- Health-care providers should use "cough etiquette" to prevent the spread of respiratory infection (cover the mouth during cough or sneeze, dispose of used tissue, etc.).
- Patient care areas and equipment that may come into contact with multiple patients should be properly cleaned.
- The use of a mouthpiece or guard during CPR is strongly encouraged.

DOCUMENTATION

Physical therapy documentation standards are set forth in the APTA's Guidelines for Physical Therapy Practice. The APTA defines documentation as "any entry into the client record, such as a consultation report, initial examination report, progress note, or flow sheet/checklist that identifies the care/service provided, re-examination, or summation of care." The physical therapist or physical therapist assistant who provides the care should sign the documentation.

Documentation Guidelines

- Handwritten documentation should be made in ink with the therapist's original signature.
- Document informed consent.
- Deletion of errors (i.e., with eraser, liquid correction fluid, etc.) is unacceptable. Use a single line through an error, with initials and date. If electronic documentation is used, mark errors with another appropriate method of identification.
- Include the client's name and identification number.
- Date and sign the therapist's name and designation (Physical Therapist, Physical Therapist Assistant, etc.).
- Co-signature of a licensed physical therapist is needed when a graduate or student of a physical therapy program does the documentation.
- Document the source of the referral (i.e., physician order or direct access).

Initial Evaluation Documentation

Initial documentation is expected with the onset of each episode of physical therapy and should include the following:

- History (including medical history, complaints, other treatments of same problem, comorbidities, and goals of the client)

- Review of systems of the body
- Objective tests and measures performed
- Evaluation, with clinical judgments
- Diagnosis
- Prognosis
- Goals
- Plan of care, including frequency, duration, and client involvement in the establishment of the plan of care
- Authentication (signature) and designation

Documentation of the Continuation of Care

Treatment interventions performed and client response to interventions should be included in the documentation. Documentation of each treatment—including client self-report, interventions provided, equipment provided, modification of interventions and reasons for the modification, and communication with the client—are all necessary components of documentation. Any reexamination, including interpretation of findings and changes in the plan of care and/or the goals, should also be included.

Summation and Discharge Documentation

At the end of the episode of physical therapy, documentation is required and should include the following elements:

- Criteria for discontinuation of physical therapy services
- Current status of the patient
- Status of goals, including reasons any goals were unmet
- Plan after discharge, including communication with client/family

SOAP Notes

The acronym SOAP stands for **S**ubjective, **O**bjective, **A**ssessment, **P**lan, and it gives the therapist a simple map to follow in documentation. The information that should be included in of each of these components is listed here.

S: Subjective

Subjective information is gained from interviewing the client and/or the client's family.

- Prior level of function
- Patient's goals
- Complaints
- Response to treatment
- Any other information that the client or family tells the therapist

O: Objective

Objective information is observable, measurable, and able to be repeated.

- Results of tests and measures performed by the physical therapist(s)
- Treatment provided to the client

- Education given to the client and/or client's family
- Chart review information

A: Assessment

- Physical therapy assessment of the client's problem(s)
- Short-term and long-term goals or outcomes, with time frames
- Address the client's progress toward goals due to physical therapy treatment

P: Plan

- Frequency and duration of physical therapy treatment
- Specific treatment approaches
- Discharge plans

Physical therapy goals

- Who will be involved (client, family)?
- What action(s) will be performed?
- What accommodations/assistance will be used?
- To what extent will action be performed (i.e., measurement)?
- What is the time frame in which the goal will be accomplished?

Goals are used to focus treatment toward functional outcomes; to measure treatment effectiveness; to revise treatment; to monitor progress; and to convey the client's goals of treatment to other therapists, assistants, and referral sources. Goals are often based on function and the client's own goals for treatment. For example, if the client needs help to move from supine to sit, a goal for independence with this action in a measurable time frame is appropriate.

Medicare initial evaluation and plan of treatment forms (forms 700, 701, and 702) are available. These forms include client data and most of the information listed above in a SOAP note.

COMMUNICATION

Physical therapists provide coordination, communication, documentation, client instruction, and procedural interventions. Coordination, communication, and documentation are integral components of this list. Coordination is defined as the responsibility of everyone who is involved in the client's care to work together. Communication is the exchange of information with the health-care team and the client/family. Documentation refers to entries to the client's chart or medical record.

Physical therapists are involved in expressive and receptive communication with clients, family, peers, and other health-care professionals. Physical therapists must communicate effectively during an examination, at discharge from therapy, when a change occurs in a client's plan of care, and in other situations.

Communication includes mandatory abuse reporting and patient advocacy. Physical therapists must communicate both expressively and receptively when involved in client-related instruction and coordination with other members of the health-care team.

NAGI DISABLEMENT MODEL

- **Disease:** Pathological condition that interrupts homeostasis and is demonstrated by signs and symptoms
- **Impairment:** Change in anatomic or physiologic structure or function
- **Functional limitation:** Limitation in performance that is a manifestation of an impairment. Examples are loss of range of motion and decreased strength.
- **Disability:** Limitation in performance of normal age-specific roles and tasks within the social or physical environment
- **Handicap:** Societal disadvantage of disability

INTERNATIONAL CLASSIFICATION OF FUNCTIONING, DISABILITY, AND HEALTH

The International Classification of Functioning, Disability, and Health (ICF) was developed by the World Health Organization. This classification divides health information into three levels: body structure and function, activities (tasks of an individual) and participation (involvement in life situations), and society level (information on environment and severity).

Impairment

An impairment is a deficit in body structure or function.

Activity limitation

Activity limitation was formerly called disability. This refers to an individual's partial inability to complete a task.

Participation restriction

Participation restriction was formerly called handicap. This is a restriction of an individual's involvement in life situations.

Disability

Disabilities include impairments, activity limitations, and participation restrictions.

LEARNING THEORIES AND TEACHING STRATEGIES

Much of what physical therapists do could actually be classified as teaching clients. Thus, physical therapists must be familiar with characteristics of learners and methods of teaching. Learning is defined as "the relatively permanent change in behavior that occurs as a result of practice." Teaching and learning are integral parts of many procedural interventions provided by physical therapists.

Learning

Learning is **specific**. People learn precisely what they are taught. Physical therapists must consider the physical and social environment in which the learning occurs.

Specificity of learning

Specificity of learning refers to the fact that the transfer and generalization of what is learned to different situations and environments is difficult. Patients learn specifically what they are taught. Specificity of learning must be addressed throughout the plan of care.

Transfer of learning

Transfer of learning means that what is learned in the clinical setting may or may not be done in other settings. The patient may be able to perform a task being taught in the clinic, but may not be able to perform the same task at home.

Generalization

Generalization of learning is defined as the client being able to perform a task that is similar to what is being taught. If a patient can perform a task that is related to the original task that was taught, the patient is capable of generalization.

Procedural Knowledge

Procedural knowledge is the knowledge of how to do something, including the sequence and set of components of the task.

Declarative Knowledge

Declarative knowledge is the knowledge of facts and information. At times a person can possess procedural knowledge but not declarative knowledge. The importance of each type of knowledge must be considered. Is it more important for a client to know how to do a task (procedural knowledge) or to be able to recite facts about the task (declarative knowledge)?

Explicit and Implicit Knowledge

Declarative knowledge is also known as **explicit knowledge**. **Implicit knowledge** includes procedural knowledge but also includes automatic behaviors and motor skills that have been learned. An example of implicit knowledge is the automatic adjustments a person makes in force production when picking an object up (i.e., how hard does the patient need to grasp something in order to maintain a grip on it?).

Practice

Motor learning refers to learning a motor task. This includes practice, organization, and feedback. Practice can be blocked together or random. An example of **blocked practice** is five repetitions of the first task, five repetitions of the second task, and so on. **Random practice** involves a less orderly sequence. Often blocked practice results in quicker achievement of the task but less preservation of the knowledge, whereas random practice results in improved preservation of knowledge but slower achievement of the task.

Feedback

Feedback is of major importance in learning. The learner has both internal and external feedback. **Internal feedback** is how the learner feels that he performed, whereas **external feedback** comes from an outside observer. One goal of therapy is for the internal feedback to approximate the external feedback, so the client can be correct in his assessments of his own performance.

Feedback can be constant, summary, faded, or client controlled. **Constant feedback** is given continuously and frequently. **Summary feedback** is provided only after a certain number of performances of the task. **Faded feedback** means feedback is provided frequently at first and then is decreased as learning occurs. In **client-controlled feedback**, feedback is provided only when requested by the client.

Learning Theories

Cognitive learning

The cognitive learning theory says that in order to learn, a person's cognition must be changed. Cognition includes a person's perception, thought, memory, processing, and organization of information. During learning, a person perceives the information, interprets the information based on past learning, and organizes it into new understanding. With the cognitive learning theory, reward is not required. Motivations toward learning, including the learner's goals, are important. Diverse personal factors must be accounted for during the learning and teaching process. Learners have different experiences, thoughts, goals, outlooks, and ways of processing information.

Behaviorist learning theory

Respondent conditioning and operant conditioning are largely the basis for behaviorist learning theory.

Respondent conditioning

Respondent conditioning takes a neutral stimulus and pairs it with a natural unlearned stimulus and unlearned response. After a few trials of the neutral stimulus paired with the unlearned stimulus, the neutral stimulus elicits the unlearned response. Learning has taken place and is often unknowingly or unconsciously done. This is classic **Pavlovian conditioning**.

Operant conditioning

Operant conditioning focuses on the behavior of the learner and the consequences that happen after the response. Applying a stimulus after the behavior can increase the probability that the desired behavior will be performed again and therefore will reinforce a behavior. Responses can be increased or decreased with this method. Behaviors can be decreased through penalty or nonreinforcement.

HEALTH BEHAVIOR CHANGE MODELS

Physical therapists use procedural interventions to cause behavior changes in their clients. There are many health behavior change models that conceptualize how people change their health behavior. These models help shape physical therapy interventions to encourage health-related change. Five health behavior change models are explained below.

Health Belief Model

The health belief model is one of the oldest models of behavior change. It accounts for why people decide to make changes and how to assist them in making those changes. The health belief model consists of five personal factors:

- Perception of the severity of the problem
- Perception of the threat or susceptibility of the problem
- Perception of the benefit of the health behavior change
- Perception of the barriers to changing the behavior
- Self-efficacy, or the person's perception of her own ability to make the change

The physical therapist's role in the health belief model is to provide education about the perceived threat and the benefits of the health behavior change. The physical therapist should also help to promote the client's self-efficacy. The health belief model is the predominant model used to explain the client's use or nonuse of preventative health services.

Transtheoretical Model

The transtheoretical model is also known as the **readiness to change model**. This model emphasizes that changing one's behavior is a process and occurs in stages. This model accounts for a person's readiness to change. It is helpful in designing procedural interventions for clients at different stages of change or readiness for change. The five stages are:

- Precontemplation: Not planning on change in the next six months
- Contemplation: Thinking of changing behavior, weighing the pros and cons
- Preparation: Preparing to change behavior in the next 30 days
- Decision or action: Implementation of changing behavior
- Maintenance of change

People do not move through these stages at the same rate or in the same sequence. Moving forward and backward between the stages is common, as is repeating several stages. The model is a continuum, and individuals can start or stop at any stage. Assessing a person's stage on this continuum and then choosing the procedural interventions that are appropriate for this stage are important in affecting change in the person.

The transtheoretical model includes three other variables. The first is a decisional balance: what are the pros and cons of the health behavior change? The second is: how confident is the person in his ability to change? The third is: what are the potential temptations that will threaten the behavior change?

Social Cognitive Theory

The social cognitive theory suggests that behavior is affected by a person's environment, by personal factors, and by the qualities of the behavior. Each of these affects and is affected by the others. This theory outlines several constructs of the learning process. Some of these constructs are:

- **Self-efficacy:** The person's belief in her own ability to change her behavior
- **Outcome expectations:** The outcome that a person expects with a change of behavior

- **Expectations:** The value that the person places on the result of the behavior change
- **Reinforcement:** Can be either positive or negative
- **Behavior capability:** The person's ability to learn the behavior and how to perform it
- **Reciprocal determinism:** The relationship between the person and his environment

Self-efficacy is of paramount importance in the social cognitive theory; a person's outcomes are affected by her environment, expectations, and beliefs. The social cognitive theory was formerly known as the social learning theory.

Theory of Reasoned Action

The theory of reasoned action focuses on the person's attitude toward the behavior and weighs that with his attitudes toward his social environment, peers, and influential persons. In this model, the person's attitudes toward the health behavior and toward important persons (or referents) are a better predictor of health behavior change than the person's attitude toward the outcome of the behavior.

Attribution Model

The attribution model of health behavior change assumes that individuals assign causes to events. Physical therapists must then help to increase an individual's control of events. This model emphasizes four attributes: locus of control, controllability, stability, and globality.

Locus of control

A person's locus of control can be either internal or external. Where does the individual believe her control is located?

Controllability

The controllability of the attribute refers to the behavior being in or out of the individual's control.

Stability

The stability or consistency of the attribute is an important attribute to consider, as the individual assigns causes to events.

Globality

Finally, does the individual feel that the event or behavior is generally applicable to other events or situations? What is its globality?

PRINCIPLES OF RESEARCH

Research Design

There are different methods of research and different research designs. Included in this group are three research paradigms: quantitative, qualitative, and single system. Clinical physical therapists should have an understanding of the types of research in order to critically examine research studies and literature. A **paradigm** is the assumptions and ideas that researchers use to direct their work. **Methods** are the techniques that researchers use to execute their studies.

Quantitative paradigm

The quantitative paradigm is the one most often used in traditional research. It relies on measurement, control groups, and reproducibility. Quantitative research assumes five basic axioms:

1. There is a single objective reality that can be determined and predicted or controlled. Research is aimed at empirically establishing rules of reality so that these rules can be used to predict or control reality.
2. Independence between the researcher and the subject is key to quantitative research. Objectivity is of utmost importance.
3. Quantitative research is thought to be generalizable. The outcome of the research can be applied to other situations and subjects.
4. Cause-and-effect relationships are established with quantitative research. Researchers manipulate independent and dependent variables while controlling all other factors to determine cause and effect.
5. Quantitative research is value-free, meaning that investigators do not influence the investigation with their opinions or beliefs.

Quantitative researchers begin with a working theory that is to be tested and then proved or disproved. A **theory** is a working model of principles and views of natural phenomena. It is able to be tested. Quantitative research establishes groups with inclusion and exclusion criteria. These are randomly assigned to experimental or control groups. Factors within the different groups are manipulated and controlled by researchers. Measurements are taken and numerical data is gathered.

Qualitative paradigm

The qualitative paradigm can be contrasted with the quantitative paradigm.

- Qualitative research maintains that multiple realities exist. Not only do multiple realities exist, but they are also shaded by how individuals attach meaning to their reality.
- In qualitative research, interdependence of the tester and the subject is inevitable and acceptable.
- The outcome of qualitative research is particular to the situation and subject and is not necessarily generalizable across different situations.
- Cause and effect cannot be established with qualitative research. Instead, description and interpretation of phenomena are established.
- Values of the researchers are inherent in the qualitative research design and experiment and therefore shade the outcomes.

Qualitative researchers do not begin with a theory to prove or disprove. A set of ideas and constructs are thought to be important, and the experiment and subjects add further realities. Subjects are not chosen on the basis of strict exclusion criteria, and groups are often smaller than those in quantitative research. Data that is collected is descriptive in nature and not numerical. The experimental groups are not manipulated or controlled by the researcher. Qualitative research occurs in a more natural setting, where influence from the researcher is part of the research design.

Single-system paradigm

Single-system research is also referred to as single-subject or single-case experimental design. It is much like the quantitative paradigm in the five axioms given above, however a single subject and setting are researched. The methods are also similar to quantitative research except for flexibility in the control of the experiment. This flexibility of the variables being studied can better approximate treatment given in the clinic.

Measurement Science

There are four standard levels of measurement: nominal, ordinal, interval, and ratio.

Nominal level

The nominal scale is a classification scale that assigns no value or order to the categories. Data is simply placed in categories that have no order. An example is grouping subjects together based on eye color.

Ordinal level

Ordinal scales possess order, but the distances between the categories are not necessarily equal. An example is minimum, moderate, and maximum levels of assistance.

Interval level

Interval scales possess order and equal distances between the intervals. Addition and subtraction are appropriate for this scale, but multiplication and division are not. An example is the Celsius scale of temperature.

Ratio level

Ratio scales possess order, distance, and a meaningful origin or true zero. All mathematical functions are appropriate for this scale. Examples include measurements of length, time, and weight.

Terminology of Measurement Science

- **Correlation coefficient:** Statistic of the level of relationship between two or more variables. The range of correlation coefficients is between 0.0 (no relationship) and 1.0 (perfect relationship). A negative correlation coefficient indicates an inverse relationship, and a positive correlation coefficient indicates a direct relationship.
- **Frequency distribution:** A count of the actual number of times that a specific measurement is found in the data set
- **Mean:** The average of a set of scores. This is calculated as the total of the scores divided by the number of scores.
- **Normal curve:** Standard bell-shaped curve that represents the numerical mean and distribution of standard deviations of a set of scores
- **Standard deviation:** Square root of the variance
- **Standard error of measurement:** Mathematical equation for establishing reliability between repeated measurements and the exact measurement being tested
- **Variance:** The degree of variation from the mean of a set of data. To calculate variance, first subtract the mean score from each score in the set. Then square each of those results. Finally, total these squares and divide by the number of scores in the data set.

Reliability

Reliability is the extent to which a measurement is dependable, repeatable, and accurate. Reliability conveys consistency and precision. There are different types of reliability.

Intra-rater reliability

Intra-rater reliability measures the reliability of one tester taking measurements on two occasions. Intra-rater reliability refers to how consistently a tester measures a variable.

Inter-tester reliability

Inter-tester reliability is the consistency between two or more testers in measuring a variable. Generally, intra-rater reliability is greater than inter-tester reliability. One tester measuring a variable more than once is more reliable than two or more testers measuring the same variable.

Instrument reliability

Instrument reliability refers to the accuracy of the instrument that is being used to measure a variable.

Intra-subject reliability

Intra-subject reliability is related to reproducibility of a performance by the same person on different occasions. For example, a person's knee flexion range of motion may be different at different times or on different days.

Validity

Validity is how well a test measures what it is used to measure. For example, the validity of a goniometer measuring knee flexion range of motion would depend on what the actual knee flexion is. Validity is specific to each instrument or test.

Common Statistical Methods

Descriptive statistics

Descriptive statistics organize and summarize data collected. Mean, median, standard deviation, and variance are descriptive. These statistics are used to describe a group using only one or two numbers.

Inferential statistics

Inferential statistics are used to determine if there are significant differences between groups, if groups are correlated, and if more than two variables can be compared. **Significant difference** is a statistic that identifies any statistically significant difference between two or more groups of measurement. **Tests for correlation** help to determine if one variable is related to another variable.

Outcome Measures

An outcome measure is defined as a measurement tool used to document change in one or more patient characteristics. Outcome measures are continually being researched for efficacy, and this relates directly to evidence-based practice. As the profession of physical therapy continues to make advances in the realm of research, evidence-based practice will come more to the forefront.

Suitability and Applicability

As a physical therapist, you must critically interpret research studies and determine if the study's outcomes are applicable to your own patients. Analyze the study's patient characteristics, including inclusion and exclusion criteria. Determine if the treatment and the treatment parameters used in the study can be replicated in the clinic. Also, consider the importance of the treatment outcomes researched in the study. A study of treatment interventions used for patients in the intensive care unit may not be applicable to a physical therapist who treats in an outpatient sports medicine setting.

Data Collection Techniques

Data can be collected via six methods: observation, interviews, surveys, records review, hardware instrumentation, and tests and measures.

Observation

Observation is used when the researcher looks at data objectively. Data can be observed in live subjects, video or audio recordings, and inanimate objects.

Interviews

Interviews with subjects can provide researchers with both verbal and nonverbal feedback. Interviews can be structured or unstructured and either face-to-face or by telephone.

Questionnaires and surveys

Questionnaires and surveys may include two different types of questions: closed-ended and open-ended. Closed-ended questions have a finite answer, such as a yes-or-no or multiple-choice answer. Open-ended questions have an infinite number of answers and wordings. Open-ended questions can allow for explanation of closed-ended answers.

Records review

Records review includes the obvious: a review of medical records. But this data collection technique also includes reviewing journals, machine readouts, audio/video recordings, and other physical material that is examined retrospectively.

Hardware instrumentation

Hardware instrumentation includes all instruments used to take measurements, such as goniometers, tape measures, and dynamometers.

Tests, measures, and inventories

Tests, measures, and inventories include child development stages, fine motor tests, and other physical or nonphysical scales. If a test is standardized, validity and reliability have been established in comparison to the population.

Hierarchy of Evidence

The hierarchy of evidence indicates the strength of evidence. The following list is ordered from the strongest form of evidence to the weakest:

1. **Randomized controlled trials:** The researcher controls the independent variable by randomly assigning subjects to a treatment group or control group. The researcher measures the dependent variable in a controlled setting.
2. **Cohort designs:** A prospective design that identifies subjects with a risk factor for the development of a condition, then follows them to establish which subjects develop the condition
3. **Case-control designs:** A retrospective design that identifies subjects with and without a specific condition and each group's exposure to supposed risk factors or causes
4. **Case study:** A nonexperimental design that follows a single case over time
5. **Expert opinion:** An opinion from a practitioner or researcher; the opinion is not based on scientific research and is not applied to a clinical setting. Included in this is anecdotal observation.

A FINAL WORD

To remain current in the methods and techniques of physical therapy and to provide evidence-based practice, the physical therapist must remain updated on current research. To provide patients with the finest level of care and safety, the therapist must also be cognizant of factors that affect the safety of patients, the physical therapist, and the therapist's staff. Finally, the physical therapist must be knowledgeable about different learning styles and teaching strategies that work best for each patient.

The next pages offer an end-of-chapter practice quiz to test your knowledge of some these principles. It is not necessary to time this, as it is a chapter review quiz.

Safety Issues, Professional Responsibilities, Learning, and Research Chapter Quiz

1. A researcher is studying edema following rotator cuff surgery. To eliminate error, the researcher has each subject measured in the same room, with the room being the same temperature each time, with the same lighting, same humidity, and same length of time of being in the room prior to measurement. The research is trying to eliminate what type of error?
   (A) Observer variability
   (B) Subject variability
   (C) Instrument variability
   (D) Environmental variability

2. A physical therapist provides feedback to a client who is performing several trials of a new, complicated lower-body exercise. The therapist provides the feedback after every third trial of the exercise. What type of feedback schedule is this physical therapist providing?
   (A) Constant feedback
   (B) Faded feedback
   (C) Client-controlled feedback
   (D) Summary feedback

3. A researcher decides to use an interview to study patients' attitudes about nursing homes. What is one disadvantage of using an interview for research?
   (A) An interview can obtain personal opinions of the subjects.
   (B) An interview can be guided by the interviewer based on responses of the subjects.
   (C) An interview can include the interviewer's personal views and biases.
   (D) An interview can establish a rapport with the subjects.

4. Borg's Rating of Perceived Exertion (RPE) scale is used to measure a person's rating of the amount of work that he or she is performing. It has descriptors such as very light, somewhat hard, and very hard; and it includes numbers that fit in with these descriptors. What is an advantage of using a scale such as the RPE?
   (A) Information is subjective in nature.
   (B) There is a tendency for each patient to give an above- or below-average rating.
   (C) There is an ease of use of the scale.
   (D) Elderly patients may have a difficult time rating exertion.

5. What learning theory focuses on changing the learner's thoughts, perceptions, and information processing?
   (A) Behaviorist learning theory
   (B) Cognitive learning theory
   (C) Social learning theory
   (D) Humanistic learning theory

6. A researcher uses inferential statistics to describe the results of his study. What is an example of inferential statistics?
   (A) Significant difference
   (B) Mean
   (C) Median
   (D) Range

7. A physical therapist is working with a 78-year-old patient, following a cerebrovascular accident. The patient is having difficulty remembering how to stand up from a chair. The physical therapist writes down four steps to instruct the patient on how to stand up, starting with "First, lock the brakes on your wheelchair." After studying the written directions, the patient is able to recite the four steps in order but is still unable to perform the task. What type of learning may be impaired in this patient?
   (A) Explicit learning
   (B) Implicit learning
   (C) New learning
   (D) Declarative learning

8. One outcome measure is a hand dynamometer. What type of measurement is the reading of pounds on the hand dynamometer?
   (A) Nominal
   (B) Ordinal
   (C) Interval
   (D) Ratio

9. Which health behavior change model incorporates a patient's readiness to change?
   (A) Health belief model
   (B) Theory of reasoned action
   (C) Transtheoretical model
   (D) Attribution model

10. A physical therapist working in a skilled nursing facility develops laryngitis. Most of her patients are able to read her lips and hand gestures to complete proper treatment. Some patients can read her written or visual cues. One of her patients, however, is a 75-year-old man who is legally blind and extremely hard of hearing. How should the therapist communicate with this patient?
   (A) Guide his extremities through passive range of motion only
   (B) Skip treatment
   (C) Have a coworker tell the patient to walk and perform exercise on his own
   (D) Ask another physical therapist to treat the patient until the laryngitis disappears

11. Which governing organization has been established to set regulations to protect workers and the public from the risk of exposure to infectious disease transmission through contact with blood-borne pathogens?
   (A) JCAHO
   (B) APTA
   (C) OSHA
   (D) CDC

12. A physical therapist is documenting information from a treatment session. The patient's active range of motion following manual stretching was 120° of flexion. Under which portion of the SOAP note does this information fit *BEST*?
   (A) Subjective
   (B) Objective
   (C) Assessment
   (D) Plan

13. Which one of the following situations does *NOT* fall under the umbrella of risk management?
   (A) A physical therapist observing signs and behaviors of domestic abuse in a patient
   (B) A tech injuring her back lifting a patient
   (C) A patient's spouse falling at the hospital
   (D) A patient straining her quad doing physical therapy exercises at home

14. The Equal Employment Opportunity Commission is a federal agency that was established to protect workers from discrimination in the workplace. Which of the following could be considered a type of discrimination?
   (A) A coworker sharing an off-color, gender-based joke
   (B) A physical therapist choosing a specific exercise based on its simplicity for a patient's home program
   (C) A patient requesting to see only a female physical therapist
   (D) A physical therapist requesting an interpreter to be present during treatment with a Hispanic patient

15. Which one of the following would be an appropriate short-term goal?

    (A) The patient should be dressing herself independently by the time she is discharged.

    (B) The patient should have 0–90° of active knee flexion within two weeks.

    (C) The patient should demonstrate an improved gait pattern within one week.

    (D) The patient should have less pain in her shoulder within two weeks.

Answers

1. **D.**

   Environmental variability refers to changes in the environment; for example, ambient temperature, humidity, lighting, and/or noise.
   (Helewa, page 62)

2. **D.**

   With summary feedback, external feedback is provided after a preset number of trials. This allows the patient to acquire some internal feedback and then compare it to the therapist-provided external feedback.
   (Christiansen, page 434)

3. **C.**

   An interview has the disadvantage of possibly including the interviewer's personal beliefs due to interaction between the subject and the interviewer.
   (Currier, page 123)

4. **C.**

   A scale is easy to use, is quick to use, and can offer a variety of choices.
   (Currier, page 127)

5. **B.**

   Cognitive learning theory emphasizes changes in thought processing, organization, and perceptions of the learner.
   (Bastable, page 50)

6. **A.**

   Inferential statistics are used to infer results obtained from a group of subjects for the population as a whole. Significant difference is an example of inferential statistics. Mean, median, and range are examples of descriptive statistics, which are used to summarize and organize data.
   (Currier, page 204)

7. **B.**

   Explicit learning is learning of facts and information, like declarative knowledge. This patient is able to recite a list from memory. Implicit learning is learning procedural knowledge like motor skills. It is implicit learning that is impaired in this patient.
   (Christiansen, page 430)

8. **D.**

   Weight in pounds is a ratio level of measurement. The distance between 1 lb and 2 lb is the same as the interval between 20 lb and 21 lb. There is a true zero point.
   (Currier, page 89)

9. **C.**

   The transtheoretical model lists five stages of change: precontemplation, contemplation, preparation, action, and maintenance. It is also called the readiness to change model.
   (Christiansen, page 425)

10. **D.**

    Coordination, communication, and documentation are integral components of physical therapy. The patient and the physical therapist need to be able to interact maximally to achieve maximal benefit of physical therapy.
    (Guide, page S100)

11. **C.**

    OSHA, the Occupational Safety and Health Administration, is responsible for the procedural establishment of working with and handling bloodborne pathogens.
    (Gabard, page 215)

12. **B.**

Information gathered, such as range of motion or any other objective measures, should be entered under the objective portion of the note. Skilled interpretations of a patient's response to treatment should be written under the assessment portion of the note.
(Shamus, page 35)

13. **D.**

Risk management is in place to identify and prevent the risk of harm or injury to patients, staff, and visitors in the health-care organization. The patient's home exercise program is the only choice given that is not an example of a situation addressed by risk management; the other three choices do fall under risk management. The provider should make sure the patient is performing exercise appropriately at home.
(Nosse, page 259)

14. **A.**

Any kind of gender-based or off-color joke can be considered sexual harassment, which is a form of discrimination in the workplace based on gender.
(Nosse, page 263)

15. **B.**

Short-term goals should be objective and usually should be met within several visits—up to four weeks, depending on the total treatment duration. These goals do not need to be functional but should be measurable. Choices C and D are not easily quantified or measured; particularly, choice C is not specific enough.
(Shamus, page 129)

PART IV

Practice Tests

Instructions

You have 5 hours to complete the National Physical Therapy Examination. The exam consists of 250 questions, divided into 5 sections. Once you complete one section, you cannot return to any previous section. Be sure to answer each question and review your answers before moving on to any subsequent section. Good Luck!

Exam 1

Section 1

1. A physical therapist is treating a patient in a nursing home with ROM and gait training, following knee surgery. Today, the patient refuses physical therapy, stating she is in too much pain. The physical therapist informs the patient of the benefits of treatment and the risks of missing treatment, but the patient still refuses. What would be the therapist's *MOST* appropriate action?

   (A) Continue on with ROM only, since the patient refuses further treatment

   (B) Explain to the patient she is making a big mistake, and leave the room

   (C) Discharge the patient

   (D) Document the refusal and try again later

2. A physical therapist is performing manual cervical traction on a patient. The patient's head is known to weigh approximately 10 lb. Since the therapist is holding the patient's head, the coefficient of friction is nearly 0. What amount of force should the physical therapist apply to achieve joint distraction?

   (A) 5 lb

   (B) 10 lb

   (C) 15 lb

   (D) 25 lb

3. A patient referred to physical therapy has been diagnosed with pulmonary edema. What is the *BEST* description of pulmonary edema?

   (A) Output from the right side of the heart is greater than output from the left side of the heart, resulting in accumulation of fluid in the lungs.

   (B) Output from the left side of the heart is greater than output from the right side of the heart, resulting in accumulation of fluid in the lungs.

   (C) Output from the left side of the heart is greater than output from the right side of the heart, resulting in edema in extremities.

   (D) Output from the heart is minimal and results in accumulation of fluid in the heart itself.

4. A patient has been referred to physical therapy for evaluation and treatment of knee pain. The patient is also undergoing chemotherapy for breast cancer. Which of the following treatment interventions would *NOT* be appropriate for this patient?

   (A) Cryotherapy

   (B) Cycling for 20 minutes at 50 percent max heart rate

   (C) Joint mobilization to the tibia-femoral joint

   (D) Moderate-resistance strength training

5. A physical therapist is instructing a patient in proper body mechanics when lifting a 40 lb box of paper from the floor to the desk. When attempting to lift the box, the patient should follow which of the following principles of mechanics?

   (A) Wide base of support, bend at the waist, neutral spine
   (B) Wide base of support, bend at the knees, neutral spine
   (C) Wide base of support, bend at the knees, slight increase in lumbar lordosis
   (D) Narrow base of support, bend at the knees, slight increase in lumbar lordosis

6. A patient presents to physical therapy with difficulty with gait. Upon inspection of the skin of the lower extremities, the physical therapist finds dark-brown staining of the skin. The patient complains of leg pain that worsens throughout the day. There is edema of bilateral lower extremities. The skin is moist to the touch through the lower extremities. The physical therapist takes a thorough health history, in which the patient relates that she has had a deep vein thrombosis in the past. The physical therapist places the patient at risk for what type of wound?

   (A) Pressure ulcer
   (B) Arterial ulcer
   (C) Venous ulcer
   (D) Neoplastic ulcer

7. A researcher is writing a questionnaire that is to be sent to patients after discharge from outpatient physical therapy. The researcher would like to use open-ended questions in the questionnaire. Which of the following is an example of an open-ended question?

   (A) Did you have a good outcome following physical therapy?
   (B) Did your symptoms improve due to your physical therapy?
   (C) Did physical therapy help to decrease your pain?
   (D) How have your symptoms changed since you first were seen by a physical therapist?

8. A physical therapist is evaluating a woman who has mid-scapular pain that began when her body shape went through pregnancy-related changes. Which of the following components of posture is the correct change during pregnancy?

   (A) Base of support narrows.
   (B) Center of gravity moves posterior.
   (C) Weight-bearing shifts toward the heels of the feet.
   (D) The plumb line for posture moves posterior.

9. A physical therapist is helping an orthotist cast a mold for an ankle-foot orthosis. Which of the following is the correct position for the foot?

   (A) Subtalar neutral
   (B) Subtalar inversion
   (C) Subtalar eversion
   (D) Dorsiflexion

10. A patient who lives in a senior retirement village is having trouble with recurrent bladder infections. Her physician has recommended a referral to physical therapy for evaluation of muscle imbalance contributing to the infections. Which of the following muscles, when displaying soft-tissue tightness, can contribute to increased urinary frequency and urgency?

   (A) Quadriceps
   (B) Hamstrings
   (C) Quadratus lumborum
   (D) Obturator internus

11. A physical therapist is assisting the front desk in filling out paperwork before patient appointments. He is presenting paperwork regarding informed consent to each patient to allow physical therapy evaluation and intervention. For which one of the following patients is the informed consent done legally?

   (A) The Hispanic patient who reads no English
   (B) The patient who is unable to communicate
   (C) The patient who is 17 years old
   (D) The patient who does not have insurance

12. A patient has been referred to physical therapy with shoulder pain and a diagnosis of chronic rotator cuff tendonitis. Prior to the referral, the patient received his third injection of hydrocortisone. Which of the following is *NOT* a physiologic effect of hydrocortisone on the body?

(A) Decreases bone formation

(B) Delays healing

(C) Decreases the inflammatory response

(D) Decreases the muscle's ability to contract

13. A physical therapist is evaluating a patient in the hospital 24 hours after a right total hip replacement. The physician's orders are for gait training. On evaluation of the patient in his bed, the physical therapist notes redness and edema present in the right calf. The patient complains of pain and tightness there also. What plan of action should the therapist take?

(A) Assisting the patient to sit at the edge of bed, and reassessing the pain

(B) Postponing gait training for the time being and checking back later that day

(C) Assisting the patient to sit at the edge of bed, and performing gait training with a walker

(D) Notifying the patient's nurse of the findings, and postponing any activity

14. A physical therapist has chosen to issue a TENS unit for home pain management. According to the gate control theory, electrical stimulation affects large sensory nerve fibers to decrease the awareness of pain. If treatment is successful, how long after treatment do the analgesic effects of TENS last?

(A) Up to 30 minutes

(B) 30–60 minutes

(C) 2–6 hours

(D) 24 hours

15. An outpatient physical therapist is treating a patient after a cerebrovascular accident. A patient presents with weakness of the left side and difficulty maintaining dynamic sitting balance. The therapist decides to have the patient perform a proprioceptive neuromuscular facilitation technique of D1 flexion and extension. What is the starting position of D1 flexion when used for the left upper extremity?

(A) Left elbow flexion, shoulder flexion and adduction

(B) Left elbow extension, shoulder extension and abduction

(C) Left elbow flexion, shoulder extension and adduction

(D) Left elbow extension, shoulder flexion and abduction

16. A patient is being seen for physical therapy evaluation and treatment three days post–ACL reconstruction with a hamstring graft. Which of the following would be the *MOST* appropriate home exercise program to give this patient on his initial surgical follow-up visit?

(A) Quad sets and straight leg raises

(B) Heel slides and quad sets

(C) Heel slides and short arc quad exercise

(D) Heel slides and wall squats to 90°

17. What is an example of declarative knowledge?

(A) The temperature of the pool is 82°F.

(B) To get into the pool, walk down the steps.

(C) To tread water, alternate upper- and lower-extremity motion.

(D) To test the temperature of the water, look at the thermometer that is tied to the ladder rail.

18. A physical therapist is evaluating a woman who is 20 weeks pregnant. He suspects she may have a cervical disc herniation. Which of the following diagnostic tests is *NOT* contraindicated during pregnancy?

(A) Plain X-ray

(B) Computed tomography scan

(C) Magnetic resonance imaging

(D) Magnetic resonance imaging with contrast

19. A physical therapist is explaining to a patient the mechanics of glenohumeral joint impingement. What role does the rotator cuff play in lessening the occurrence of shoulder impingement?

    (A) Provides an inferior pull on the humeral head
    (B) Provides a superior pull on the humeral head
    (C) Provides an anterior pull on the humeral head
    (D) Aids in humeral elevation

20. A physical therapist is treating a patient for low back pain using interferential current (IFC). When administering the IFC for sensory level pain management, what sensation should the patient be expected to feel?

    (A) No sensation at all
    (B) Strong, comfortable tingling
    (C) Strong, noxious tingling
    (D) Strong muscular contraction

21. A physical therapist is examining a patient that he suspects may have nerve root irritation. When performing manual muscle testing, what is the *BEST* way to identify myotomal weakness?

    (A) Hold the contraction for five seconds
    (B) Hold the contraction for ten seconds
    (C) Hold the contraction for three seconds
    (D) Hold the contraction until it breaks

22. A physical therapist is working with a patient in a home health setting. The physical therapist is treating a patient who has had a recent myocardial infarction. During the physical therapist's second treatment with the patient, the patient starts to complain of severe chest pain, then becomes diaphoretic and weak. The physical therapist calls 911. Which drug (if prescribed and available to the patient) should the patient take in this situation?

    (A) Corticosteroid
    (B) Diuretic
    (C) Nitroglycerin
    (D) Drugs are contraindicated in this situation.

23. A physical therapist is treating a patient following a cerebrovascular accident with left-sided hemiplegia. The patient complains of pain in the left upper extremity. The therapist examines the shoulder and finds the humerus to be inferiorly displaced within the glenoid fossa. The patient's complaints of pain decrease with superior pressure on the humerus. What does the therapist suspect is the patient's problem?

    (A) Increased tone
    (B) Shoulder subluxation
    (C) Complex regional pain syndrome
    (D) Upper extremity edema

24. A patient is seen by a physical therapist following a contusion injury to the hand. The patient describes the pain as "sharp and pricking" and well localized to the dorsum of his hand. Which peripheral neuron relays localized sharp pain sensation?

    (A) C fibers
    (B) A-beta fibers
    (C) A-delta fibers
    (D) A-gamma fibers

25. What is the thickest layer of the heart wall called?

    (A) Epicardium
    (B) Pericardium
    (C) Myocardium
    (D) Endocardium

26. A patient in a skilled nursing facility has a stage II pressure ulcer on her mid-thoracic spine. The wound has no exudate and no necrotic tissue. The physical therapist performs wheelchair positioning and supplies the patient a back cushion to prevent pain and further skin breakdown. The physical therapist recommends the use of a hydrocolloid on this wound. What purpose is the hydrocolloid serving in this patient?

    (A) Exudate absorption
    (B) Treatment of infection
    (C) Mechanical debridement
    (D) Protection of the wound from contamination

27. What does an ECG measure?

    (A) Electrical activity of the heart
    (B) Electrical activity of the brain
    (C) Electrical activity of the entire body
    (D) Electrical activity of the skin

28. A 62-year-old male has been referred to physical therapy for evaluation and treatment of adhesive capsulitis. He is generally deconditioned and clinically obese. When asked about any other recent changes in his health, he admits that his vision has been blurred and that he also gets occasional numbness in his feet. What differential diagnosis could explain this presentation?

    (A) Full-thickness rotator cuff tear
    (B) Urinary tract infection
    (C) Type II diabetes mellitus
    (D) Type I diabetes mellitus

29. A physical therapist is hired at a hospital to start a pulmonary rehab program. One decision she has to make is what tests and measures the team will use to assess and monitor each patient. She decides that blood pressure, heart rate, and oxygen saturation will be checked every five minutes during exercise. What other tool could she use to determine how hard the patients are working during their exercise sessions?

    (A) Arterial blood gas
    (B) Borg's Rating of Perceived Exertion
    (C) Pitting edema scale
    (D) Lung volume testing

30. A physical therapist is designing a strengthening program for a patient who is able to bench press 225 lb in a predetermined ten-repetition maximum (10-RM). According to the Oxford technique, what should his lifting regimen be?

    (A) Ten reps 225 lb, ten reps 170 lb, ten reps 112 lb
    (B) Ten reps 112 lb, ten reps 170 lb, ten reps 225 lb
    (C) Ten reps 225 lb, eight reps 170 lb, four reps 112 lb
    (D) Ten reps 112 lb, eight reps 170 lb, four reps 225 lb

31. A physical therapist working in a pulmonary rehab clinic notices that when completing the stepping exercise, a patient always holds onto the rail next to the steps. The protocol for the clinic is that the patient should not hold onto the rail. The patient, however, insists on holding the rail for support. What is the appropriate response from the physical therapist?

    (A) Discharging the patient from the program
    (B) Not allowing the patient to complete the stepping activity unless he performs it without using the rail
    (C) Asking the patient to perform the stepping activity for a longer period of time, since he is holding the rail
    (D) Allowing the patient to continue with the use of the rail, offering standby assistance, and assessing the need for an assistive device

32. A physical therapist tests a patient's cranial nerves. What nerve is the physical therapist testing by asking the patient to perform different facial expressions and to close the eyes?

    (A) Cranial nerve VI
    (B) Cranial nerve VII
    (C) Cranial nerve VIII
    (D) Cranial nerve IX

33. A physical therapist is evaluating a patient who has left hip pain. On evaluation, the therapist notices that during the manual muscle test for hip flexion, the patient is initially able to hold against maximal resistance for three seconds. There is no pain with this testing. What could this finding indicate?

    (A) Muscle strain of the iliopsoas complex
    (B) L3 nerve root involvement
    (C) Hip joint pathology
    (D) L4 nerve root involvement

34. An infant normally demonstrates a positive Babinski sign. What is the stimulus for this reflex?

(A) Stroking the lateral part of the sole of the foot from the heel to the ball and then across the ball of the foot

(B) Stroking the medial part of the sole of the foot from the heel to the ball several times

(C) Stroking the Achilles tendon with a reflex hammer

(D) Stroking the plantar surface of the foot from the distal tibia to the toes along the medial side

35. A child is referred to physical therapy for evaluation and treatment of acute-onset knee pain. He does not recall any injury and says he has not even participated in physical education class at school for the last week due to restrictions from recent removal of his wisdom teeth. On evaluation, he has localized erythema, tenderness just above the patella, and localized edema. He has also been running a low-grade fever. What primary pathology may be causing his knee pain?

(A) Patellofemoral pain

(B) Osteomyelitis

(C) Osteoarthritis

(D) Osgood-Schlatter syndrome

36. An infant is born with a vertebral abnormality of the lumbar spine that is covered by a cyst. The cyst contains part of the spinal cord. What is the term that describes this condition?

(A) Meningocele

(B) Myelomeningocele

(C) Anencephaly

(D) Encephalocele

37. A physical therapist is evaluating a high-school pitcher who is having right shoulder pain during the deceleration phase of his throw. Which muscle group must be strengthened to assist with decelerating the shoulder during a throw?

(A) Deltoid and pectoralis

(B) Deltoid and latissimus dorsi

(C) Supraspinatus, infraspinatus, subscapularis, and teres minor

(D) Triceps, deltoid, and latissimus dorsi

38. Following a traumatic brain injury, a patient suffers from ataxia. How is ataxia defined?

(A) Lack of movement

(B) Weakness of one side of the body

(C) Slow movement

(D) Uncoordinated movement

39. During treatment for selective debridement of a necrotic wound, a physical therapist should remove which type of tissue?

(A) Granulation tissue

(B) Slough

(C) Pink or red tissue

(D) Macerated tissue

40. A physical therapist is treating a patient with left-sided C4 facet impingement. She plans to use manual cervical traction to attempt to open the left facet. Which position of the cervical spine would maximally open the left facet?

(A) Flexion, left side-bending, left rotation

(B) Flexion, left side-bending, right rotation

(C) Flexion, right side-bending, left rotation

(D) Flexion, right side-bending, right rotation

41. A patient is referred to physical therapy following a class 3 complete neurotmesis of the radial nerve. The patient asks the physical therapist, "Will my wrist ever work again?" What should be the physical therapist's response?

(A) "Yes, I expect full recovery of your strength and sensation. You will have full return of wrist function."

(B) "I expect that you will recover some of your strength and sensation. You will regain some of your wrist function."

(C) "No, you will have no return of your strength and sensation. You will not have any function of your wrist."

(D) "I anticipate that you may have no to minimal return of the strength and sensation of your wrist, but I anticipate that you will be able to gain some function of your wrist with continued physical therapy."

42. A physical therapist is designing an exercise program. Which of the following motions would be an example of an econcentric muscle exercise?

(A) Resisted elbow flexion
(B) Resisted elbow extension while flexing
(C) Resisted elbow flexion with the shoulder extended
(D) Resisted elbow flexion with the shoulder flexed

43. A 22-year-old construction worker spends most of his workday outdoors in high humidity and high heat. A physical therapist is contacted to give the construction worker and his crew some education on skin protection. The physical therapist talks about the skin's functions. Thermoregulation is achieved through many mechanisms; but in the heat, what are the main mechanisms that dissipate heat?

(A) Dilatation of skin blood vessels and decrease in sweat production
(B) Constriction of skin blood vessels and decrease in sweat production
(C) Dilatation of skin blood vessels and increase in sweat production
(D) Constriction of skin blood vessels and increase in sweat production

44. A physical therapist uses functional training in the treatment of a patient with neurological impairments. What is the *BEST* example of functional training?

(A) Demonstration, instruction, and performance of bed mobility
(B) Performance of ten repetitions of knee extensions while sitting with 1 lb ankle weight
(C) Sitting on a stability ball for ten minutes with minimum assistance
(D) Active assistive D1 upper-extremity flexion pattern

45. A patient with a right transtibial amputation and prosthesis ambulates with excessive knee flexion at the right knee. What is the *MOST* likely intrinsic cause of this gait deviation?

(A) Excessive hip extension
(B) Knee flexion contracture
(C) Knee cruciate ligament insufficiency
(D) Instability of the knee joint

46. A patient is referred to physical therapy after rupture of the transverse ligament of the shoulder. What structure is held in place with an intact transverse humeral ligament?

(A) Supraspinatus tendon
(B) Triceps tendon
(C) Infraspinatus tendon
(D) Biceps tendon

47. A health behavior change model purports that a person progresses and fluctuates through six stages of change: precontemplative, contemplative, preparation, action, maintenance, and termination. Which health behavior change model does this describe?

(A) Transtheoretical model (stages of change model)
(B) Health belief model
(C) Social cognitive theory
(D) Theory of reasoned action

48. A patient is evaluated in the hospital for a knee injury following a fall on the ice. During the acute inflammatory process, what is the role of prostaglandin?

(A) Vasoconstrictor
(B) Maintains the acid-base balance
(C) Dissolves clots
(D) Vasodilation

49. An outcomes measure is a measurement tool used to establish change in a patient trait over time. What is one example of an outcomes measure?

(A) Berg Balance Scale
(B) Proprioceptive neuromuscular facilitation
(C) Neurodevelopmental treatment
(D) Craniosacral therapy

50. A patient has just finished physical therapy treatment and is leaving the facility when she slips on a patch of ice in the parking lot and lands on her knee. When asked if she is hurt, she responds, "I'm fine," and walks toward her car. What is the appropriate action for the physical therapist to take?

(A) Document the patient's fall in a SOAP note
(B) Fill out an incident report
(C) Immediately send the patient to the emergency department to rule out any major trauma
(D) Since the patient feels fine, no action is necessary.

End of Section 1

IF YOU FINISH BEFORE TIME IS CALLED, YOU MAY CHECK YOUR WORK ON THIS SECTION ONLY. DO NOT TURN TO ANY OTHER SECTION IN THE TEST. **STOP**

Section 2

51. A physical therapist is performing an active range of motion assessment of the lumbar spine. During active flexion, what accessory motion is happening at the facet joints?

(A) Both sides open.

(B) Both sides close.

(C) The left side opens, the right side closes.

(D) The right side opens, the left side closes.

52. A five-year-old boy demonstrates these signs and symptoms: weakness of the shoulder and hip girdles, contractures, scoliosis, and respiratory impairments. The boy's mother states that he began walking much later than his older brother did. What pathology do you suspect?

(A) Parkinson's disease

(B) Osteogenesis imperfecta

(C) Guillain-Barré syndrome

(D) Duchenne muscular dystrophy

53. A physical therapist is assessing a patient's ankle edema with volumetric water displacement. The volume of the water displaced on the initial assessment was 17 oz. Two weeks later the volume displaced was 19 oz. What does this indicate?

(A) Ankle edema has increased.

(B) Ankle edema has decreased.

(C) Ankle edema has remained the same.

(D) Unable to assess a change in edema with these measures.

54. A physical therapist is reviewing the past medical history of a home health patient he is going to evaluate. The physician's referral indicates she has multi-joint pain, decreased functional mobility, and decreased lung function. Which of the following secondary pathologies could be considered a disorder that affects multiple body systems?

(A) Rheumatoid arthritis

(B) Osteoarthritis

(C) COPD

(D) Fibromyalgia

55. A patient presents to physical therapy with diagnosis of a countercoup head injury. Her hearing is impaired and she has difficulty understanding spoken communication. Which lobe of the cerebral cortex is *MOST* likely injured?

(A) Frontal lobe

(B) Parietal lobe

(C) Temporal lobe

(D) Occipital lobe

56. A physical therapist is designing a home exercise program for a patient with chronic knee pain. The patient also has a past medical history of irritable bowel syndrome (IBS). What is the physical therapist's recommendation for moderate-intensity exercise for this patient?

    (A) Exercise only when symptoms of IBS are absent.
    (B) Exercise only when symptoms of IBS are present.
    (C) Exercise regularly whether or not symptoms are present.
    (D) Moderate-intensity exercise is not recommended for this patient.

57. A woman is referred to physical therapy for pelvic floor muscle strengthening to aid in urinary incontinence. She describes her incontinence as being stress-related and reports that she cannot get to the bathroom in time. She is unfamiliar with pelvic floor exercise. Teaching the patient to feel which muscles need to contract to slow or stop the flow of urine is an example of what kind of activity?

    (A) Motor learning
    (B) Resistive strengthening
    (C) Eccentric loading
    (D) Proprioception

58. A physical therapist has given six treatments to a woman with rotator cuff tendonitis. She does not appear to be responding as expected to the intervention techniques. When asked about other symptoms, she describes a slight tremor, weight loss (although hungry), poor coordination, and unusual swelling in the front of her neck. What underlying pathology may be contributing to her wrist pain and stiffness?

    (A) Hypothyroidism
    (B) Hyperthyroidism
    (C) Hyperparathyroidism
    (D) Addison's disease

59. A patient demonstrates 0/5 strength of the left tibialis anterior muscle. She ambulates with a steppage gait of the left lower extremity. The patient has had recent surgery of the left hip. She had a prolonged course of bed rest in which her left leg was held in abduction and external rotation. She does not complain of any pain of the left lower leg. With what condition is this patient presenting?

    (A) Deep vein thrombosis
    (B) Compartment syndrome
    (C) Injury to the common peroneal nerve
    (D) Ankle fracture

60. A patient who calls himself a "weekend warrior" is being evaluated by a physical therapist after he injured his right ankle while sliding into third base two days ago. He states he immediately iced the ankle for one hour after his injury and then one hour again later that night. Today he complains of pain and numbness on the lateral side of his right foot. On evaluation, he is found to have weakness with ankle aversion but no pain. What is the *MOST* probable cause of this patient's presentation?

    (A) First-degree anterior talofibular ligament sprain
    (B) Distal fibular fracture
    (C) Peroneal nerve anastomosis
    (D) Talocrural dislocation

61. A patient with a complete spinal cord needs preservation of what motion to use tenodesis grasp to replace active grasping?

    (A) Wrist extension
    (B) Wrist flexion
    (C) Elbow flexion
    (D) Elbow extension

62. A physical therapist is positioning a patient for mechanical cervical traction. What position of the neck provides the greatest amount of intervertebral foraminal separation?

    (A) 25° flexion
    (B) 45° flexion
    (C) Neutral
    (D) 5° extension

63. A five-year-old boy demonstrates these signs and symptoms: weakness of the shoulder and hip girdles, contractures, scoliosis, and respiratory impairments. The boy's mother states that he walked much later than his older brother did. What pathology do you suspect?

(A) Parkinson's disease
(B) Osteogenesis imperfecta
(C) Guillain-Barré syndrome
(D) Duchenne muscular dystrophy

64. A physical therapist is evaluating a patient following a shoulder scope. The patient's medication list includes recent short-term use of a corticosteroid. What impact does this have on the patient's outcome?

(A) It will expedite the healing process.
(B) It will offer better pain relief after the surgery.
(C) It will allow the patient to tolerate aggressive passive range of motion by the therapist.
(D) It will increase the risk of infection at the scope/surgical site.

65. A patient presents to physical therapy with cervical and upper thoracic pain following a motor vehicle accident five weeks ago. She says the pain is much less than it was initially but that she has nagging tightness in her mid-scapular region and neck. Which response to pain could account for her complaints?

(A) Muscle weakness
(B) Muscle guarding
(C) Localized edema
(D) Joint hypomobility

66. A patient is referred to physical therapy for right buttock and posterior leg pain. Even before any assessment, the physical therapist makes a mental list of possible differential diagnoses. Which of the following would *NOT* be on the therapist's list?

(A) L5 nerve root irritation
(B) L4 facet irritation
(C) L5 facet irritation
(D) L4 nerve root irritation

67. A physical therapy school keeps track of the states in which applicants live. This data would be classified as what level of measurement?

(A) Nominal
(B) Ordinal
(C) Interval
(D) Ratio

68. A physical therapist is evaluating a patient with shoulder pain. Evaluation reveals decreased scapulothoracic motion during active flexion on one side more than the other. What is the normal ratio of glenohumeral to scapulothoracic joint motion of the shoulder?

(A) 3:1
(B) 1:1
(C) 2:1
(D) 1:3

69. A physical therapist provides education on lung disease to a freshman health class at a local college. The physical therapist describes chronic obstructive pulmonary disease (COPD) and the risk factors for developing this disease. What should the physical therapist tell the students is the biggest risk factor for developing COPD?

(A) Sedentary lifestyle
(B) High blood pressure
(C) Obesity
(D) Cigarette smoking

70. A physical therapist is developing an exercise program focused on endurance training of postural stabilizers. Which one of the following is *NOT* considered to be primarily a postural stabilizer made of mostly type I muscle fibers?

(A) Tibialis anterior
(B) Rhomboids
(C) Deep cervical flexors
(D) Gastrocnemius

71. A patient is referred to physical therapy for evaluation and treatment of right-sided low back pain with radiculopathy to the anterolateral thigh. Her radicular pain is reduced with manual lumbar traction. Where would be the *BEST* area to apply the ultrasound using a 5 cm sound head?

    (A) Over a 20 cm area of her lateral thigh
    (B) Over a 10 cm area of her lateral thigh
    (C) Over a 10 cm area of her right low back
    (D) Over a 20 cm area of her right low back

72. A physical therapist is preparing a list of home exercise for a patient who is 3.5 weeks post–left shoulder dislocation. Which of the following exercises is *MOST* appropriate for the patient at this stage?

    (A) Cane-assisted shoulder flexion
    (B) Cane-assisted shoulder abduction
    (C) Cane-assisted shoulder external rotation
    (D) Cane-assisted shoulder internal rotation/adduction

73. A physical therapist and her patient are mutually setting goals for physical therapy. The patient is four days post–total knee replacement. Which of the following would be the *BEST* example of a short-term goal?

    (A) The patient will have 100° of active knee flexion in two weeks.
    (B) The patient will have less pain in one week.
    (C) The patient will be independent with ambulation by discharge.
    (D) The patient will ambulate better with a walker in two weeks.

74. A physical therapist working with a 75-year-old patient in a phase II cardiac rehab takes an initial blood pressure measurement of 130/70 mm Hg. After five minutes of walking on a treadmill, the patient's blood pressure is 142/76 mm Hg. Normally, the systolic blood pressure rises with submaximal exercise. How does the diastolic blood pressure normally respond with submaximal exercise?

    (A) Increases significantly
    (B) Remains the same
    (C) Decreases significantly
    (D) Can possibly increase slightly, remain the same, or decrease slightly

75. What techniques can be used to increase the rate of return of a mailed questionnaire that asks about patients' experience with physical therapy?

    (A) Long, complicated survey form
    (B) No follow-up mailings
    (C) Sending the survey during the summer
    (D) Including a gracious and informative cover letter

76. A physical therapist examines a patient who is hospitalized secondary to an acute exacerbation of chronic obstructive pulmonary disease. Upon assessment of the patient's vital signs, the physical therapist notes his respiratory rate is 30 breaths per minute. What word should the therapist use to describe the patient's breathing?

    (A) Eupneic
    (B) Bradypneic
    (C) Tachypneic
    (D) Apneic

77. A physical therapist is examining a patient who has been hospitalized with severe low back pain. Radiological reports are negative for bony or disc pathology. The physician has written orders for pain management by physical therapy for mechanical low back pain. Which mobilization technique would be *MOST* appropriate for this patient?

(A) Prone grade I PAIVMs

(B) Side-lying rotation mobilization

(C) Side-lying grade III PAIVMs

(D) Prone transverse mobilization

78. A hospitalized patient begins to complain of weakness and moderately productive cough following a colon resection surgery. Lung sounds are coarse and the patient's temperature is 101.5°F (38.6°C). What test is the physician *MOST* likely to run first to diagnose possible pulmonary condition?

(A) Chest X-ray (radiograph)

(B) ECG

(C) EEG

(D) Urinalysis

79. A physical therapist tests a patient's cranial nerve XII (hypoglossal nerve). What motion does the physical therapist ask the patient to perform?

(A) Turn the head

(B) Abduct the eye

(C) Chew

(D) Move the tongue

80. A physical therapist is evaluating a patient in a nursing home after a hip fracture from a fall. The patient has dementia but is motivated and agreeable to participate in physical therapy. Which of the following would be the *MOST* appropriate treatment goal for this patient?

(A) The patient will progress to ambulation with supervision within the nursing home using a wheeled walker.

(B) The patient will be independent with home exercises for hip strengthening.

(C) The patient will be independent in understanding fall precautions in her room.

(D) The patient will obey weight-bearing restrictions with all mobility in her room.

81. A patient living in a nursing home has Alzheimer's disease. The patient's ability to understand and perform spoken commands is severely impaired. He is unable to follow directions for range-of-motion measurements. The physical therapist receives a referral for this patient for left shoulder pain. Since the patient is unable to follow spoken directions, what alternative does the therapist have to performing standardized active range-of-motion (ROM) measurements?

(A) Observing the patient as he performs activities of daily living such as dressing and eating to see if any functional ROM restrictions are present

(B) Performing passive ROM and assuming that active ROM is of the same quality

(C) Using ROM measurements from a previous physical therapy evaluation one year ago

(D) Skipping ROM measurements or observation

82. To treat a patient with COPD and increase his oxygen saturation level, the physical therapist uses pursed-lip breathing training. What description can this physical therapist use to train the patient on pursed-lip breathing?

(A) Breathe in and out quickly through pursed lips.

(B) Breathe in through pursed lips, breath out through the nose.

(C) Breathe in and out quickly through the nose.

(D) Breathe in through the nose, and breathe out slowly through pursed lips.

83. A physical therapist is reviewing the labs of a patient in an acute care setting who was admitted with symptoms of dizziness and dehydration. The therapist notes that the nonfasting plasma glucose levels are indicative of diabetes mellitus. What plasma glucose concentration is diagnostic of diabetes mellitus?

(A) <100 mg/dL
(B) >100 mg/dL
(C) >200 mg/dL
(D) >220 mg/dL

84. After a cerebrovascular accident, a patient holds her right arm in scapular retraction, elbow flexion, forearm supination, and wrist flexion. She holds her right leg in hip flexion/external rotation and knee flexion/ankle inversion. What Brunnstrom's synergy patterns describe this position?

(A) Upper extremity flexion and lower extremity flexion
(B) Upper extremity flexion and lower extremity extension
(C) Upper extremity extension and lower extremity flexion
(D) Upper extremity extension and lower extremity extension

85. A physical therapist is working with a patient on the burn unit of the hospital. The therapist provides education to the patient on the functions of the skin. She explains to him that burns can destroy sudoriferous glands. To what skin function are sudoriferous glands *MOST* closely related?

(A) Protection
(B) Thermoregulation
(C) Sensation
(D) Vitamin D production

86. A patient enters the clinic with a complaint of neck pain. On evaluation, she has weakness with myotomal testing of the biceps. Which reflex would be impaired?

(A) Biceps reflex
(B) Triceps reflex
(C) Brachioradialis reflex
(D) Brachialis reflex

87. A patient is hospitalized due to arterial ulcers. The physician is *MOST* likely to perform what test for the patient?

(A) Magnetic resonance imaging (MRI)
(B) X-ray
(C) CT scan
(D) Ankle-brachial index (ABI)

88. A physical therapist is treating a patient with left hip flexion contracture following surgical removal of a brain tumor. The physical therapist decides to use proprioceptive neuromuscular techniques to address this patient's impaired range of motion. The physical therapist asks the patient to isometrically contract his hip flexors maximally. The therapist does not allow any motion to occur. After this maximal contraction, the patient is then stretched into a lengthening position of increased hip extension. What proprioceptive neuromuscular facilitation (PNF) technique is the therapist using?

(A) Hold-relax
(B) Rhythmic initiation
(C) Alternating isometrics
(D) Slow reversals

89. A physical therapist is using a wet-to-dry dressing to debride a patient's wound. What should the physical therapist consider prior to changing the dressing?

(A) Mechanical debridement may be painful for the patient; the therapist may want to consider premedication.
(B) Wet the old dressing before removing it.
(C) Wet-to-dry dressings should not be used with another treatment.
(D) Wet-to-dry dressings remove only necrotic tissue.

90. A 65-year-old patient is hospitalized following right total hip arthroplasty. The orthopedic surgeon has ordered physical therapy with the following restrictions: right lower extremity TWB (touch weight-bearing) and hip flexion restriction of 60°. The physical therapist determines that wheelchair positioning is his first goal for this patient. What is the *MOST* important feature on a wheelchair for this patient?

    (A) Hemi-height wheelchair
    (B) Sport wheelchair
    (C) Reclining-back wheelchair
    (D) One-arm-drive wheelchair

91. A physical therapist wishes to conduct a test for neural provocation of the median nerve, specifically at the wrist. Which of the following special tests would be *MOST* appropriate to confirm the suspected origin of the patient's symptoms?

    (A) Tinel test
    (B) Phalen test
    (C) Upper limb tension testing
    (D) Slump test

92. A patient who weighs 360 lb is admitted to a nursing home. He is dependent for transfers. The physical therapist is asked to train the nursing staff on the safest mode of transfer for the patient. What type of transfer would be the *BEST* for this patient?

    (A) Two-person lift
    (B) Stand-pivot transfer
    (C) Hydraulic lift
    (D) Sliding board transfer

93. A therapist who is working with a patient with a traumatic brain injury always plays soothing music when working on sit-to-stand mobility. One day, a visitor turns the radio on to the same soothing music that the therapist uses. The patient immediately tries to stand up from his wheelchair, without anyone asking him to do so. What type of learning has happened in this situation?

    (A) Operant conditioning
    (B) Respondent conditioning
    (C) Cognitive learning
    (D) Social learning

94. A physical therapist in a busy outpatient office finds himself with two patients needing treatment at the same time. To keep himself on schedule and avoid making his next patient wait, he needs assistance in starting one of the patients with active range-of-motion exercise. Who should be delegated this duty?

    (A) The physical therapy assistant
    (B) The physical therapy aide
    (C) The graduate-student physical therapist
    (D) The patient himself

95. A patient wears a left solid, non-articulating ankle-foot orthosis. The patient also has weak left quadriceps muscles. What effect does this orthosis have at the knee?

    (A) Prevents knee hyperextension
    (B) Increases knee extension
    (C) Prevents medial knee rotation
    (D) Prevents lateral knee rotation

96. A physical therapist is conducting an assessment of lower-extremity muscle tightness with the patient in the supine position. Which position would *BEST* assess hamstring flexibility?

    (A) Straight leg raise with the opposite leg extended
    (B) Hip and knee flexed to 90°, then knee extended with the opposite leg extended
    (C) Hip and knee flexed to 90°, then knee extended with the opposite leg flexed
    (D) Straight leg raise with the opposite leg flexed

97. A physical therapist is preparing to evaluate a patient who is on droplet precautions. The patient does well covering his mouth while coughing. What personal protective equipment must the therapist put on before entering the room?

    (A) Gloves
    (B) Gloves and mask
    (C) Gloves, gown, and mask
    (D) None necessary

98. Which of these is an example of explicit learning?

    (A) Automatic adjustments in force generation after attempts to pick up a small weight are unsuccessful

    (B) Reciting the name of the company who makes the weight

    (C) Giving the name of the physical therapy clinic

    (D) Learning that the weight is 5 lb

99. A researcher is studying the effect that rate chest percussion has on heart rate in patients with cystic fibrosis. What is the dependent variable in this study?

    (A) Rate of chest percussion

    (B) Cystic fibrosis

    (C) Number of patients in the study

    (D) Heart rate

100. A physical therapist is examining a female patient who is referred for hip pain from a fall. Upon observation, the therapist notices that the woman has multiple contusions on her back and hip and forearms. The therapist is suspicious of domestic abuse. What would be the *MOST* appropriate plan of action?

    (A) Report her findings to the Department of Human Services

    (B) Ask the woman if she is in a harmful relationship

    (C) Report her findings to her clinic supervisor

    (D) Provide the woman with information about domestic violence without asking questions

End of Section 2

IF YOU FINISH BEFORE TIME IS CALLED, YOU MAY CHECK YOUR WORK ON THIS SECTION ONLY. DO NOT TURN TO ANY OTHER SECTION IN THE TEST. **STOP**

Section 3

101. A physical therapist is evaluating a patient with neck pain. On evaluation, he finds pain and limited range of motion on rotation to the right. Which mobilization technique would be *MOST* appropriate to specifically restore right rotation range of motion?

(A) Anterior glides of the uncovertebral joint
(B) Joint distraction with manual cervical traction
(C) Rotational mobilization of the right facet joint toward the right (or laterally)
(D) Side gliding mobilization of the right facet joint toward the left (or medially)

102. To treat a patient with atelectasis, the physical therapist uses a technique involving manual pressure to a localized area of the lung to increase expansion of that area of the lung. This treatment intervention is known as what?

(A) Diaphragmatic breathing exercises
(B) Pursed-lip breathing exercises
(C) Segmental breathing exercises
(D) Relaxation exercises

103. A physical therapist is preparing a patient for discharge from the hospital following a total knee replacement. As part of patient education, she is instructing the patient on what to look for in infection. Which of the following is *NOT* a cardinal sign of inflammation?

(A) Erythema
(B) Loss of function
(C) Pain
(D) Low-grade fever

104. A physical therapist is evaluating a patient for vestibular rehabilitation. On evaluation, the patient shows upbeating (ageotropic) nystagmus with Dix-Hallpike testing on the left. Which of the following would be the correct repositioning technique?

(A) Epley maneuver beginning with the head toward the left
(B) Epley maneuver beginning with the head toward the right
(C) Roll maneuver beginning with the head toward the left
(D) Roll maneuver beginning with the head toward the right

105. A physical therapist has been asked to address a community education group on the benefits of exercise for the obese population. He has been told that all of the attendees are clinically obese themselves. Which of the following would be the *BEST* information to present to this population?

(A) The benefits of exercise in improving cardiovascular health and preventing diabetes
(B) The benefits of exercise in weight loss
(C) The benefits of exercise in improving athletic skill
(D) The benefits of exercise in improving walking speed and endurance

106. A young man is referred to physical therapy for left anterior hip pain. Three weeks ago he was tackled during a football game. Then last week he was helping a friend lift a TV when the pain became sharp. The pain is worse when he is exerting, such as during weightlifting or going to the bathroom. There is no change in pain with walking or running. On inspection, there is a nickel-sized bulge just above the inguinal crease. What differential diagnosis would account for this presentation of symptoms?

(A) Inguinal hernia
(B) Hip avulsion fracture
(C) Hip flexor strain
(D) Appendicitis

107. A physical therapist is treating a patient following a right cerebrovascular accident. The patient is working on self-propulsion of the wheelchair but often runs into the wall and other objects on the left side. The physical therapist needs to give the patient frequent verbal cues for her to advance her left leg with gait training. The patient is unaware of painful stimuli on the left leg. What phenomenon is this patient demonstrating?

(A) Pusher syndrome
(B) Neglect
(C) Spasticity
(D) Synergy

108. A patient presents with a complaint of hip pain for the past three months. She described it as bad for one week, then better for three to four weeks. On evaluation, she had pain with manual muscle testing of the hip flexors and hip flexor tightness. What differential diagnosis should be considered?

(A) Endometriosis
(B) Pelvic floor muscle dysfunction
(C) Urinary tract infection
(D) Colon cancer

109. A physical therapist is working with a patient with a spinal cord injury who has weak grip strength. One goal of treatment is to assist the patient to pre-position his thumb toward the palm of his hand. Which type of orthosis is appropriate for this patient?

(A) Assistive
(B) Substitutive
(C) Protective
(D) Corrective

110. A physical therapist is reviewing the past medical history of a patient she is evaluating. The patient reports a history of cancer. Which one of the following cancers is *MOST* likely to metastasize to the musculoskeletal system?

(A) Lung
(B) Cervical
(C) Colon
(D) Ovarian

111. A physical therapist is treating a patient who has had a cerebrovascular accident. In the patient's treatment plan, the physical therapist includes alternating isometrics, slow reversals, and agonistic reversals as treatment techniques. In what global treatment technique are these approaches used?

(A) Proprioceptive neuromuscular facilitation
(B) Neurodevelopmental treatment
(C) Brunnstrom's stages of recovery
(D) Therapeutic positioning

112. A patient presents to a physical therapy clinic with tennis elbow that has been ongoing for two weeks. In addition to stretching and patient education, the physical therapist will use iontophoresis to manage pain and inflammation. Which of the following medications used for iontophoresis would be *MOST* appropriate for analgesic benefits?

(A) Lidocaine
(B) Dexamethasone
(C) Acetic acid
(D) Sodium diclofenac

113. Which of the following is a random practice schedule?

(A) Four repetitions of Task A, then four repetitions of Task B, then four repetitions of Task C
(B) Repeat Task A only until it is mastered
(C) One repetition of Task A, then one repetition of Task B, then one repetition of Task C; repeat this sequence four times
(D) Task A, Task C, Task B, Task C, Task A, Task A, Task B

114. A physical therapy student receives a 97 percent on her first anatomy test. What level of measurement is this score?

(A) Nominal
(B) Ordinal
(C) Interval
(D) Ratio

115. A 50-year-old woman is referred to physical therapy for sharp pain in her hip that began suddenly one week ago. She has a family history positive for osteoporosis but has not had a bone scan herself. Prolonged use of which medication could also affect this patient's risk for bone loss?

(A) Acetaminophen

(B) NSAIDs

(C) Heparin

(D) Hydrocodone

116. A physical therapist is examining a patient who complains of low back pain. During active range of motion of the lumbar spine, the patient has pain and difficulty with extension and side-bending to the left. The physical therapist suspects facet joint involvement. Which of the following *BEST* describes the facet joint dysfunction?

(A) Left facet joint cannot open

(B) Left facet joint cannot close

(C) Right facet joint cannot close

(D) Both facet joints cannot close

117. A patient with chronic bronchitis presents to the pulmonary rehab clinic for evaluation. Upon evaluation, the physical therapist notes the motion of the diaphragm upon inspiration. In what motion does the rib cage move normally with inspiration?

(A) Equal and upward motion of the lower ribs

(B) Equal and inward motion of the lower ribs

(C) Lower ribs move laterally

(D) No motion of the rib cage

118. A physical therapist is making a home health visit to a patient he has been treating for gait dysfunction. When the therapist arrives, the patient states he is just starting to feel better from a three-day bout with the flu. On this day, he has increased muscle weakness, tingling in his legs, and complaints of leg cramps. What secondary pathology may be contributing to these new symptoms?

(A) Electrolyte imbalance

(B) Diabetes mellitus

(C) Cardiac myopathy

(D) Stomach ulcer

119. A patient has an L4-L5 disc herniation. Which position would put the *LEAST* amount of intradiscal pressure on the disc?

(A) Sitting

(B) Standing

(C) Walking

(D) Lying supine

120. A patient is in need of physical therapy treatment interventions to assist with quad atrophy following ACL reconstruction. The patient is ten days postsurgery and unable to elicit a good quad contraction. What would be the *BEST* electrode configuration for muscle education to the vastus medialis oblique (VMO)?

(A) Four electrodes surrounding the distal, medial aspect of the quadriceps

(B) One small electrode over the anterior thigh and one large electrode over the VMO motor point

(C) One small electrode over the VMO motor point and one large electrode over the anterior thigh

(D) Two electrodes over the anterior thigh

121. A patient who has been treated by a physical therapist for the last four weeks is now being discharged. On her last scheduled treatment session, she brings a thank-you card and two free movie passes as a token of gratitude for the physical therapist. What would be the *MOST* appropriate response by the physical therapist?

(A) Graciously accept the card and gift

(B) Graciously refuse the gift because it is over a $10 value

(C) Graciously refuse the gift, explaining to the patient that it is against professional conduct policies

(D) Graciously refuse the gift, knowing the patient does not have much money

122. A patient is seen in physical therapy six weeks post-immobilization of humeral shaft fracture. On evaluation, wrist flexion is 3+/5 with manual muscle testing. There is also impaired sensation along the middle finger. There is no tenderness in the lumbar spine. Which of the following would be the *MOST* likely differential diagnosis?

(A) Disuse atrophy

(B) Radial nerve palsy

(C) C7 nerve root impingement

(D) Carpal tunnel syndrome

123. A physical therapist is evaluating a patient who has left shoulder pain following an MVA. The patient was the driver in a vehicle that slid into a light pole during a snowstorm. The airbags were deployed. The patient says he felt achy everywhere. Since then, he has felt bloated and weak and has had this diffuse shoulder pain. Which of the following could be the cause of these symptoms?

(A) Injury to the spleen

(B) Injury to the kidney

(C) Lower GI injury

(D) Injury to the lung

124. A physical therapist reviews the pulmonary function tests of a patient with chronic obstructive pulmonary disease. What is the definition of tidal volume (V_T)?

(A) Volume of air that can be inspired after normal inspiration

(B) Volume of air that can be expired after normal expiration

(C) Volume of air remaining in the lungs after maximal expiration

(D) Volume of air inspired or expired during normal breathing

125. A patient who is being evaluated for gait dysfunction demonstrates a Trendelenburg gait. Which one of the following positions would be *BEST* for improved control by the weakened muscle during the stance phase?

(A) Standing hip abduction

(B) Side-lying hip abduction with ankle weights

(C) Hook-lying hip abduction/external rotation with Thera-Band

(D) Single-leg standing

126. What is the pathophysiology of pulmonary emphysema?

(A) Viral infection

(B) Destruction of lung tissue that results in large airspaces

(C) Genetic disorder affecting lung secretions

(D) Hyperreactive smooth muscle of the bronchioles

127. A physical therapist is designing an exercise program to be offered by a senior center. He has been asked to highlight some of the benefits of exercise. Which one of the following is *NOT* a benefit of exercise for the elderly?

(A) Decreases the progression of osteoporosis

(B) Decreases resting blood pressure

(C) Increases walking speed

(D) Increases resting heart rate

128. A patient who resides in a nursing home has a VO_2 max of four METS and is very deconditioned. The patient is hospitalized due to multiple medical problems and ordered to bed rest for two weeks. Upon return to the nursing home and discharge of the bed rest order, her VO_2 max has decreased to three METS. What treatment intervention will the physical therapist *MOST* likely need to employ?

(A) Aggressive strength training with heavy weights

(B) Supine passive ROM only; sitting and standing are not indicated.

(C) No physical therapy is indicated.

(D) Progress the patient's position to sitting and standing as tolerated, checking vital signs for each position change and to allow for acclimation

129. A patient presents to physical therapy after a head injury that affects his sensation. He has difficulty perceiving sensory stimulus and also demonstrates short-term memory loss. Which lobe of the cerebral cortex is *MOST* likely injured?

(A) Frontal lobe

(B) Parietal lobe

(C) Temporal lobe

(D) Occipital lobe

130. A physical therapist plans to use manual joint mobilization of the tibia-femoral joint to increase knee flexion ROM on a patient. He is mobilizing the tibia on the stationary femur. According to the concave-convex rule, in which direction is the slide motion of the tibial surface occurring?

(A) Superior

(B) Inferior

(C) Anterior

(D) Posterior

131. A patient experiences homonymous hemianopia. How is the patient's vision affected?

(A) Double vision

(B) Loss of vision of half of the visual field

(C) Eyes rapidly move laterally and medially

(D) Inability to recognize familiar objects

132. A physical therapist is working in an acute care setting when a large-scale emergency occurs in her city with a need for more patient rooms to be available for triage. The physical therapist has been instructed to move some of the patients who are now in single rooms into group areas. How should patients be grouped?

(A) Those on precautions in one room; those not, in another

(B) Those on droplet or airborne precautions in one room; those not, in another

(C) Those who have the same precautions grouped in a room together except for those on airborne precautions, who should stay in single rooms

(D) Those on precautions intermixed with those who are not

133. Which condition can a physical therapist diagnose?

(A) Cerebrovascular accident

(B) Parkinson's disease

(C) Sensory integrative dysfunction

(D) Peripheral nerve injury

134. A patient is burned in a house fire. His burns completely cover his entire left arm and his entire posterior trunk. What percentage of his skin is burned?

(A) 18 percent

(B) 27 percent

(C) 36 percent

(D) 45 percent

135. A patient is seeing a physician for lower-extremity venous testing. What test is the physician *MOST* likely to utilize?

(A) Ankle-brachial index (ABI)

(B) Plethysmography

(C) X-ray

(D) CT scan

136. A patient is hospitalized with severe back pain from an acute compression fracture at T7 36 hours ago. The physician indicates that the fracture is stable and the patient may begin exercise. The *MOST* appropriate activity for the patient to begin with is which of the following?

(A) Supine knee-to-chest stretch
(B) Prone leg extensions
(C) Seated transverse abdominis isometrics
(D) Supine posterior pelvic tilts

137. The posterior columns of the spinal cord cross in the brain stem. What information do these tracts convey?

(A) Pain and temperature
(B) Proprioception and vibration
(C) Motor impulses
(D) Orientation of the head toward a sound

138. A physical therapist determines that a patient is positive for upper-limb neural tension with an ulnar nerve bias. Which position would have an increased response if the tension is originating proximally?

(A) Extending the elbow and wrist with the head in neutral
(B) Extending the elbow and wrist with the head sidebent away from the affected side
(C) Extending the elbow and wrist with the head sidebent toward the affected side
(D) Flexing the elbow and wrist with the head sidebent toward the affected side

139. A person with a diagnosis of chronic venous insufficiency asks her physical therapist why she has been prescribed leg exercises. What is the reason for leg exercises for a person with chronic venous insufficiency?

(A) Maintain muscle length
(B) Increase isometric muscle strength
(C) Aerobic conditioning
(D) Increase muscle pump activity

140. A physical therapist is treating a patient who has a traumatic brain injury. The patient exhibits hypertonicity of the left trunk and upper extremity that makes sitting difficult. The therapist selects an initial goal of normalizing muscle tone. The therapist feels that once tone is normalized, then stability will occur and mobility can be superimposed. The physical therapist is using the theory of what treatment technique?

(A) Proprioceptive neuromuscular facilitation
(B) Neurodevelopmental treatment
(C) Craniosacral therapy
(D) Brunnstrom's synergy patterns

141. A patient with a right transtibial amputation complains of pain. The pain is described as burning and cramping of the right foot. The therapist determines that the pain is which of the following?

(A) Phantom limb pain
(B) Nonpainful phantom limb sensations
(C) Residual limb pain
(D) Back pain

142. A physical therapist is looking through a journal, reading the titles of the research articles. One article is entitled "Effectiveness of pulsed ultrasound in wound healing of decubitus ulcers." The therapist works full-time in an outpatient sports medicine clinic on a college campus. Only students of the college are treated at the clinic. The therapist scans the article and then reflects on it. What is the therapist's *MOST* appropriate analysis of the article?

(A) She should evaluate the validity of the research.
(B) She should study what brand of ultrasound was used in the study and compare it to the ultrasound in her clinic.
(C) She should read more articles about decubitus ulcers.
(D) She should ask if this article is applicable to her clinical practice and the clientele she serves.

143. A patient with a traumatic brain injury is diagnosed with increased intracranial pressure. How is increased intracranial pressure defined?

(A) Decreased blood flow to the brain
(B) Bleeding of blood vessels in the brain
(C) Cell death due to infection
(D) Swelling of the brain or ventricles resulting in increased forces on the brain against the skull

144. A patient has been referred to physical therapy for exercise prescription concurrent with chemotherapy. Which of the following is *NOT* a benefit of exercise during cancer treatment using chemotherapy?

(A) Reduced nausea
(B) Reduced fatigue
(C) Increased stamina
(D) Reduced bone marrow suppression

145. A hospitalized patient who weighs over 350 lb and has limited mobility poses a risk for pressure ulcer development. A specialized bariatric bed is needed to accommodate this patient. The physical therapist should request what feature to optimize the patient's mobility and transfer ability?

(A) Bed scale
(B) Foot exit
(C) Cardiac chair conversion
(D) Continuous passive movement

146. A physical therapist follows the cognitive learning theory. What is this therapist *LEAST* likely to do to assist patients in achieving goals?

(A) Reward the patient with candy after each goal is achieved
(B) Change the patient's beliefs and attitudes toward the goals
(C) Establish goals with the input of the patient
(D) Interview the patient to discover the patient's past experiences with physical therapy

147. A physical therapist is treating a patient who has a spinal cord injury. The therapist is addressing wheelchair positioning. The therapist's goal is to maintain skin integrity and prevent pressure ulcers. For a patient with paraplegia, what motion is needed to perform independent pressure relief while sitting in a manual wheelchair?

(A) Scapular elevation
(B) Scapular depression
(C) Shoulder abduction
(D) Shoulder flexion

148. Prior to beginning a research study, what should be a scientist's first step?

(A) Establish control groups
(B) Outline a proposal
(C) Create a hypothesis
(D) Perform a literature review

149. A newly hired physical therapist is concerned about the safety of the work site to which he has been assigned. Which of these governing agencies' primary function is to ensure a safe workplace for employees?

(A) JCAHO
(B) OSHA
(C) APTA
(D) CDC

150. When routinely checking the ultrasound head for wave emittance, a physical therapist at a hospital-based clinic notices that there is no water displacement. Who should be contacted to further check the function of the equipment?

(A) Hospital maintenance
(B) Biomedical department
(C) JCAHO
(D) OSHA

End of Section 3

IF YOU FINISH BEFORE TIME IS CALLED, YOU MAY CHECK YOUR WORK ON THIS SECTION ONLY. DO NOT TURN TO ANY OTHER SECTION IN THE TEST. STOP

Section 4

151. A physical therapist has chosen to use ice as a means of vasoconstriction to decrease the patient's post-exercise soreness and inflammation. Which method of temperature exchange is ice considered?

(A) Conduction
(B) Convection
(C) Conversion
(D) Evaporation

152. A physical therapist is evaluating a patient who has abnormal gait. She observes the patient demonstrating ankle instability and loss of balance during mid to late stance phase. Which exercise would be *MOST* appropriate to address this gait deficit?

(A) Heel walking
(B) Toe raises
(C) Resistive ankle eversion
(D) Resistive ankle inversion

153. A physical therapist is evaluating a patient with low-level, nearly constant dizziness. On evaluation, the patient has no visible nystagmus but has mildly increased symptoms with Dix-Hallpike testing of both sides. Which of the following home exercises would be *MOST* appropriate for this patient?

(A) Brandt-Daroff exercises
(B) Convergence-divergence oculomotor exercise
(C) Visual tracking exercise
(D) Fixation exercise

154. A physical therapist examines a patient three days post–total knee arthroplasty. On evaluation, his AROM is 5–95°, the girth is 7 cm greater than the unaffected side, and there is localized erythema. There is localized redness around the incision and a nonpurulent, clear discharge on the bandage. What type of response is this patient having?

(A) A normal inflammatory response to surgery
(B) An abnormal infectious response at the incision site
(C) An abnormal infectious response to the prosthesis
(D) An allergic reaction to the anesthesia used in surgery

155. What is the *MOST* serious potential outcome of a deep vein thrombosis?

(A) Pneumonia
(B) Lower-extremity edema
(C) Pulmonary embolism
(D) Asthma

156. A physical therapist is designing an exercise program for a patient with chronic patellofemoral syndrome. The patient is also clinically obese and is interested in beginning a long-term exercise program. Which of the following would *NOT* be the most beneficial for the patient to start with?

(A) Resistance exercise with weights
(B) Stationary bicycle
(C) Walking on the treadmill
(D) Aquatic therapy

157. A patient is referred to physical therapy for treatment of nagging lower thoracic pain. During evaluation, the physical therapist is unable to provoke or eliminate painful symptoms with range of motion or positional changes. The patient states he has also had low-level nausea in the last week. Which of the following differential diagnoses should the physical therapist be considering as a potential causative factor in this presentation?

(A) Cardiac pathology
(B) Gastric pathology
(C) Genitourinary pathology
(D) Endocrine pathology

158. A child is diagnosed with meningitis. What is the innermost layer of meninges called?

(A) Dura mater
(B) Arachnoid mater
(C) Pia mater
(D) Epidural space

159. A physical therapist is treating a patient for hip pain that has been ongoing for several months and is cyclic in nature (on one week, gone three weeks). The pain is unrelated to activity or positioning. The patient does not recall any mechanism of injury. Which patient demographic could lead the physical therapist to suspect endometriosis?

(A) A 10-year-old gymnast
(B) A 63-year-old grandmother
(C) A 23-year-old mother
(D) A 30-year-old single woman

160. A physical therapist is designing a general strengthening program for a woman with osteoporotic changes in her hip and femur. Which of the following exercises would provide the greatest buildup of bone density in her hip and thigh?

(A) Cycling on a stationary bike for ten minutes
(B) Walking in the shallow end of the arthritic pool
(C) Seated knee extension with ankle weights
(D) Hip abduction with Thera-Band

161. A physical therapist determines that a patient has humeroradial joint restriction for elbow flexion. What accessory joint movement would be *MOST* appropriate to improve elbow flexion?

(A) Lateral radial glides
(B) Dorsal radial glides
(C) Volar radial glides
(D) Rotational mobilization

162. Some motor-control theories purport that the learner must be involved through the problem-solving process. The learner/patient can then learn via what technique?

(A) Experience of only normal movement
(B) Repetitive practice of one specific joint movement
(C) Trial and error
(D) Maximal immediate feedback from the teacher/therapist

163. A physical therapist is developing exercise recommendations for a 32-year-old patient who is pregnant. Her obstetrician has cleared her for exercise. Her preference is to walk or to ride a stationary bicycle. Which of the following would be her *MOST* appropriate intensity, duration, and frequency?

(A) Target heart rate 135 bpm, 20 minutes, 2x/wk
(B) Target heart rate 140 bpm, 15 minutes, 3x/wk
(C) Target heart rate 110 bpm, 30 minutes, 4x/wk
(D) Target heart rate 125 bpm, 20 minutes, 4x/wk

164. A physical therapist is designing a strengthening program for a patient who has general lower-extremity weakness. Which type of muscular contraction recruits the *MOST* motor units?

(A) Isometric
(B) Concentric isotonic
(C) Eccentric isotonic
(D) Isokinetic

165. A physical therapist has been treating a patient for hip pain from a fall. The patient also has type 1 diabetes mellitus. As part of the planned treatment interventions, the physical therapist uses moist heat to warm the hip and thigh prior to stretching. Upon removing the heat pack, the therapist notices the patient has become drowsy and unsteady when standing up from the table. What adverse reaction could have taken place?

(A) Hyperglycemic response
(B) Hypoglycemic response
(C) Heat exhaustion
(D) Dehydration

166. A physical therapist is examining a patient with left knee pain and finds the patient to have limited knee flexion. The therapist wishes to mobilize the tibiafemoral joint. In which direction should he mobilize the tibia on the femur?

(A) Anterior
(B) Posterior
(C) Medial
(D) Lateral

167. When a physical therapist removes a moist hot pack from the elbow of a patient after application for 20 minutes, he notices mottling of the patient's skin. The patient reports no discomfort with the heat treatment. What would be the physical therapist's plan of action with the hot pack on the next treatment session?

(A) Continue using it as done previously
(B) Discontinue use of the hot pack
(C) Add extra layers of towels with the next treatment
(D) Remove layers of towels with the next treatment

168. A patient has been referred to physical therapy for adhesive capsulitis, a complication of type 1 diabetes mellitus. Which of the following is correct information regarding type 1 diabetes mellitus?

(A) Insulin-dependent
(B) Non-insulin dependent
(C) Controlled with diet and exercise
(D) Most often adult-onset

169. A patient presents with a complaint of numbness in his left little finger and the lateral side of his ring finger. During evaluation, which upper-limb tension test would be *MOST* likely to re-create his symptoms?

(A) Median nerve bias
(B) Radial nerve bias
(C) Ulnar nerve bias
(D) Brachial plexus bias

170. A physical therapist is evaluating a patient in a nursing home for pain and joint stiffness associated with Graves' disease. Graves' disease is the hyperfunctioning of what endocrine gland?

(A) Pituitary
(B) Thyroid
(C) Parathyroid
(D) Adrenal

171. If a patient has a heart rate of 60 beats per minute and a stroke volume of 0.1 L, what is the patient's cardiac output?

(A) 60 L/min
(B) 6 L/min
(C) 10 L/min
(D) 600 L/min

172. A patient is referred to physical therapy for evaluation and treatment of his right shoulder for pain and decreased function after a fall. What position of the shoulder would put maximal stress on tightened ligaments of the glenohumeral joint?

(A) Abduction and internal rotation
(B) Abduction and external rotation
(C) Extension and internal rotation
(D) Adduction and external rotation

173. A physical therapist is monitoring a patient during aerobic warm-up in the clinic. The patient's medication list includes tricyclic antidepressants. Given this information, which response can the physical therapist expect when the patient begins to exercise?

(A) Heart rate does not increase as it should.
(B) Blood pressure does not increase as it should.
(C) Heart rate increases greater than normal.
(D) Heart rate and blood pressure rises as expected during exercise.

174. A physical therapist is going on a home visit with a patient about to be discharged from a skilled nursing facility to determine if he is safe to go home independently. His primary means of mobility is a wheelchair. He can transfer independently but does not walk. Which of the following is the correct modification of the patient's home setting?

(A) A handrail on the stairs leading into the home
(B) A 34-inch-wide doorway into the bathroom
(C) A toilet that is 14 inches high
(D) A recliner that is 16 inches high

175. A physical therapist receives a referral for a patient with a C5 spinal cord injury. What motion should the physical therapist test for strength to determine the anticipated highest level of function for this patient?

(A) Elbow flexion
(B) Wrist extension
(C) Elbow extension
(D) Finger flexion

176. A physical therapist is performing a chart review for a patient new to pulmonary rehab. At discharge from the hospital, the patient's pulse oximetry measurement was 95 percent on 2 L of supplemental oxygen via nasal cannula. The patient asks the therapist what this number measures. How should the physical therapist respond?

(A) "This is a measurement of the volume of oxygen in your lungs."
(B) "This is a measurement of the amount of oxygen that is saturated in the blood of your arteries."
(C) "This is a measurement of the percentage of carbon dioxide in your lungs."
(D) "This is a measurement of the amount of hemoglobin in your blood."

177. A physical therapist examines a patient with a referral diagnosis of leg pain. Subjectively, the patient reports pain and sensation changes along the front and inner thigh. On evaluation, she has weakness with resisted hip flexion. Which nerve root is *MOST* likely involved?

(A) L2
(B) L3
(C) L4
(D) L5

178. Preferred practice pattern 6A is the primary prevention and risk reduction for cardiovascular/pulmonary disorders. What strategy can a physical therapist use to initiate this pattern?

(A) Treatment of a hospitalized patient with recent myocardial infarction and history of CABG and who is a graduate of cardiac rehab; treatment interventions include ongoing cardiac rehab.
(B) Treatment of a patient with newly diagnosed diabetes, a history of smoking, and family history of heart disease; treatment interventions include progression of an exercise program and extensive patient education on the risk factors of heart disease.
(C) Treatment of a patient with end-stage COPD in a nursing facility; medical treatment interventions include palliative care.
(D) Treatment of a six-year-old patient with cystic fibrosis; treatment interventions include airway clearance techniques.

179. A patient is evaluated in physical therapy for right knee pain that is present when walking and descending stairs. The physical therapist observes the patient's gait and sees decreased stance time on the painful knee. What consequence would this have in the patient's step length?

(A) Increased left step length
(B) Decreased left step length
(C) Increased right step length
(D) Decreased right step length

180. Following a traumatic brain injury, a patient is evaluated by a physical therapist. The therapist notes a grade of 3 on the Modified Ashworth Scale. What is the physical therapist seeing?

(A) Poor strength
(B) Hyperreflexia
(C) Joint laxity
(D) Increased muscle spasticity

181. Which of the following is a contraindication to using postural drainage accompanied by manual percussion?

(A) Increased intracranial pressure

(B) Presence of secretions

(C) Cystic fibrosis

(D) Mechanical ventilation

182. A physical therapist performs an initial evaluation for a patient following a traumatic brain injury. After the chart review and patient interview, the physical therapist starts to assess the autonomic nervous system. What assessment is the physical therapist *MOST* likely to perform in evaluating the autonomic nervous system?

(A) Vital signs

(B) Deep tendon reflexes

(C) Sensation testing

(D) Balance testing

183. A physical therapist has just finished performing PROM on a patient who is non-ambulatory in the ICU. He is placing the patient in supine position but wants to make sure that there are no pressure areas that could be susceptible to breakdown. Where should he place pillows for positioning?

(A) Under the knees and under the elbows

(B) Lengthwise under the knees and under the shoulder and forearm

(C) Under the head and under the feet

(D) Under the thighs and under the shoulders

184. A physical therapist is planning treatment interventions (TIs) for a patient who has significant upper trapezius guarding and spasticity. Along with manual TIs and stretching, he would like to use an electrical modality for spasticity reduction. In choosing NMES, what parameters would be *MOST* beneficial for spasticity reduction?

(A) 200 μs width, 50 Hz, 15 sec on/30 sec off, sensory intensity

(B) 200 μs width, 50 Hz, 15 sec on/15 sec off, motor intensity

(C) 200 μs width, 50 Hz, 15 sec on/45 sec off, motor intensity

(D) 200 μs width, 100 Hz, 15 sec on/30 sec off, motor intensity

185. A patient presents to physical therapy with difficulty rising from a chair. The physical therapist provides a home exercise program for strengthening and also performs neurodevelopmental treatment to facilitate the patient's sit-to-stand motion. The therapist asks the patient to sit on the side of the treatment mat. The therapist then places her hands on the patient's lateral pelvis. What motion should be facilitated?

(A) Anterior weight shift

(B) Posterior weight shift

(C) Posterior pelvic tilt

(D) Anterior pelvic tilt

186. A frail resident of a nursing home has a stage III pressure ulcer on the left ischial tuberosity. He is dependent for transfers and has been sitting in a wheelchair for much of the day. The physical therapist prescribes frequent position changes and increased time in bed to relieve pressure on the ischial tuberosity. What should be considered prior to increasing the amount of time the patient spends in bed?

(A) Respiratory status

(B) Nutritional status

(C) Presence of infection

(D) Cognition

187. A physical therapist is treating a patient in the hospital therapy gym. The patient has had a spinal cord injury at the T1 level. During physical therapy treatment, the patient suddenly becomes hypertensive, complains of a massive headache, and becomes diaphoretic. What condition does the physical therapist suspect?

(A) Postural hypotension
(B) Deep vein thrombosis
(C) Spasticity
(D) Autonomic dysreflexia

188. A 79-year-old patient suffered a CVA with resulting left-sided weakness. Physical therapy was initiated. The physical therapist notes only 1/5 muscle strength of the left dorsiflexors. He also notes that the patient drags his left foot during the swing phase of gait. The patient's knee extension strength is 5/5, and he also has good hip control. Which orthosis is the physical therapist's *BEST* choice for this patient?

(A) Foot orthosis
(B) Ankle-foot orthosis
(C) Knee-ankle-foot orthosis
(D) Hip-knee-ankle-foot orthosis

189. A researcher is conducting a study on the use of electrical stimulation to increase strength of the quadriceps muscle in subjects without quadriceps pathology. What would be considered unethical for the researcher to require of the subjects?

(A) Obtaining informed consent for the electrical stimulation protocol
(B) Discussing with the subjects the risks of treatment
(C) Not allowing the subjects to withdraw from the study
(D) Forming a control group that receives a placebo

190. A physical therapy student reads about multiple sclerosis. She reads that multiple sclerosis is a progressive demyelinating neurological disease. What is disrupted with demyelination of the neurons?

(A) Decreased neurotransmitters
(B) Impaired sensory neuron transmission
(C) Impaired integration of impulses
(D) Decreased speed of nerve impulses

191. A patient presents to physical therapy with a diagnosis of left lateral epicondylitis. The physical therapist establishes a goal of decreasing the stress on the forearm extensors through use of an orthosis. What orthosis would be *BEST* to decrease stress on the forearm extensors?

(A) Basic opponens orthosis
(B) Forearm cuff
(C) Wrist-hand stabilizer
(D) Wrist flexion control orthosis

192. A physical therapist who works in a nursing home is treating an 82-year-old patient with multiple fractures that resulted from a motor vehicle accident. Five months post-trauma, the patient has improved tremendously. She requires minimum assistance with bed mobility. At home, the patient will only perform bed mobility when she is not wearing shoes on her feet and her bed does not have a bed rail. For this patient to learn this specific task of bed mobility, what treatment interventions should the physical therapist use?

(A) Asking the patient to practice bed mobility on the hard adjustable plinth in the therapy room
(B) Asking the patient to practice bed mobility with shoes on, using a bed rail
(C) Asking the patient to practice bed mobility on a therapy-room bed that is the same height as her home bed, without shoes on and without using the bed rail
(D) Teaching the patient to crawl into bed

193. A physical therapist is treating a patient who is in the intensive care unit following a surgical removal of a brain tumor. The patient is not medically stable and is not easily arousable. The patient has ventricle drain, catheter, and supplemental oxygen via nasal cannula. There are multiple monitors that measure heart rate, pulse oxygen saturation, and intracranial pressure. What is the *MOST* likely treatment intervention to be used for this patient?

(A) Quick movement of supine to sit, then sitting on the edge of the bed for 15 minutes during the first treatment
(B) Trendelenburg position
(C) Chest percussions
(D) Passive range of motion of all extremities

194. During a treatment session, a physical therapist provides feedback to the patient after every trial of a new task or motor skill. What type of feedback is this?

(A) Constant feedback
(B) Summary feedback
(C) Faded feedback
(D) Client-controlled feedback

195. The standard deviation is a valuable measurement that is used in research. What is its definition?

(A) Difference between the highest and lowest score in a set of data
(B) Average score in a set of data
(C) Middle score in a set of data
(D) Average amount that a set of scores deviates from the mean

196. A patient is receiving physical therapy following a total knee replacement. The incision is healed, but the scar is raised and extends beyond the original incision. The physical therapist documents that the patient has what type of scar?

(A) Normotrophic scar
(B) Hypertrophic scar
(C) Keloid scar
(D) Hyperkeratotic scar

197. A physician tells a patient that he has a countercoup lesion following a head injury. The patient asks his physical therapist to explain what this means. What is the *MOST* appropriate response?

(A) Damage to the same side of the brain as the impact to the head
(B) Damage to the opposite side of the brain
(C) Damage to both sides of the brain after impact to the head
(D) Diffuse damage to the brain after impact to the head

198. A physical therapist is seeing a patient for wound care. The wound has necrotic tissue present. The patient's physician discusses with the physical therapist selective debridement of the wound. Which of the following is a selective debridement technique?

(A) Wet-to-dry dressings
(B) Whirlpool
(C) Sharp debridement via tweezers
(D) Wound irrigation

199. A research study finds that the age of a person is positively correlated with the number of days that the person spends in the hospital each year. What does this mean?

(A) As the patient's age increases, the number of days spent in the hospital decreases.

(B) As the patient's age increases, the number of days spent in the hospital increases.

(C) There is no relation between patient age and number of days spent in the hospital.

(D) Increased age of the patient is a direct cause of number of days spent in the hospital.

200. A physical therapist has been asked to evaluate the workstation of an administrative assistant to see if it is ergonomically correct. As the administrative assistant sits in his chair looking directly at his computer monitor, it appears that his seat height is incorrect. What should the position of his seat be relative to his knees?

(A) The knees should be slightly higher than the seat.

(B) The knees should be slightly lower than the seat.

(C) The knees should be straight out with feet supported on a stool.

(D) The legs should dangle off the edge of the chair.

End of Section 4

IF YOU FINISH BEFORE TIME IS CALLED, YOU MAY CHECK YOUR WORK ON THIS SECTION ONLY. DO NOT TURN TO ANY OTHER SECTION IN THE TEST. STOP

Section 5

201. A physical therapist is reading the chart of a patient admitted to the hospital with severe back pain. The chart indicates the patient has a spondylolisthesis at L3-L4. Which of the following *MOST* accurately describes what has happened to the vertebrae?

    (A) The two vertebrae have begun to fuse.
    (B) The two vertebrae are showing degenerative changes that appear "anvil-like" on X-ray.
    (C) There is a pars defect.
    (D) There is forward slippage of one vertebra on the vertebra below.

202. A physical therapist chooses to use electrical stimulation in the healing of an abdominal surgical wound. What is a contraindication to using electrical stimulation in this patient?

    (A) Recent surgery
    (B) Presence of edema
    (C) Decreased blood flow
    (D) Presence of a pacemaker

203. A patient is diagnosed with pericarditis following bypass surgery. What treatment interventions should *NOT* be included in the physical therapist's treatment plan?

    (A) High-level exercise
    (B) Ankle pumps
    (C) Skin protection via bed positioning
    (D) Patient education

204. A physical therapist has chosen to use a moist hot pack on a patient's knee at the beginning of her treatment session. Which of the following is *NOT* a treatment intervention goal to be accomplished with the use of heat early in the treatment?

    (A) Increased tissue extensibility
    (B) Decreased pain
    (C) Decreased muscle spasm
    (D) Increased muscle endurance with activity

205. A physical therapist is designing a home exercise program for a patient with vestibular pathology. He instructs the patient to perform Cawthorne exercises twice daily. Cawthorne exercises would be an example of what type of treatment intervention technique?

    (A) Adaptation
    (B) Habituation
    (C) Repositioning
    (D) Remodeling

206. A 72-year-old woman is referred to physical therapy with left thigh pain that is thought to be radicular in nature. She does not recall any injury or any activity that aggravates her pain. She does say that it wakens her at night and she cannot fall back to sleep. In the clinic, her symptoms are unable to be reproduced with assessment of the low back, hip, or knee. What differential diagnosis must be ruled out?

    (A) Metastatic cancer
    (B) Osteoarthritis
    (C) Lumbar disc herniation
    (D) Hip fracture

207. A physical therapist is educating a patient on the anti-inflammatory effects of ice after an injury. Which of the following is a secondary effect of inflammation following an injury?

    (A) Vasodilation in the area
    (B) Damage to surrounding viable tissue
    (C) Ligamentous laxity
    (D) Joint capsule tightness

208. A healthy 28-year-old patient has been instructed by his physician to maintain non-weight-bearing status on his left leg following an ankle fracture. He is preparing to return home independently and needs to be able to get from his bed to his chair. Which transfer technique would be *MOST* appropriate for him?

    (A) Slide board transfer
    (B) Stand-pivot transfer
    (C) One-person assist transfer
    (D) Hoyer lift transfer

209. A physical therapist examines an arterial wound of a patient's right lower extremity. Adjacent to the wound, the skin is white in appearance, is very thin, and has a soggy texture. The physical therapist documents this surrounding tissue as having what quality?

(A) Maceration
(B) Callus
(C) Scar tissue
(D) Slough

210. In an acute-care setting, a physical therapist is treating a patient who was recently diagnosed with a hiatal hernia. When exercising, which position should be avoided with a hiatal hernia?

(A) Supine
(B) Prone
(C) Right side-lying
(D) Left side-lying

211. A physical therapist is treating a patient for musculoskeletal pain who also has an underlying endocrine system dysfunction. Although the two may be completely unrelated, what is the significance of an endocrine pathology in treatment considerations?

(A) Acid-base imbalance
(B) Electrolyte imbalance
(C) Hormone imbalance
(D) Fluid imbalance

212. A physical therapist has been asked to give recommendations for appropriate exercise frequency and duration to a women's community group that is hosting a beginning exercise program. The women are all 30–45 years of age and have all been cleared to exercise by their family physicians. What would be the *MOST* appropriate recommendation for their program?

(A) 3x/week resistance training alternating with 3x/week aerobic exercise
(B) 5x/week resistance training alternating with 2x/week aerobic exercise
(C) 3x/week resistance training followed by 4x/week aerobic exercise
(D) 5x/week aerobic exercise

213. A physical therapist is directing his assistant and an aide in the transfer of a patient from a tilt table to the hospital bed. In a draw-sheet slide transfer from a cart to a bed, if there are three people available, where should each person be?

(A) Two on the pull side, one on the push side.
(B) Two on the push side, one on the pull side
(C) One at the head and one on each side
(D) One at the head, one at the feet, and one at the pull side

214. Following a cerebrovascular accident, a patient holds her right upper extremity in scapular retraction, elbow flexion, forearm supination, and wrist/finger flexion. What should the physical therapist use to document this position?

(A) Brunnstrom's classification of synergy
(B) Proprioceptive neuromuscular facilitation
(C) Neurodevelopmental treatment
(D) Modified Ashworth Scale

215. A physical therapist is working on gait training with a patient who is two months post-stroke. The patient is needing some assistance with ankle dorsiflexion, and the therapist has chosen to use functional electrical stimulation. Which of the following are the *MOST* appropriate parameters to assist with foot drop during gait?

(A) 30 μs width, 20 Hz, foot switch, motor intensity
(B) 30 μs width, 20 Hz, 10 sec on/30 sec off, motor intensity
(C) 30 μs width, 80 Hz, 10 sec on/30 sec off, motor intensity
(D) 30 μs width, 80 Hz, foot switch, motor intensity

216. A physical therapist is designing an exercise program for a patient with chronic low back pain and instability. Which of the following muscle groups should be strengthened to work together to stabilize the lumbar spine?

(A) Rectus abdominis, erector spinae, pelvic floor
(B) Rectus abdominis, multifidus, pelvic floor
(C) Transverse abdominis, erector spinae, pelvic floor
(D) Transverse abdominis, multifidus, pelvic floor

217. A group of patients who are all three months post–total knee arthroplasty are in a supervised strengthening program following discharge from physical therapy. They have all been cleared by their physicians to continue to exercise following discharge from therapy. Which member of the health-care team would be *BEST* suited to lead this group?

(A) A new-grad physical therapist
(B) An orthopedic surgical nurse
(C) A PTA with six years of long-term care experience
(D) A PT aide with three years of orthopedic experience

218. A physical therapist performs an initial evaluation on a patient at a skilled nursing facility. The patient's current diagnosis is exacerbation of COPD. Her goal is to return to her home, where she lives by herself. Currently, she requires minimum assistance for bed mobility, moderate assistance to transfer, and stand-by assistance for gait with a walker. What treatment intervention(s) can specifically address her physical impairments?

(A) Airway clearance techniques
(B) Diaphragmatic breathing exercises
(C) Functional training
(D) Pursed-lip breathing exercise

219. A patient suffers from demyelinating disease of the nervous system. What function does myelin have?

(A) Decreases the speed of impulse conduction
(B) Increases the speed of impulse conduction
(C) Transmits impulse across the synapse
(D) Organizes impulses

220. A physical therapist has chosen to use therapeutic ultrasound to decrease pain and increase tissue healing on a patient with acute lateral epicondylitis. The patient's symptoms have been present for the last two days and there is visible edema present. Which of the following parameters would be *MOST* appropriate for this patient?

(A) 1.0 W/cm^2, 3 MHz, continuous × ten minutes
(B) 1.0 W/cm^2, 1 MHz, continuous × ten minutes
(C) 1.0 W/cm^2, 3 MHz, pulsed 20 percent × ten minutes
(D) 1.0 W/cm^2, 1 MHz, pulsed 20 percent × ten minutes

221. A physical therapist is observing the posture of a woman with low back pain who is also 27 weeks pregnant. As her pregnancy progresses, what happens to the woman's center of gravity?

(A) It moves anterior/superior.
(B) It moves posterior/superior.
(C) It moves anterior/inferior.
(D) It moves posterior/inferior.

222. A female patient requests that a female physical therapist evaluate her. Her referring physician indicates she should be seen as soon as possible. The one female on staff is out on vacation for the next week, but there are many openings with other staff. What would be the appropriate action to take?

(A) Scheduling the patient with the next available appointment with any staff
(B) Scheduling the patient with the female staff next week
(C) Giving the patient the option of the next available appointment with a male therapist or next week with the female therapist
(D) Telling the patient there is no appointment available with a female therapist this week and referring the patient to another clinic

223. A physical therapist receives a referral to perform chest percussions on the right upper lobe of a child with cystic fibrosis. What are the lobes of the right lung?

(A) Upper and lower lobes
(B) Upper, middle, and lower lobes
(C) Anterior and posterior lobes
(D) Apical, upper, and lower lobes

224. A patient is receiving physical therapy for care of a wound. The physical therapist chooses whirlpool as a treatment technique. When should the whirlpool be discontinued?

(A) When the patient does not complain of pain in the wound
(B) When the wound stops bleeding
(C) When the signs of infection are gone
(D) When there is no necrotic tissue present in the wound bed

225. A physical therapist assistant reading the prior documentation for a patient that she is about to treat notices that the patient has dysphagia. What should the PTA do?

(A) Speak loudly to the patient
(B) Describe to the patient where things are located in the clinic
(C) Speak to the patient in simple words
(D) Be cautious when giving the patient food or drink

226. A physical therapist is treating two different patients following traumatic hip fractures. Patient A is a married female with a healthy, strong husband who is very eager to help. Patient B is a widowed female who has minimal family support and lives independently. Both patients have difficulty moving from sit to supine due to having trouble getting their legs into bed. Each patient requires moderate assistance with sit-to-supine at initial evaluation. The discharge plan is for both patients to return home. If the patients' strength and cognition are assumed to be the same, which patient would the physical therapist guess will be the first to learn how to get her legs into bed independently?

(A) Patient A will be the first to achieve independence with sit to supine.
(B) Patient B will be the first to achieve independence with sit to supine.
(C) The two patients will attain independence in sit-to-supine at the same time.
(D) Neither will be able to perform this activity independently.

227. A physical therapist is examining a patient whom he suspects has lower-limb neural tension. Which one of the following special tests would be *MOST* appropriate to confirm this diagnosis?

(A) Tinel test
(B) Phalen test
(C) Slump test
(D) Straight leg raise test

228. A hospitalized patient has been diagnosed with pleural effusion. How is this condition defined?

(A) Increased amount of pleural fluid
(B) Free air leaked into the pleural space
(C) Collapse of lung tissue
(D) Viral infection

229. A physical therapist evaluates a patient who has a traumatic brain injury. The therapist documents that the patient is demonstrating "Level IV—confused/agitated: maximal assistance." What scale is the physical therapist using?

(A) Modified Ashworth Scale
(B) Glasgow Coma Scale
(C) Rancho Los Amigos Cognitive Functioning Scale
(D) Brunnstrom's stages of recovery

230. A physical therapist is reviewing the past medical history of a 54-year-old patient who was referred to physical therapy for right shoulder pain. The patient has a 30-year history of smoking. He reports that recently he has also had trouble dropping things with his right hand. During evaluation, he has palpable tenderness of the right mid-scapular region. What differential diagnosis is the physical therapist concerned about?

(A) Pancoast tumor
(B) Spinal tumor
(C) Cervical nerve root irritation
(D) Brachial plexus injury

231. A physical therapy researcher plans to study the degree of agreement between clinicians measuring the range of motion of elbow flexion using a goniometer. What is this researcher examining?

(A) Validity
(B) Inter-rater reliability
(C) Intra-rater reliability
(D) Instrument reliability

232. A patient with cerebellar dysfunction may have difficulty performing rapid alternating movements such as rapid supination and pronation of the forearm. What term *BEST* describes this problem?

(A) Ataxia
(B) Bradykinesia
(C) Dysdiadochokinesia
(D) Dysphagia

233. A physical therapist working in a skilled nursing facility is treating a 72-year-old patient following a right total knee arthroplasty. The patient's medical history includes left total knee arthroplasty and prior postoperative deep vein thrombosis. The patient is currently taking a pain medicine and an anticoagulant. What does the physical therapist expect this patient's maximal heart rate to be?

(A) 220 beats per minute
(B) 148 beats per minute
(C) 120 beats per minute
(D) 144 beats per minute

234. A physical therapist is treating a patient who has neurological impairment and at initial evaluation is unable to sit on the side of the treatment mat independently. Two weeks later, the patient progresses to sitting on the side of the treatment mat independently, but only statically. One goal of physical therapy is to achieve independent dynamic sitting balance. Which treatment technique can be used to reach this goal?

(A) Increasing static sitting time by 20 minutes
(B) Having the patient perform fine motor tasks of the hands while supine
(C) Supine lower-extremity passive range of motion
(D) Multidirectional weight-shifting in sitting

235. A patient presents to physical therapy with a rash on his forearm following application of hydrocortisone gel the previous day. The skin is red with raised bumps. The physical therapist documents that the outer layer of skin is affected. What is the correct term for this layer of skin?

(A) Epidermis
(B) Dermis
(C) Hypodermis
(D) Subcutaneous layer

236. A patient with Alzheimer's disease sees a physical therapist who prescribes a home therapeutic exercise program to increase the strength of the lower extremities. What would be the *MOST* appropriate method of issuing the exercise program?

(A) Having the patient memorize the exercises
(B) Giving the patient written instructions for the exercise program
(C) Giving the patient time to practice the exercises twice in the clinic and giving the patient written instructions for the exercise program
(D) Having the patient practice the exercises several times with a caregiver present and providing written and pictorial instructions

237. A physical therapist is working with a patient with a transradial amputation. The patient, the prosthetist, and the physical therapist are determining the kind of terminal device with which the patient is to be fitted. The patient's goals are cosmesis and being able to open and close the terminal device without using the opposite, sound hand. Which terminal device is *BEST* suited to the patient?

(A) Active hook
(B) Active hand
(C) Passive hook
(D) Passive hand

238. A patient is referred to physical therapy for evaluation and treatment of carpal tunnel syndrome. The patient gives a subjective report of general fatigue and occasional body muscle soreness despite cutting back on her exercise routine and physical demands. She also reports that she gets worn out trying to sit up at her desk and feels that her legs weigh a ton when walking. What could be the *MOST* likely cause for this presentation?

(A) Neuromuscular pathology
(B) Musculoskeletal pathology
(C) Cardiovascular pathology
(D) Endocrine system pathology

239. A physical therapist is examining a patient who is found to have a left-rotated, left side-bent and flexed lumbar vertebra. When palpating that vertebral segment in extension, what structure should be prominent?

(A) The right transverse process
(B) The left transverse process
(C) The spinous process more posterior than the adjacent segments
(D) The spinous process more anterior than the adjacent segments

240. A patient with polio ambulates with Lofstrand crutches. He advances one crutch, then the opposite leg, then the other crutch, and finally the other leg. How would the physical therapist document this gait pattern?

(A) Two-point pattern
(B) Three-point pattern
(C) Four-point pattern
(D) Five-point pattern

241. How is generalization of learning defined?

(A) Learning is specific.
(B) It is the transfer of performance of a skill to a different environment.
(C) It is the carryover of learning from one learned skill to another related skill.
(D) All learning is the same.

242. A physical therapist takes an informal poll of patients in the physical therapy clinic. He asks each patient to classify his or her impairment as to what body system the patient feels is most affected. He asks them to classify their impairment into one of four categories; musculoskeletal, cardiopulmonary, neurological, or other. What type of information is the physical therapist gathering?

(A) Quantitative
(B) Qualitative
(C) Observational
(D) Statistical

243. A physical therapist is evaluating passive ROM of a patient's shoulder. He is trying to determine if a capsular pattern is present. What pattern of restriction would indicate a capsular pattern for the glenohumeral joint?

(A) Limitation of flexion > external rotation > internal rotation
(B) Limitation of external rotation > abduction > internal rotation
(C) Limitation of internal rotation > external rotation > abduction
(D) Limitation of external rotation > internal rotation > abduction

244. A research report states that an outcome measure is statistically significant. What does this mean?

(A) The sample size is too small.
(B) The treatment is not effective.
(C) The difference in the outcome measure is not likely due to chance.
(D) The studied treatment is not clinically important.

245. A patient is being evaluated at the clinic after being hit in the shin with a ground ball during a softball game. She describes pain and numbness on the lateral side of her lower leg and foot. On evaluation, she has weakness with ankle dorsiflexion and eversion. She has increased anthropometric measures at the mid-calf by 4 cm compared to the uninvolved side. What differential diagnosis *BEST* describes the subjective and objective findings?

(A) Tibialis anterior strain
(B) Lower-leg contusion
(C) Anterior compartment syndrome
(D) Tibial fracture

246. A physical therapist has been treating a patient in a nursing home for gait dysfunction. The patient has been making excellent progress, requiring only supervision with walking. For the past two days, the patient has had the flu. He is feeling better today but says his legs feel "worthless." Depletion of which electrolyte has a significant effect on muscle contraction and relaxation?

(A) Potassium
(B) Magnesium
(C) Calcium
(D) Iron

247. A physical therapist evaluates a patient after a cerebrovascular accident. The therapist has the patient close his eyes. The therapist then places the patient's big toe into dorsiflexion and asks the patient if the toe is up or down. What is the therapist evaluating?

(A) Light touch
(B) Reflexes
(C) Vibration
(D) Proprioception

248. A physical therapist working at an outpatient clinic has noticed that many of the patients she sees following knee replacement surgery at Hospital X tend to have decreased range of motion three weeks after surgery as compared to patients who had the same surgery at Hospital Y. What is one of the first actions the physical therapist should take?

(A) Calling Hospital X and complaining

(B) Discussing with each of her coworkers what she is seeing and refusing to treat patients from Hospital X

(C) Not discussing the problem with another physical therapist, but asking another physical therapist to measure the range of motion of these patients

(D) Using a different goniometer for the patients from Hospital X

249. An elderly female patient demonstrates an external locus of control regarding her health behavior. What technique would work *BEST* in getting this patient to change a health-related behavior?

(A) Asking another patient to share his related story with the patient

(B) Giving the patient several research articles with conflicting information and allowing her to draw her own conclusions

(C) Allowing the patient to direct her own treatment, with little guidance from medical staff

(D) Asking the patient's physician to offer expert advice and direction directly to the patient regarding the health behavior

250. A physical therapist is evaluating the range of motion of a patient's painful hip. Which one of the following orders of restriction would indicate capsular involvement?

(A) extension, abduction, medial rotation

(B) flexion, abduction, medial rotation

(C) flexion, abduction, lateral rotation

(D) flexion, adduction, medial rotation

End of Section 5

IF YOU FINISH BEFORE TIME IS CALLED, YOU MAY CHECK YOUR WORK ON THIS SECTION ONLY. DO NOT TURN TO ANY OTHER SECTION IN THE TEST. STOP

Exam 2

Section 1

1. A physical therapist is assisting a patient with some advanced gait activities to improve balance and mobility. When guarding the patient, the physical therapist should be in which of the following positions?

   (A) Directly in front of the patient
   (B) Directly behind the patient
   (C) At a 45° angle in front of the patient
   (D) At a 45° angle behind the patient

2. The lymphatic system drains into two large ducts. What are these terminal lymphatic vessels called?

   (A) Right and left lymphatic ducts
   (B) Thoracic and cervical ducts
   (C) Right lymphatic duct and thoracic duct
   (D) Superior vena cava and inferior vena cava

3. A physical therapist is reviewing the medication list of a current patient. He notices a list of medications the patient has taken or is currently taking to manage his back pain, which is extensive. Which one of the following pain medications could produce tolerance and physical addiction?

   (A) NSAIDs
   (B) Aspirin
   (C) Codeine
   (D) Acetaminophen

4. A physical therapist is evaluating a women's health patient with a chief complaint of involuntary leakage of urine. The patient describes it as occurring when she coughs, sneezes, or runs on the treadmill. Which diagnosis would *BEST* fit these symptoms?

   (A) Stress incontinence
   (B) Urge incontinence
   (C) Neurogenic bladder
   (D) Spastic bladder

5. A researcher decides to design a cohort study that examines the development of cerebral palsy in infants born to overweight mothers. He decides to study the children from birth to eight years of age. What type of research design is this?

   (A) Randomized clinical trial
   (B) Cohort study
   (C) Case study
   (D) Descriptive study

6. An 80-year-old resident of a nursing home has a stage I pressure ulcer on her coccyx. She is incontinent and needs moderate assistance with toileting. She is unable to reliably complete perianal hygiene herself. The physical therapist recommends what treatment interventions by the nursing staff?

   (A) Toileting schedule and application of protective ointment to the perianal area
   (B) Allowing the patient to complete toileting herself
   (C) Referral to a surgeon
   (D) Bathing the patient only biweekly

7. A physical therapist is treating a patient who has balance deficits. The therapist asks the patient to stand with her feet together and maintain standing balance with therapist-initiated challenges to balance. The therapist places her left hand at the patient's right anterior shoulder and her right hand at the patient's left hip and then increases pressure. If balance is maintained, the therapist places pressure on the posterior shoulder and anterior hip. What treatment technique is this therapist using?
   (A) Proprioceptive neuromuscular facilitation
   (B) Craniosacral therapy
   (C) Range of motion
   (D) Therapeutic exercise

8. Following a mastectomy, a female patient has lymphedema of the right arm. She is referred to physical therapy for the management of the lymphedema. What treatment intervention is appropriate for this patient?
   (A) Keeping the right arm in a sling
   (B) Limiting range of motion to passive
   (C) Compression wraps of the entire right arm
   (D) Keeping the right arm in a dependent position

9. A patient uses a manual wheelchair for independent mobility. The patient presents to physical therapy with complaints of difficulty propelling the wheelchair with the upper extremities, difficulty negotiating narrow hallways, and leaning to one side. The physical therapist determines that the wheelchair is which of the following?
   (A) Too narrow
   (B) Too wide
   (C) Too high
   (D) Too low

10. A physical therapist is researching what percentage of patients who have had a total knee arthroplasty at the local hospital received follow-up outpatient physical therapy. He obtains a list of people who have had this surgery in the last year. He intends to call each person on the list to obtain this information. How should he word this question when speaking with each patient?
   (A) "Did you seek the services of a licensed physical therapist following your total knee arthroplasty for increased range of motion and strength?"
   (B) "Didn't you need to go to a physical therapist after your knee surgery?"
   (C) "How many physical therapy treatments did you receive following your total knee arthroplasty?"
   (D) "Did you attend outpatient physical therapy services after your recent knee surgery?"

11. A physical therapist has just completed an initial evaluation on a patient who was referred with shoulder pain from a rotator cuff tear. As part of his intervention, the therapist performed manual therapy and instructed the patient in therapeutic exercise. Which of these would he use as his CPT code(s)?
   (A) Shoulder pain
   (B) Rotator cuff tear
   (C) Initial evaluation
   (D) Initial evaluation, manual therapy, and therapeutic exercise

12. A patient enters the clinic with low back pain. On evaluation of gait, there is a unilateral drop foot. Which reflex should the physical therapist test to confirm the level of nerve root involvement?
   (A) Patellar tendon reflex
   (B) Posterior tibial reflex
   (C) No reflex at this level
   (D) Achilles tendon reflex

13. A patient is referred to physical therapy for pelvic floor muscle retraining for urinary incontinence. She describes her incontinence as occurring when she sneezes or coughs or when she lifts her grandson. Which type of pelvic floor muscle exercise would be *BEST* suited for this patient?

    (A) Ten reps of pelvic floor isometrics, holding for seconds
    (B) Ten reps of quick pelvic floor contractions
    (C) Five reps of pelvic floor isometrics to fatigue
    (D) Five reps of pelvic floor resistive strengthening with vaginal weights, to fatigue

14. A physical therapist suspects development of endocrine disease in a patient he is treating. Which tissues would be *MOST* likely to be influenced by endocrine dysfunction?

    (A) Bony tissues
    (B) Connective tissues
    (C) Nervous tissues
    (D) Vascular tissues

15. A stabbing victim is in the hospital's intensive care unit. Besides suffering an incomplete C6 spinal cord injury, he also has other internal organ injuries. The knife caused damage to his pleura, which allowed air to leak into the pleural space. What is the *BEST* term for his condition?

    (A) Pleural effusion
    (B) Pneumothorax
    (C) Atelectasis
    (D) Pneumonia

16. Which major nerve is *NOT* included in the brachial plexus?

    (A) Radial nerve
    (B) Musculocutaneous nerve
    (C) Median nerve
    (D) Obturator nerve

17. Which of the following is an example of procedural knowledge?

    (A) The spinal level tested in the Achilles tendon reflex is S1-S2.
    (B) The Achilles tendon is attached to the gastrocnemius muscle.
    (C) To perform the test for the Achilles tendon reflex, tap the Achilles tendon.
    (D) The Achilles tendon reflex involves the tibial nerve.

18. A physical therapist has received a physician order for nonselective debridement of a 2 cm wound on a patient's coccyx. The patient is non-ambulatory but is transferred to a chair and repositioned regularly throughout the day. Which method of hydrotherapy would *BEST* suit this patient?

    (A) Hubbard tank
    (B) Highboy whirlpool
    (C) Irrigation
    (D) Pulsatile lavage

19. A physical therapist is evaluating a patient who has complaints of hip pain and tightness. Which functional test of the hip would *BEST* provide a quick screen for a capsular pattern of the hip?

    (A) Squat to the floor
    (B) Backward walking
    (C) Side-stepping
    (D) Bridging

20. A physical therapist is treating a patient in a nursing home for low back pain. On his third physical therapy session, the patient begins to complain of right flank pain and generally not feeling well. His chart shows that his temperature was 100°F yesterday and 102°F (39°C) today. He has also been calling for assistance to the bathroom more frequently. What may be the reason for the new symptoms?

    (A) Urinary tract infection
    (B) Colon cancer
    (C) Neurogenic bladder
    (D) Diverticulitis

21. A physical therapist decides to incorporate energy conservation techniques into the treatment of a patient with post-polio syndrome. What is the goal of this intervention?

    (A) Increase muscular strength
    (B) Decrease the work of muscles
    (C) Decrease pain
    (D) Improve posture

22. A physical therapist suspects that a patient has an electrolyte imbalance that is affecting muscular contractions and causing muscle cramping during exercise. Which of the following ions is *NOT* an electrolyte needed for peak muscular function?

    (A) Potassium
    (B) Magnesium
    (C) Calcium
    (D) Selenium

23. A patient presents to a physical therapy clinic with low back and buttock pain. The physical therapist has chosen to use mechanical lumbar traction for pain management and centralization of symptoms. Which clinical finding would be a contraindication for the use of lumbar traction?

    (A) Spinal nerve root irritation
    (B) Segmental joint hypomobility
    (C) Segmental joint hypermobility
    (D) Guarding of lumbar paraspinals

24. A physical therapist has been treating a patient for neck pain for seven weeks. The patient is no longer in need of skilled therapy services but really likes the soft-tissue mobilization he has been getting. On his final scheduled appointment, the patient brings in two free movie passes and suggests he continue for one more week. What would be the *MOST* appropriate plan of action?

    (A) Accepting the gift and agreeing to one more week of therapy
    (B) Graciously declining the gift but agreeing to one more week of therapy
    (C) Graciously declining the gift and explaining again the reason for discharge
    (D) Accepting the gift and explaining again the reason for discharge

25. A football player is cutting to one side to make a tackle when he tears his anterior cruciate ligament. What type of injury is this an example of?

    (A) Microtrauma
    (B) Macrotrauma
    (C) Transection
    (D) Compression

26. A physical therapist evaluates a wound that has hard black tissue throughout the open area. The therapist documents the amount of this tissue in the patient's chart. What term should the therapist use to correctly identify this tissue?

    (A) Slough
    (B) Eschar
    (C) Exudate
    (D) Granulation

27. A physical therapist is seeing a patient who is lacking terminal right elbow range of motion. What type of orthosis is appropriate for this patient?

    (A) Assistive
    (B) Substitutive
    (C) Protective
    (D) Corrective

28. A patient presents to physical therapy with a complaint of pain in the L5-S1 area with no radicular symptoms. Palpation and ROM assessment of the lower lumbar spine do not reproduce any of the patient's symptoms. What other musculoskeletal structure can refer pain to the lumbar spine?

    (A) T12 disc
    (B) T12 nerve root
    (C) L2 nerve root
    (D) L2 facet

29. A patient is referred to physical therapy for chronic low back pain. On evaluation, the physical therapist finds generally decreased trunk stability and poor postural awareness. The patient also has past medical history of diverticulosis. Which exercise may be *MOST* beneficial in controlling pain without irritating this GI disease?

(A) Diaphragmatic breathing techniques
(B) Posterior pelvic tilt
(C) High-load resistance training
(D) Bridging

30. A physical therapist performs a chart review of a hospitalized patient referred to physical therapy. The medical chart states the patient has a history of seizures. What medical test is used to diagnose seizures?

(A) X-ray
(B) Doppler ultrasound
(C) CT scan
(D) Electroencephalogram

31. A physical therapist working in a skilled nursing facility notes edema, warmth, and redness of a patient's right calf. The patient's gallbladder was removed, with a complicated postoperative course. The patient winces in pain when she squeezes her own calf. What test or measure is the next step for the physical therapist to perform?

(A) Thomas's test
(B) Thompson's test
(C) Speed test
(D) Homan's test

32. A patient is being treated for patellofemoral pain in both knees. Evaluation reveals that she has bilateral poor proprioception when performing single-leg balance tasks. Her physical therapist plans to strengthen the dynamic stabilizers of the knee. Which one of the following is *NOT* a dynamic stabilizer of the knee?

(A) The anterior cruciate ligament
(B) The popliteus
(C) The quadriceps femoris
(D) The semimembranosus

33. A physical therapist has been asked to evaluate and treat a patient who is in ICU with multiple organ dysfunction syndrome (MODS). Which of the following would be an appropriate goal for treatment intervention with this patient?

(A) Ambulation with a walker
(B) Active range of motion exercise
(C) Bed mobility
(D) Bed positioning to prevent skin breakdown

34. A physical therapist is planning intervention for a patient who presents with significant chronic suboccipital muscle tightness. Which of the following ultrasound parameters is *MOST* appropriate to decrease muscle spasm and reduce pain for this patient?

(A) 3 MHz, 1.0 W/cm^2, continuous × ten minutes
(B) 1 MHz, 1.0 W/cm^2, continuous × ten minutes
(C) 3 MHz, 0.8 W/cm^2, pulsed × ten minutes
(D) 1 MHz, 0.8 W/cm^2, pulsed × ten minutes

35. A physical therapist is designing an exercise program for a patient with a history of falls and gait dysfunction. Which of the following would be the *BEST* exercise program for this patient?

(A) Standing ankle dorsiflexion, standing ankle plantar flexion, standing hip abduction
(B) Seated long-arc quads, seated ankle dorsiflexion, hip adductor squeeze
(C) Side-lying hip abduction, straight leg raise, resisted ankle dorsiflexion
(D) Standing hamstring curls, standing hip flexion, standing hip abduction with weight

36. A senior center has asked a physical therapist to give its members a presentation on preventing falls. Which of the following recommendations would be the *LEAST* appropriate instruction for this group?

(A) Practice single-leg standing in the middle of the room to improve balance.
(B) Remove any throw rugs that may trip you.
(C) Provide adequate lighting in any high-traffic areas.
(D) Wear skid-resistant shoes or socks while walking around the house.

37. Which patient is the *MOST* likely candidate for an immediate postoperative prosthesis (IPOP)?

    (A) A frail 80-year-old woman with a transfemoral amputation and history of CVA
    (B) A 55-year-old man with good balance and a history of slow-healing wounds and incisions
    (C) A 21-year-old woman with a transtibial amputation due to a motor vehicle accident
    (D) A newborn with bilateral congenital transtibial deficiency of the left thigh

38. A physical therapist wants to test a patient's balance. Which of the following tests is the *MOST* appropriate?

    (A) Functional reach test
    (B) Nine-hole peg test
    (C) Mini-Mental State Exam
    (D) Frenchay arm test

39. A physical therapist must decide which types of tissue respond best to which type of intervention. To do this, it is necessary to understand tissue makeup. Which tissue type has the greatest percentage of elastin as a component?

    (A) Ligament
    (B) Tendon
    (C) Meniscus
    (D) Nucleosis propulsus

40. A physical therapist is reading a scientific journal. Which research design has the *MOST* scientific power in predicting treatment efficacy?

    (A) Randomized clinical trial
    (B) Case study
    (C) Descriptive study
    (D) Cohort studies

41. A physical therapist is addressing physical therapy students on wound care. With a wound that is draining and non-necrotic, what are the primary goals of treatment?

    (A) Add moisture and debride
    (B) Absorb moisture and debride
    (C) Add moisture and do not debride
    (D) Absorb moisture and do not debride

42. Following a cerebrovascular accident, a patient exhibits contralateral pelvic drop with left stance phase of gait. What should the physical therapist evaluate first?

    (A) Strength of left plantar flexors
    (B) Length of right hamstrings
    (C) Strength of left hip abductors
    (D) Strength of right hip abductors

43. A patient is seen at a sports medicine physical therapy clinic following an acute anterior talofibular ligament sprain. The initial goals of modality use are to lessen edema formation and manage pain. Which one of the following would be the *MOST* appropriate electrical modality to use?

    (A) Transcutaneous electrical nerve stimulation
    (B) Interferential current
    (C) Negative high-volt pulsed current stimulation
    (D) Positive high-volt pulsed current stimulation

44. A 27-year-old woman is being seen for low back pain; she is also 20 weeks pregnant. While riding the recumbent bicycle, after ten minutes her heart rate has increased from 90 bpm to 120 bpm. What is the correct action to have the patient take?

    (A) Continue exercising at the current intensity
    (B) Decrease the intensity
    (C) Increase the intensity
    (D) Stop all exercise

45. A physical therapist is treating a patient for patellar tendonitis. The patient's pain is most aggravated with the activities of playing basketball and running. The therapist has chosen to progress exercise to plyometrics and squats as long as they are pain-free. This is an example of what principle of exercise?

(A) Overload
(B) Specificity of training
(C) Fatigue
(D) Periodization

46. A patient is receiving physical therapy for gait training with a cane. The patient has a diagnosis of Parkinson's disease. What limitations can the physical therapist expect from this patient?

(A) Bradykinesia and rigidity
(B) Bradykinesia and paresthesias
(C) Chorea and rigidity
(D) Flaccidity and neglect

47. What is one purpose of the use of outcome measures in clinical practice?

(A) To document progress and goal attainment
(B) To decrease the efficiency of the therapist
(C) To decrease the time available for therapeutic intervention during patient visits
(D) To increase the number of therapy visits

48. One perspective of learning theory places emphasis on self-efficacy in health behavior change. An overweight patient discusses weight-loss strategies with her physical therapist. The patient relates that she has been on several diets, with only minimal success. Her mother and her husband have tried exercise and diet and lost some weight, but gained the weight back. Her family appears unsupportive in her weight-loss efforts. The patient states that she does not want to try to lose weight because she does not think the attempt will be successful. Does this person *MOST* likely have high or low self-efficacy?

(A) High self-efficacy
(B) Low self-efficacy
(C) Impossible to tell
(D) Fluctuating self-efficacy

49. A patient with Guillain-Barré syndrome (acute inflammatory demyelinating polyradiculopathy) presents with lower motor neuron impairments. What symptoms would be anticipated in a patient with Guillain-Barré syndrome?

(A) Hyporeflexia and spasticity
(B) Hyperreflexia and spasticity
(C) Hyporeflexia and flaccidity
(D) Hyperreflexia and flaccidity

50. As a treatment intervention for a patient with COPD, a physical therapist plans to educate the patient on proper body position to decrease the work of breathing. What position tends to decrease the work of breathing?

(A) Trendelenburg position
(B) Supine on flat surface, no pillows
(C) Forward-flexed with arms supported in front, with the patient in a sitting position
(D) Standing upright without arm support

End of Section 1

IF YOU FINISH BEFORE TIME IS CALLED, YOU MAY CHECK YOUR WORK ON THIS SECTION ONLY. DO NOT TURN TO ANY OTHER SECTION IN THE TEST. STOP

Section 2

51. A physical therapist is performing a canalith repositioning technique on a patient with positional vertigo. Partway through the maneuver, the patient becomes increasingly nauseated and dizzy. What is the *MOST* appropriate action for the therapist to take?

    (A) Stop the maneuver altogether
    (B) Continue the maneuver while the patient is dizzy and nauseated
    (C) Stop the maneuver, sit the patient up, wait for symptoms to lessen, and continue the maneuver where it was stopped
    (D) Wait for the symptoms to subside in the current position, then continue the maneuver

52. A physical therapist is evaluating a patient who presents with bilateral knee pain that he describes as arthritis. He states that he has never been officially diagnosed with arthritis and wonders if it could be osteoarthritis (OA) or rheumatoid arthritis (RA) or neither. Which of the following is a similarity between osteoarthritis and rheumatoid arthritis?

    (A) Both involve inflammation around the joints.
    (B) Both are symmetrical in joint presentation.
    (C) Both are prevalent in weight-bearing joints.
    (D) Both can be genetically linked.

53. While evaluating a patient, a physical therapist finds weakness in the patient's postural stabilizers that causes her to fatigue quickly with prolonged sitting at her computer. Which muscle fiber type primarily makes up the postural stabilizer muscles?

    (A) Type I
    (B) Type IIa
    (C) Type IIb
    (D) Type IIc

54. A patient presents to physical therapy five days post–ACL reconstruction. On evaluation, the physical therapist determines there is poor VMO activation with quad setting. He has given the patient NMES for home exercise, but the patient is fatiguing quickly with exercise. What parameter should be adjusted to decrease the onset of fatigue?

    (A) Decreasing the pulse rate
    (B) Decreasing the treatment duration
    (C) Decreasing the duty cycle
    (D) Increasing the duty cycle

55. A physical therapist is filling out his charge sheet following evaluation and intervention of a patient with knee pain from a medial meniscal tear. His charges included PT evaluation, therapeutic exercise, and manual therapy. In this case, which one would be considered the ICD-9 code(s)?

    (A) PT evaluation only
    (B) Knee pain
    (C) Therapeutic exercise and manual therapy
    (D) Medial meniscal tear

56. A physical therapist reads a research article that states that two variables are strongly and positively correlated. In this experiment the correlation coefficient is closest to what number?

    (A) –1.0
    (B) –0.5
    (C) 0
    (D) +1.0

57. A physical therapist is designing a patient's exercise program. His goal with this program is to increase the recruitment of type IIa, fast-twitch oxidative-glycolytic muscle fibers. Which exercise regimen and duration would be *MOST* appropriate for this type of training?

    (A) A 70-minute moderate-intensity circuit training workout
    (B) A 45-minute low-intensity bicycle workout
    (C) Ten repetitions of moderate-intensity 100-meter sprints
    (D) A 30-minute moderate-intensity jog

58. A patient has a tumor that is placing pressure on the cerebellum. The physical therapist is telling the patient where the cerebellum is located. How should the physical therapist explain this to the patient?

(A) The cerebellum is in the superior (or top) part of the brain.

(B) The cerebellum is in the posterior (back) and inferior (lower) part of the brain.

(C) The cerebellum is in the anterior (front) part of the brain.

(D) The cerebellum is in the lateral (side) area of the brain.

59. After a cerebrovascular accident, a patient is hospitalized in the intensive care unit with several fractures of the extremities, cervical vertebrae, and two ribs. The patient has atelectasis of the left lower lobe. He has a halo/vest orthosis to stabilize the cervical fracture. What is an appropriate treatment intervention for this patient?

(A) Postural drainage, Trendelenburg position

(B) Chest percussion

(C) Vibration

(D) Pursed-lip breathing

60. Which armrest style is *MOST* appropriate for a patient who plans to use sliding board transfers?

(A) Fixed armrests

(B) Adjustable armrests

(C) Desk armrests

(D) Removable armrests

61. A physical therapist uses an alginate to treat a patient with a wound. What type of wound is an alginate *BEST* used for?

(A) Shallow with no exudate

(B) Shallow with moderate exudate

(C) Deep with no exudate

(D) Deep with moderate exudate

62. A physical therapist is examining a patient with low back hypomobility and has chosen to do accessory joint mobilization of the lumbar spine. Which grade of mobilization would be large-amplitude oscillations into the range of resistance?

(A) Grade II

(B) Grade III

(C) Grade IV

(D) Grade V

63. A physical therapist who practices in the sports medicine setting with college-aged athletes is an avid reader of research articles. What outcome measure is *MOST* suitable to this physical therapist's clinical setting?

(A) The respiratory rate of retirement community residents after an 800-meter walk

(B) The Berg balance scores of people with Parkinson's disease

(C) The isometric strength of 20-year-old males following hamstring strain

(D) Modified Ashworth scores of spinal cord–injured patients

64. A physical therapist is treating a four-year-old boy who has cerebral palsy. The therapist has found that faded feedback is best suited for this patient. How should feedback be given to this patient?

(A) Providing feedback after every trial

(B) Providing feedback after every three trials

(C) Providing extensive feedback after the first few trials, but then decreasing the amount of feedback and increasing the time between feedback sessions

(D) Providing feedback only upon the patient's request

65. A 77-year-old woman has been referred to physical therapy for chronic knee pain. The physician has suggested she receive aquatic therapy in a heated pool to avoid joint irritation. Which of the following medications on her list might necessitate the suggestion of another option for physical therapy?

(A) Tricyclic antidepressants
(B) Beta-adrenergic blockers
(C) Insulin
(D) Anticoagulants

66. A physical therapist is evaluating a patient who is hospitalized with a compression fracture in the thoracic spine. The patient is a 77-year-old Caucasian female. She was transported to the hospital from the long-term care facility where she resides. Each morning she has two cups of regular coffee, then she crochets until lunchtime. What differential diagnosis must be considered with these demographics?

(A) Osteoarthritis
(B) Osteoporosis
(C) Osteosarcoma
(D) Rheumatoid arthritis

67. An 85-year-old woman is referred to physical therapy with a recent history of falls at the senior living center where she resides. She is generally deconditioned and appears frail but is able to walk safely with a walker in the clinic. Which exercise is *MOST* appropriate for her first day?

(A) Isometric strengthening
(B) Resistance strengthening with Thera-Bands
(C) Active range of motion
(D) Walking on the treadmill

68. A patient is three weeks post–ACL reconstruction and is having trouble gaining good quadriceps muscle activation. The treating physical therapist plans to implement the use of electrical stimulation to make further gains in quad strength. The *MOST* appropriate machinery and parameters are which of the following?

(A) Battery-powered stimulator, 300 μs width, 55 Hz, 15 seconds on/45 seconds off
(B) Battery-powered stimulator, 300 μs width, 55 Hz, 45 seconds on/15 seconds off
(C) Clinical stimulator, 200 μs width, 55 Hz, 15 seconds on/45 seconds off
(D) Clinical stimulator, 200 μs width, 55 Hz, 45 seconds on/15 seconds off

69. A 33-year-old female is running in her first marathon. The conditions at the start of the race are 80°F (27°C) and high humidity. At mile 20, the runner becomes disoriented and overly fatigued. She complains of a dry mouth and dry, cracked lips. She must sit down and cannot finish the race. From what is she *MOST* likely suffering?

(A) Allergic reaction
(B) Dehydration
(C) Deep vein thrombosis
(D) Asthma

70. Proprioceptive neuromuscular facilitation places emphasis on what type of movement?

(A) Flexion
(B) Extension
(C) Diagonals
(D) Single-joint

71. How can the bronchial secretions of a five-year-old boy with cystic fibrosis *BEST* be described?

(A) Absent
(B) Normal
(C) Abnormally thick
(D) Abnormally thin

72. A patient with a complete C7 spinal cord injury has a dual goal: to maintain bone strength to avoid future fractures and to maintain good respiration function to avoid lung infections. Which orthosis would be the *MOST* appropriate to achieve these goals?

(A) Knee-ankle-foot orthosis (KAFO)
(B) Standing frame
(C) Knee immobilizer
(D) Hip-knee-ankle-foot orthosis (HKAFO)

73. A patient is referred to physical therapy for a whiplash injury from a motor vehicle accident. The physician calls it a torticollis. What muscle remains in a shortened position, causing rotation and side-bending of the head?

(A) Levator scapulae
(B) Scalene
(C) Sternocleidomastoid
(D) Upper trapezius

74. A new instrument used to measure range of motion of the spine is being studied to test its validity. What is the *BEST* definition of validity?

(A) Likelihood for random error of a set of results
(B) Degree to which there is agreement between examiners
(C) Degree to which the instrument measures what it is intended to measure
(D) The same examiner obtaining the same measurement on different attempts

75. The health belief model is a health behavior change model that proposes the idea that the likelihood of a person making a health change is related to the person's thoughts about the health threat. A physical therapist should use this information in what way in treating a patient with postoperative total hip arthroplasty who refuses to follow prescribed hip position precautions?

(A) Refusing to treat the patient if he does not follow the precautions
(B) Educating the patient on the severity and cost of consequences of disobeying the hip position precautions
(C) Asking the patient's wife to remind him of precautions
(D) Not addressing this issue; it is the patient's choice

76. A physical therapist notes edema in a patient's left lower extremity following an abdominal surgery. As part of the evaluation, the therapist measures the edema. What procedure should the therapist follow to measure the edema?

(A) Measuring the girth of the patient's left leg at the level of the malleoli
(B) Measuring the girth of the patient's left leg in several places, including at the malleoli; at 3 cm, 12 cm, and 18 cm above the malleoli; and at the patella
(C) Measuring the girth of the patient's left and right legs in several places, including at the malleoli; at 3 cm, 12 cm, and 18 cm above the malleoli; and at the patella
(D) Take a picture only

77. A patient is referred to physical therapy for hip pain secondary to trochanteric bursitis. He is treated with stretching, resistive strengthening, and iontophoresis. After four treatments there is no change in his symptoms. He is also developing paresthesia along the lateral thigh. What other structure may be overlooked?

(A) Sciatic nerve
(B) Lateral femoral cutaneous nerve
(C) Iliotibial band tendonitis
(D) Femoral fracture

78. A physical therapist has been asked to educate a patient on diaphragmatic breathing techniques to coordinate with activity and exercise. The patient has been hospitalized with what has been diagnosed as a hiatal hernia. Which activity does *NOT* increase intra-abdominal pressure for this patient?

    (A) Lifting
    (B) Coughing
    (C) Prolonged sitting
    (D) Walking

79. A patient develops lateral epicondylitis from repetitive turning of knobs in his line job at a factory. This is an example of what kind of tissue injury?

    (A) Microtrauma
    (B) Macrotrauma
    (C) Dynamic overload
    (D) Compression

80. A physical therapist is instructing a patient in a bladder control program for urge incontinence. The patient has been successful in strengthening the pelvic floor, but he continues to have the urge to urinate every 20 minutes. Which method of retraining would be *BEST* suited for this patient?

    (A) Neuromuscular reeducation of the pelvic floor using electric stimulation
    (B) Use of biofeedback with pelvic floor contractions
    (C) Progressive voiding schedules
    (D) Decreasing the amount of water consumed daily

81. A physical therapist is treating a patient for knee pain. The woman has religious beliefs that require her to wear a dress at all times. Part of her treatment intervention includes cycling on the stationary bicycle for ROM. Her dress restricts this activity. What would be the *MOST* appropriate resolution to the problem?

    (A) Explaining to the patient that she must wear shorts for medical reasons
    (B) Discharging the patient, knowing that she cannot act against her beliefs
    (C) Creating a different way of working on ROM so as not to compromise her beliefs
    (D) Moving the stationary bicycle into a room where no one will see her wearing shorts

82. A diabetic patient has recently undergone transtibial amputation of his left leg and is experiencing phantom limb pain. The physical therapist has chosen to use TENS as a method of home pain management. Which of the following would *NOT* be an option for electrode placement?

    (A) On his right lower leg
    (B) On the distal end of his residual limb
    (C) On the proximal end of his residual limb
    (D) Over the L4-L5 nerve roots

83. A physical therapist has seen several patients in the last week with ankle injuries of ligamentous sprains. Which coexisting patient condition will *LEAST* inhibit the healing of the ligamentous injury?

    (A) Obesity
    (B) Diabetes mellitus
    (C) Arteriosclerosis
    (D) Pregnancy

84. A patient who works full-time as a receptionist is referred to physical therapy with chronic medial elbow pain that has progressively worsened over the last five years. There does not appear to be any inflammation over the area. What type of tendinopathy does this patient have?

(A) Tenosynovitis
(B) Tendonitis
(C) Peritendinitis
(D) Tendinosis

85. A physical therapist at a hospital prescribes a wheelchair for a patient with a fractured pelvis. To prescribe the seat depth, the therapist ensures that the patient's pelvis is positioned to the back of the wheelchair. The therapist should recommend a seat depth that allows for support of the thighs to approximately what distance from the popliteal fossa?

(A) 0 to 0.5 inch
(B) 1.5 to 2 inches
(C) 3 to 3.5 inches
(D) 5 to 5.5 inches

86. A patient with amyotrophic lateral sclerosis presents to physical therapy for one-time evaluation and training on an exercise program. The physical therapist educates the patient on the benefits of strengthening exercise. What goal is physical therapy *MOST* likely to address with exercise for this patient?

(A) Improving flexibility
(B) Preventing disuse atrophy while avoiding overwork fatigue
(C) Improving initiation of movement
(D) Preventing disease progression

87. Cardiac output depends on what two factors?

(A) BP × HR
(B) PVR × HR
(C) SV × HR
(D) BP × SV

88. A physical therapist is performing a manual muscle test for knee extension on a patient who is in the seated position. The therapist must place the patient in what position for the test to avoid the knee's locking "screw home mechanism"?

(A) Full extension
(B) 90° flexion
(C) 45° flexion
(D) 5° flexion

89. A physical therapist evaluates a two-month-old infant with multiple medical problems. When she touches the infant's cheek, the infant turns his head toward the therapist and opens his mouth. The physical therapist has tested what reflex?

(A) Moro reflex
(B) Startle reflex
(C) Stepping reflex
(D) Rooting reflex

90. A physical therapist is instructing a patient in body mechanics for moving a 150 lb load on a cart. Which of the following puts the *LEAST* amount of strain on the low back when moving the load?

(A) Pushing the cart
(B) Pulling the cart
(C) Both put equal stress on the low back.
(D) Since the load is on the cart, there is no stress.

91. A physical therapist examines a patient after a coronary artery bypass graft. The therapist finds that the patient's resting heart rate is 48 bpm. The heart rate is of normal rhythm. What term *BEST* describes this patient's heart rate?

(A) Normal heart rate
(B) Bradycardia
(C) Tachycardia
(D) Dysrhythmia

92. A physical therapist performs reflex testing on a patient. What neurologic level is the physical therapist testing when testing the Achilles tendon reflex?

(A) C1-C2
(B) T1-T2
(C) L1-L2
(D) S1-S2

93. A physical therapist working in a skilled nursing facility evaluates a patient who was recently discharged from the hospital after an intracranial hemorrhage and seizure disorder. The patient is able to ambulate with the use of a wheeled walker and minimum assistance. The therapist notices that the patient's right foot tends to drag during the swing phase. After completion of gait analysis, what test should the physical therapist perform?

(A) Manual muscle testing of the tibialis anterior
(B) Single-leg stance with eyes closed and no assistive device
(C) Finger-to-nose testing
(D) Reflex testing

94. Following her discharge from a skilled nursing facility, a patient experiences difficulty rising from her recliner chair. At the skilled nursing facility, she was independent with transfers and with sit-to-stand from her wheelchair, but she never had the opportunity to practice from other chairs. This patient has had decreased transfer of learning. What technique should have been used to avoid this?

(A) Bringing in her chair from home and practicing sit-to-stand prior to discharge
(B) Having the patient practice functional tasks, such as transfers, in a variety of environments
(C) Recommending a lift chair for the patient
(D) Increasing the number of repetitions of lower-extremity exercise

95. A physical therapist working at an inpatient brain injury rehabilitation center is treating a patient who has a traumatic brain injury. The patient initially had normal, pain-free range of motion of the right hip; however, he starts to complain of pain of the right hip, and the physical therapist notes a decrease in the range of motion. The hip is warm to palpation. What condition is this patient possibly exhibiting?

(A) Autonomic dysreflexia
(B) Heterotopic ossification
(C) Gout
(D) Flaccid paralysis

96. A physical therapist suspects that a patient is showing symptoms of an electrolyte imbalance. He is reviewing the patient's medication list to see if there is anything that may add to his assessment. Which of the following drugs can cause electrolyte imbalance?

(A) NSAIDs
(B) Diuretics
(C) Beta-blockers
(D) Corticosteroids

97. A patient who sprained his ankle stepping off a curb chooses to see a physical therapist as a primary entrance into health care in a direct access state. On evaluation, the physical therapist notes grade II laxity of the man's anterior talofibular ligament. What would be the *MOST* appropriate treatment intervention?

(A) Immobilization of the ankle in a walking boot
(B) AROM in a non-weight-bearing position
(C) AROM in a weight-bearing position
(D) Heel raises off the edge of a step

98. A child with cerebral palsy presents to the physical therapy clinic, where the physical therapist performs an evaluation. The therapist notes problems with posture and impaired timing and coordination of movement of the child's extremities. The child's movements appear to be poorly controlled. What word *BEST* describes this type of movement pattern?

(A) Hypotonicity
(B) Spasticity
(C) Flaccidity
(D) Athetosis

99. Which exercise should a physical therapist expect will cause the *GREATEST* increase in blood pressure?

(A) Standing lower-extremity exercise
(B) Isometric supine lower-extremity exercise
(C) Passive range of motion of the upper extremities
(D) Maximally resisted upper-extremity exercises while standing

100. A physical therapist prepares to interview a patient as part of his evaluation. The patient indicates that he does not speak or understand English very well, as Spanish is his primary language. What would be the *MOST* appropriate action for the therapist to take next?

(A) Continue with the interview and evaluation, and arrange for an interpreter on the patient's next visit
(B) Reschedule the evaluation to another time when an interpreter is available
(C) Skip the patient interview for now and move directly to the evaluation
(D) Continue with the interview and evaluation, using what minimal amount of Spanish the physical therapist can speak

End of Section 2

IF YOU FINISH BEFORE TIME IS CALLED, YOU MAY CHECK YOUR WORK ON THIS SECTION ONLY. DO NOT TURN TO ANY OTHER SECTION IN THE TEST. STOP

Section 3

101. A patient shows his physical therapist a list of current medications. The patient takes levodopa. What condition is this drug *MOST* likely used to treat?

   (A) Alzheimer's disease
   (B) Parkinson's disease
   (C) Post-polio syndrome
   (D) Multiple sclerosis

102. An 88-year-old patient at a skilled nursing facility is newly oxygen-dependent. She is a frail, deconditioned woman who plans to go home after discharge. She is unsteady on her feet and at risk for falls. She states that prior to hospitalization, she walked around her apartment by grabbing onto furniture. She also plans to go outside in her yard this summer and will need to keep her supplemental oxygen with her. From what type of assistive device might she benefit?

   (A) Four-wheeled walker with a basket
   (B) Single-tip cane
   (C) Quad cane
   (D) No assistive device

103. A physical therapist is treating an athlete who has developed reflux as a result of his strenuous swim workouts while training for a triathlon. The *BEST* position to avoid irritating a gastroesophageal reflux would be which of the following?

   (A) Left side-lying
   (B) Right side-lying
   (C) Prone
   (D) Supine

104. A physical therapist is just finishing treatment with a patient in an acute-care setting. The patient is considered a fall risk when trying to ambulate or transfer and should not be out of bed without assistance. Which of the following is *NOT* an appropriate safety precaution to take with this patient?

   (A) Keeping the bed at its lowest position
   (B) Keeping the side bed rails in the lowest position
   (C) Keeping the bedside table within close reach for essentials the patient may need
   (D) Keeping the call light within close reach of the patient

105. A physical therapist asks a patient to perform a biceps curl using a 4 lb weight. As the elbow flexes, there is a shortening of the biceps muscle while it contracts. The shortening of any muscle during an isotonic contraction occurs by which of the following means?

   (A) The sliding of troponin over tropomyosin filaments
   (B) The sliding of sarcomeres over Z-lines
   (C) The sliding of actin over myosin filaments
   (D) The sliding of myofibrils within the endomysium

106. A physical therapist has chosen to use ultrasound as a means of increasing tissue extensibility and facilitating pain relief as a heat mechanism. Which method of heat exchange is ultrasound considered?

   (A) Conduction
   (B) Convection
   (C) Conversion
   (D) Radiation

107. During evaluation, a physical therapist is manually muscle testing the knee extension of a patient who is unable to move through full range of motion in the seated position. In what position should the patient be placed to further assess strength?

   (A) Standing
   (B) Supine
   (C) Side-lying
   (D) Prone

108. A patient has been hospitalized for complications related to a urinary tract infection (UTI). Which of the following is *NOT* a complication from an untreated UTI?

(A) Osteoporosis
(B) Osteomyelitis
(C) Pericarditis
(D) Pleurisy

109. A physical therapist is reviewing the chart of a patient who was recently admitted to the hospital with heat exhaustion. The patient is being referred to physical therapy for recent complaints of problems with balance and coordination. Her recent labs indicate low TSH levels. What underlying pathology do these findings indicate?

(A) Hypothyroidism
(B) Hyperthyroidism
(C) Hypoparathyroidism
(D) Adrenal insufficiency

110. A physical therapist has chosen iontophoresis for pain management and decreased inflammation in a patient with lateral epicondylitis. Iontophoresis is an example of which type of electric current?

(A) Alternating current
(B) Direct current
(C) Pulsatile current
(D) Interferential current

111. A patient has been advised by his physician to begin an exercise program to assist with weight loss. The patient is considered clinically obese. Which of the following would be the *LEAST* appropriate exercise activity for this patient?

(A) Pedaling on a recumbent bicycle
(B) Aquatic therapy
(C) Resistive Thera-Band strengthening
(D) Walking the stairs

112. A physical therapist is just finishing treatment with a patient who is on contact and droplet precautions. As the therapist leaves the room, which one of the following is the correct order of action?

(A) Exit the room, remove mask and gown, remove gloves, wash hands
(B) Remove gloves, remove mask and gown, exit room, wash hands
(C) Remove gloves, remove mask and gown, wash hands, exit room
(D) Remove mask and gown, remove gloves, wash hands, exit room

113. A physical therapist is treating a patient for patellar tendinosis. Which of the following treatment interventions would be the *LEAST* beneficial in the long term for this patient?

(A) Stretching of quadriceps and hamstrings
(B) Modifying activity to avoid negative factors
(C) Ultrasound
(D) Closed kinetic chain resistive strengthening

114. A physical therapist is treating a patient who has a traumatic brain injury. The therapist notices that the patient is able to ambulate with less assistance when the lights are dimmed and soft music is playing. She decides to write an article about the patient for her local physical therapy chapter newsletter. She includes a funny story on how the dimmed lights and soft music make her feel. What type of evidence is the therapist including in this article?

(A) Anecdotal observation
(B) Randomized control
(C) Cohort study
(D) Case-control design

115. A patient with transfemoral amputation and prosthesis ambulates with an abducted gait. The patient is complaining of pain that causes this gait pattern. Where is the patient's *MOST* likely cause of pain?

(A) Medial pubic ramus
(B) Distal residual limb
(C) Greater trochanter
(D) Ischial tuberosity

116. A hospital administrator asks a physical therapist to talk to the staff of the hospital about preventing skin tears. The therapist educates the staff on the importance of patients' nutritional and hydration status in preventing skin tears. Protection and moisturization of the skin is also discussed. The therapist also recommends physical therapy referral for the prevention of skin tears. What could be one goal of physical therapy for the prevention of skin tears?

(A) Increase mobility to improve function and blood flow

(B) Increase strength through aggressive upper-body exercise on machines

(C) Remove assistive devices from the patient's use

(D) Placement of throw rugs throughout the facility to pad the floor

117. A patient enters the clinic with a complaint of low back and left leg pain. She says the pain is better with walking, worse with standing, and unchanged with sitting. Based on her subjective positional aggravating factors, which differential diagnosis would be the *MOST* likely cause?

(A) Degenerative joint disease

(B) Vascular compromise

(C) Disc herniation

(D) Hip osteoarthritis

118. A patient had a complete spinal cord injury at the C5 level two weeks ago. A physical therapy referral is made after the patient is medically stable and his spine is stabilized. The patient has not been out of bed following the injury. What treatment technique is the therapist *MOST* likely to use initially?

(A) Standing frame

(B) Quick positioning to sitting upright at the edge of the bed

(C) Tilt table

(D) Stand-pivot transfers

119. A physical therapist is working with a patient on range of motion of the right knee following total knee arthroplasty. The patient's knee motion is poor (80° three weeks postoperatively). He has expressed an interest in working on ambulation outdoors with a walker since the weather is nice. The therapist tells the patient that every time he gains 3° of right knee range of motion, she will assist him in walking outdoors. The patient achieves 83° of AROM, and the therapist assists him to ambulate outside. On her next visit he achieves 86° of AROM and again the therapist assists him outdoors. The patient likes being outside so much that he achieves nearly 3° of increased AROM each treatment session. What type of learning theory did the therapist employ?

(A) Operant conditioning

(B) Respondent conditioning

(C) Cognitive learning

(D) Social learning

120. A physical therapist is treating a patient in a home health setting following hospitalization due to pneumonia. During initial evaluation, the patient complains of one-pillow orthopnea and an occasional unproductive cough. Two days later, the patient is dyspneic at rest. She tells the therapist that she has gained 6 lb in the past two days. Her cough is much more frequent, but still unproductive. She also states that last night she needed to use two pillows to breath easier while she slept. The patient complains of extreme fatigue from walking to answer the door. The physical therapist calls the patient's physician with her signs and symptoms. The physician recommends that the patient go to the emergency room for evaluation and treatment. The physical therapist and the physician are concerned about this patient presenting with what condition?

(A) Congestive heart failure
(B) Myocardial infarction
(C) Peripheral vascular disease
(D) Cerebrovascular accident

121. A physical therapist is examining a patient with right low back pain and radiculopathy that travels to just above the right knee. On observation, she sees that the patient is shifted toward the left. Which direction has the disc *MOST* likely herniated?

(A) Directly posterior
(B) Left posterolateral
(C) Right posterolateral
(D) Right posteromedial

122. A physical therapist receives a phone message from a patient's wife asking how her husband is progressing with his therapy. Which of the following is the *MOST* appropriate action for the physical therapist to take?

(A) Call and give the wife the information over the phone
(B) Call and let the wife know that the husband's information cannot be given out without his permission
(C) Ask the patient if it is okay to give his wife his information
(D) Call and let the wife know she must come in to receive that information in person

123. A patient is exercising during his regular physical therapy treatment session. He has a history of type 1 insulin-dependent diabetes. After his ten-minute warm-up on the bicycle, he looks flushed and feels nauseated. He has some confusion about where he is, and he has acetone breath. What abnormal response to exercise is occurring?

(A) Myocardial infarction
(B) Hypoglycemic response
(C) Hyperglycemic response
(D) Hyperhydration

124. A physical therapist receives a referral for wound care of a patient with a pressure ulcer on the left heel. The heel has an open wound that extends to the underlying subcutaneous tissue. The physical therapist documents that the wound is in what stage?

(A) Stage I
(B) Stage II
(C) Stage III
(D) Stage IV

125. A physical therapist decides to use proprioceptive neuromuscular facilitation as a treatment technique for a patient with neurologic impairment. What is the proper progression of stages of motor control that this treatment can treat, starting with the lowest stage?

(A) Stability, mobility, controlled mobility, skill
(B) Mobility, stability, controlled mobility, skill
(C) Mobility, skill, stability, controlled mobility
(D) Stability, skill, mobility, controlled mobility

126. A physical therapist is creating an exercise program for a patient with gastrocnemius weakness following a muscle strain. What type of muscular contraction is *BEST* for functional strengthening of this type of muscle?

(A) Isometric
(B) Concentric isotonic
(C) Eccentric isotonic
(D) Econcentric isotonic

127. A researcher establishes this hypothesis: "Following knee replacement, patients over the age of 80 have a more decreased knee range of motion than patients under the age of 80." What is the independent variable of this hypothesis?

(A) Knee range of motion prior to knee replacement
(B) Knee range of motion after knee replacement
(C) Age of knee replacement patients
(D) Sex of patients

128. A physical therapist is instructing a patient in pelvic floor strengthening exercise. When giving instructions on how to perform the exercise, which of the following will yield the *BEST* results in pelvic floor strengthening?

(A) "Tighten the muscles that stop the flow of urine by also contracting your gluteals."
(B) "Tighten the muscles that stop the flow of urine by also contracting your adductors."
(C) "Tighten the muscles that stop the flow of urine while allowing your gluteals and adductors to relax."
(D) "Tighten the muscles that stop the flow of urine by also contracting your gluteals and your adductors and holding for five seconds."

129. In normal, relaxed respiration of a healthy person, what is responsible for the work of expiration?

(A) Diaphragm
(B) Elastic recoil
(C) External intercostals
(D) Internal intercostals

130. A five-year-old female patient has a diagnosis of cerebral palsy. The patient has severe spasticity of all four limbs. What classification of cerebral palsy does this patient have?

(A) Spastic quadriplegia
(B) Spastic diplegia
(C) Spastic hemiplegia
(D) Flaccid quadriplegia

131. A patient is referred to physical therapy for gait training and balance assessment after several near falls. The patient denies any pain but says she just catches her toes when she walks. On evaluation, she has weakness with ankle dorsiflexion and eversion but no pain. She also has paresthesia on the lateral side of her foot. Which modifiable activity of daily living could bring on these symptoms?

(A) Crossing her legs
(B) Kneeling on the floor
(C) Prolonged standing
(D) Driving

132. A physical therapist is researching the distance ambulated by a patient on five separate treatments. He wants to find the median distance that this patient has ambulated. The distances are: 25 feet, 100 feet, 36 feet, 10 feet, and 82 feet. What is the median distance?

(A) 50.6 feet
(B) 36 feet
(C) 100 feet
(D) 10 feet

133. An infant with myelomeningocele has recently had surgical closure of the spinal defect. The infant then starts showing signs of hydrocephalus, including bulging fontanelles, increased head circumference, and downward-gazing eyes. What medical treatment is *MOST* likely to be performed for this infant?

(A) Serial casting
(B) Ventricular shunt placement
(C) Bracing
(D) Prescription glasses

134. A 45-year-old woman has been referred to physical therapy for bilateral knee pain. She presents with swelling throughout both knees, complaints of morning stiffness regardless of activity, and pain with walking. When asked about any other areas of pain, she admits to bilateral wrist and hand pain and strange little bumps on the backs of her fingers. Based on her subjective information, which of the following differential diagnoses must be suspected?

(A) Osteoarthritis
(B) Degenerative joint disease
(C) Rheumatoid arthritis
(D) Systemic lupus erythematosus

135. A physical therapist is treating a patient who was referred with shoulder pain that began as a result of a fall four months ago. The patient's next follow-up appointment with her physician to learn the results of a recent MRI is in two weeks. A copy of the MRI has been sent to the therapist's office and indicates she has a torn labrum and supraspinatus. On her visit to the clinic today, the patient asks the therapist if she has a rotator cuff tear. What would be the appropriate response?

(A) Explain that the MRI indicates a torn rotator cuff and labrum
(B) Explain that the results are known but will not be discussed
(C) Explain that discussing an MRI is beyond the scope of physical therapy practice
(D) Tell her that you know nothing about the MRI

136. A physical therapist has chosen to use high-volt pulsed current for pain management. According to the opiate pain control theory, electrical stimulation stimulates the release of what chemicals within the body?

(A) Enkephalin and beta-endorphins
(B) Prostaglandins
(C) Norepinephrine
(D) Epinephrine

137. A patient presents with vision problems, loss of balance, tinnitus, and dysphagia. Past medical history reveals a diagnosis of rheumatoid arthritis. What progression may be happening?

(A) Atlantoaxial instability
(B) Hyperfunctioning vestibular system
(C) Spondylolisthesis
(D) Transischemic attack

138. A patient with a C5 spinal cord injury and impaired sensation has a history of decubitus ulcers on his coccyx. The patient's physical therapist should recommend what type of wheelchair cushion?

(A) Foam
(B) Gel
(C) Gel/foam combination
(D) Air cell

139. A physical therapist evaluates a patient who has a burn of the right elbow. The therapist should note what key measures at the elbow?

(A) Range of motion
(B) Stage of the wound
(C) Oxygen saturation
(D) Lower-extremity strength

140. A patient asks a physical therapist about the brain stem. The therapist tells the patient that the brain stem is made up of three structures. What is the order of the three brain-stem structures, from most cephalic to most caudal?

(A) Medulla, midbrain, pons
(B) Pons, midbrain, medulla
(C) Midbrain, pons, medulla
(D) Medulla, pons, midbrain

141. Preferred practice pattern 6B involves patients with deconditioning. What is a physiologic change that is seen in patients with prolonged bed rest?

(A) Increased strength
(B) Decreased VO_2 max
(C) Decreased functional activities
(D) Hypertension

142. A patient is referred to physical therapy with shoulder pain. She reports pain with reaching overhead and out to the side. Evaluation reveals signs and symptoms that are indicative of impingement. Which of the following is *NOT* a probable cause of shoulder impingement?

(A) Forward-shoulders posture
(B) Deltoid weakness
(C) Rotator cuff weakness
(D) Scapular weakness

143. A physical therapist is teaching three new tasks to a patient with neurologic impairments. The therapist asks the patient to repeat Task #1 five times in a row. Then the therapist asks the patient to repeat Task #2 five times in a row. Finally, the patient is asked to repeat Task #3 five times in a row. What type of practice schedule has this therapist employed?

(A) A patient-directed practice schedule
(B) Unsystematic practice
(C) Blocked practice
(D) Random practice

144. Use of the Peabody Development Motor Scales are *MOST* appropriate for which patient population?

(A) Elderly patients with risks of falls
(B) Patients who have had a cerebrovascular accident
(C) Patients with chronic obstructive pulmonary disease
(D) Children with myelomeningocele

145. A 99-year-old patient fractures her pelvis due to a fall. She has a significant amount of pain with weight-bearing on the left leg and therefore self-limits her weight-bearing on the left lower extremity. During ambulation with a walker, she advances the walker, then the left leg, then the right leg. What gait pattern is this patient using?

(A) Two-point gait pattern
(B) Modified four-point gait pattern
(C) Three-point gait pattern
(D) Four-point gait pattern

146. A physical therapist examines an 80-year-old male patient in an outpatient clinic. Before reviewing his patient interview form, the therapist notices that the man is barrel-chested. His sternocleidomastoid and trapezius muscles are hypertrophic. Digital clubbing of the fingers is present. On the basis of these physical observations, in what organ system does the therapist expect to see dysfunction?

(A) Nervous system
(B) Skeletal system
(C) Urinary system
(D) Pulmonary system

147. A physical therapist documents that a patient with neurologic impairment presents with clonus of the right foot. What is the stimulus for the test for clonus?

(A) Rapid dorsiflexion of the ankle
(B) Slow dorsiflexion of the ankle
(C) Squeezing the calf
(D) Stroking the outer edge of the sole of the foot

148. A patient has been diagnosed with a positive chest X-ray for tuberculosis. What special considerations must be taken for the patient's room while he is hospitalized?

(A) Door remains closed, with ventilation to the outside

(B) Door remains open

(C) Door remains closed, with no additional ventilation

(D) Door remains open with a screen

149. A physical therapist is reviewing the medication list of a patient she is going to evaluate. She notices that the patient has been taking a beta-blocker for hypertension and was just given Relafen for its anti-inflammatory benefits. What effect does this have on the therapist's choice for treatment intervention?

(A) Indicates that heat modalities should not be used

(B) Indicates that blood pressure may not be controlled as well by the beta-blocker during exercise

(C) Indicates that activity in the supine position should be avoided

(D) Indicates that heart rate may significantly elevate during exercise

150. A physical therapist is treating a patient who has right hemiplegia due to cerebrovascular accident. The therapist uses lateral weight-shifting in sitting in order to activate the trunk musculature. With the patient sitting on the side of the mat, the therapist asks the patient to reach toward the left side. What muscle activity is the therapist addressing?

(A) Eccentric contraction of the right trunk musculature

(B) Concentric contraction of the right trunk musculature

(C) Eccentric contraction of the trunk extensors

(D) Concentric contraction of the trunk extensors

End of Section 3

IF YOU FINISH BEFORE TIME IS CALLED, YOU MAY CHECK YOUR WORK ON THIS SECTION ONLY. DO NOT TURN TO ANY OTHER SECTION IN THE TEST. STOP

Section 4

151. A physical therapist determines that a patient is experiencing symptoms consistent with impingement of the C6 nerve root. Where does the C6 nerve root exit the spine?

(A) Between C3 and C4
(B) Between C4 and C5
(C) Between C5 and C6
(D) Between C6 and C7

152. A patient is evaluated for a complaint of right foot pain that is present with walking. The physical therapist observes the patient's gait and notices decreased heel strike on the right foot. The observations would be written in which portion of the note?

(A) Subjective
(B) Objective
(C) Assessment
(D) Plan

153. A physical therapist is conducting a regular safety inspection of clinical electrical equipment. Which of the following does *NOT* meet the standards of electrical safety in the clinic?

(A) Use of an extension cord to avoid a trip hazard for patients and staff
(B) Use of a ground fault interrupter outlet
(C) Use of equipment that was checked eight months ago
(D) Use of equipment that is 20 years old but was inspected six months ago

154. A patient has made six visits to the physical therapist for treatment for pain along the lateral border of the right scapula. The pain continues to be a dull ache that does not seem to change with mobility but may increase with activities that involve bearing down. There has been no change in the symptoms since the patient started therapy, despite several different treatment interventions. What visceral pathology may be occurring?

(A) Cardiac
(B) Pancreas
(C) Peptic ulcer
(D) Kidney

155. A patient exhibits hypertonicity following a traumatic brain injury. What possible problems can exist for failing to identify and address this hypertonicity?

(A) Increased flexibility
(B) Joint contractures
(C) Shoulder subluxation
(D) Hip dislocation

156. A physical therapist is using airway clearance techniques to treat a 13-year-old girl who has cystic fibrosis. The patient's current obstructions due to her secretions are in the bilateral lower lobes. What is the ideal position for clearing secretions from the lower lobes by means of postural drainage and percussion?

(A) Supine in a flat bed
(B) Sitting
(C) Prone in a flat bed
(D) Prone, with the foot of the bed raised 18 inches higher than the head of the bed

157. A patient is referred to physical therapy with a diagnosis of pain in the anatomical snuffbox. Which of the following areas should the physical therapist palpate as the painful area?

(A) Distal to the radial styloid process
(B) Proximal to the radial styloid process
(C) Distal to the ulnar styloid process
(D) Proximal to the ulnar styloid process

158. What is an example of nonexperimental research?

(A) Oral interview
(B) Longitudinal design
(C) Cross-sectional design
(D) Blind design

159. A physical therapist is treating a female patient who has had a left hemispheric cerebrovascular accident. She has difficulty with all functional movements and requires moderate assistance for bed mobility. She cannot get her legs up into bed with sit-to-supine activity and cannot stand up from the bed once she is seated. During one treatment session, the therapist focuses on getting into and out of bed. She wants to provide the patient with some challenge and also the possibility of success. What treatment intervention could the therapist use?

(A) Using an adjustable mat, place the mat in the highest position possible and ask the patient to get on and off the mat.

(B) Using an adjustable mat, place the mat in the lowest position possible and ask the patient to get on and off the mat.

(C) Using an adjustable mat, place the mat in the lowest position possible and ask the patient to move from sit to supine. Then adjust the mat to the highest position possible and ask the patient to sit and then stand up.

(D) Using a soft, nonadjustable bed, ask the patient to get into and out of bed. Do not offer the patient any assistance.

160. A patient presents to physical therapy two weeks after a total hip replacement. The physical therapist examines the scar, which is well healed and dry. What color is the scar *MOST* likely to be?

(A) Red

(B) Pink

(C) Purple

(D) Brown

161. A patient with a spinal cord injury wants to be able to roll side-to-side on his bed. What instructions should his physical therapist give him so he can achieve his goal?

(A) "Leave your arms at your side and press down with your hands to roll."

(B) "Cross your ankles and raise your arms up toward the ceiling. Use a rocking motion to roll your body over."

(C) "Extend your head and neck to roll from your back to your front."

(D) "Ask your family to roll you."

162. A patient enters the clinic with a complaint of low back pain with radicular symptoms down the right leg. She describes the symptoms as better with sitting and worse with standing. Based on her subjective complaints, which differential diagnosis is *MOST* appropriate?

(A) Disc herniation

(B) Spinal stenosis

(C) Sciatica

(D) Degenerative disc disease

163. A physical therapist is instructing a patient in crutch training to descend a curb or step. The patient is to maintain touch weight-bearing on his left foot. What should be the first instruction given by the physical therapist?

(A) "Place the left foot on the step below."

(B) "Place the right foot on the step below."

(C) "Place both crutches on the step below."

(D) "Place the right foot and the left crutch on the step below."

164. A physical therapist is exercising a patient who has mechanical low back pain. The patient complains of worsening muscle pain with exercise and weakness that is worsening throughout the treatment session. What adverse reaction could be occurring in a patient with hypothyroidism?

(A) Ketoacidosis

(B) Hyperhydrosis

(C) Dehydration

(D) Rhabdomyolysis

165. A 21-year-old patient sustained a distal tibial fracture. The physician set and casted the patient's leg, and ordered non-weight-bearing for six weeks. The patient is referred to physical therapy for gait training with an assistive device. The physical therapist teaches the patient to use axillary crutches. The therapist teaches the patient that improper use of the device carries the risk of injury to which of the following?

(A) Axillary vessels or nerves

(B) Biceps muscle

(C) Triceps muscle

(D) Low back

166. What body part has the largest representation on the sensory homunculus compared to the actual size of the body part?

(A) Knee
(B) Elbow
(C) Face
(D) Abdomen

167. A physical therapist working in a hospital evaluates a patient with newly diagnosed COPD. At rest on room air, the patient's oxygen saturation is 92 percent. His heart rate is 82 bpm. Blood pressure is 140/70 mm Hg. The patient ambulates 300 feet with standby assistance. After this bout of ambulation, his vital signs are: oxygen saturation 86 percent, heart rate 90 bpm, blood pressure 148/70 mm Hg. The patient complains of shortness of breath. What is the therapist's next course of action?

(A) Allow the patient to use a walker for ambulation
(B) Call the physician immediately
(C) Apply supplemental oxygen and reevaluate the vital signs
(D) Ambulate the patient back to his room quickly

168. A physical therapist is treating a number of patients with low back pain. Each patient has a different diagnosis with different aggravating factors. It would be *MOST* characteristic of which diagnosis for the patient to have pain that is worse in the morning and improves within several hours of getting out of bed?

(A) Spinal stenosis
(B) Mechanical low back pain
(C) Discogenic pain
(D) Piriformis syndrome

169. A researcher expects to find a normal distribution of measurements in a research study. What is the shape of the curve of a normal distribution?

(A) Bell-shaped curve
(B) J-shaped curve
(C) Bi-peaked curve
(D) Spiked curve

170. While evaluating a patient, a physical therapist notes digital clubbing. What does this *MOST* likely signify?

(A) Arthritis
(B) Drug abuse
(C) Cardiopulmonary disease
(D) Pain

171. A 75-year-old patient is referred for physical therapy evaluation of acute-onset thoracic pain. She describes the pain as sharp in nature but does not recall any mechanism of injury. Her DXA score at age 70 was –2.0. What underlying pathology should be suspected?

(A) Diabetes mellitus
(B) Osteoarthritis
(C) Degenerative disc disease
(D) Osteoporosis

172. A physical therapist is making discharge recommendations to a patient for his home program. He has been exercising in therapy 3x/wk and at home 3x/wk for four weeks. Twice a week he exercised twice a day (resistance and aerobic). Which exercise recommendations are *BEST* to maintain the strength gains this patient has seen?

(A) 2x/week, 1x/day, same intensity/duration
(B) 3x/week, 1x/day, same intensity/duration
(C) 1x/week, 1x/day, same intensity/duration
(D) 5x/week, 1x/day, same intensity/duration

173. A physical therapist is positioning a 120 lb patient for mechanical lumbar traction. The table is not a split traction table. Assuming the coefficient of friction is 50 percent, at what amount of force should the mechanical unit be set to generate a 40 lb force?

(A) 40 lb
(B) 70 lb
(C) 80 lb
(D) 60 lb

174. A physical therapist who works in a hospital setting comes upon a liquid spill as he is working. Which would be his *MOST* appropriate plan of action?

(A) Leave the spill as it is

(B) Clean up the spill

(C) Block off the area and contact the unit supervisor

(D) Block off the area and notify housekeeping

175. A patient describes having dizziness when getting into and out of bed. She describes it as a spinning sensation that lasts ten seconds or so. Which of the following tests for vertigo would be *MOST* appropriate to further diagnose the cause?

(A) Dix-Hallpike test

(B) Roll test

(C) Vestibular-ocular reflex test

(D) Gaze stabilization test

176. A physical therapist is evaluating a patient for hip pain. During the physical assessment, he notes facial grimacing, tremors, and a shuffling gait. Which of the following psychopathological conditions may be the cause of these presentations?

(A) Nonmedicated schizophrenia

(B) Medicated schizophrenia

(C) Dementia

(D) Bipolar disorder

177. An infant is born with congenital hip dysplasia. Orthotics are used in the infant's treatment. What is the main physicaltherapy goal of these orthotics?

(A) Increase the strength of the hip musculature

(B) Decrease the tone of the hip musculature

(C) Position the femoral head in the acetabulum

(D) Provide resistance to hip movement

178. A physical therapist is treating a hospitalized patient who has a large venous ulcer on the left leg. A copious amount of exudate is draining from the wound. The physical therapist should use what treatment technique?

(A) Absorbent dressing

(B) Nonabsorbent dressing

(C) Noncompressive dressing

(D) Dependent positioning

179. A physical therapist is asked to see an infant who was diagnosed with osteogenesis imperfecta. Osteogenesis imperfecta is a congenital autosomal-dominant disease that results in brittle, easily broken bones; hyperlaxity of ligaments; and hypotonia. What should be a major intervention in treatment of this infant?

(A) Aggressive strengthening

(B) Early standing

(C) Caregiver instruction on proper handling and positioning to prevent fractures

(D) Icing

180. A patient is referred to physical therapy for low back pain that is worse with standing or with lying in the prone position. He also complains of radicular symptoms down his leg to below the knee. On evaluation, the physical therapist determines that the patient has signs and symptoms coincident with spinal stenosis. Which spinal ligament is *MOST* commonly the culprit in the narrowing of the spinal foramina?

(A) Anterior longitudinal ligament

(B) Posterior longitudinal ligament

(C) Ligamentum flavum

(D) Interspinous ligament

181. A patient is being treated for adhesive capsulitis at an outpatient physical therapy clinic. The clinician measures range of motion of shoulder flexion at each treatment. On the first five treatments, the ranges of motion are as follows: 80°, 85°, 82°, 89°, and 90°. What is the mean range of motion of these measurements?

(A) 85.2°
(B) 85°
(C) 85.6°
(D) 90°

182. Where does the normal electrical conduction of the heart begin?

(A) SA node
(B) AV node
(C) Bundle of His
(D) Purkinje fibers

183. A patient presents to physical therapy with a spinal cord injury. Specifically, the patient suffers from anterior cord syndrome. What should the physical therapist anticipate will be the patient's symptoms?

(A) Loss of movement, pain, and temperature sensation bilaterally below the level of the injury
(B) Loss of movement, proprioception, and vibration on the same side as the injury
(C) Loss of proprioception and vibration bilaterally
(D) Upper and lower motor neuron signs present

184. A patient presents weak dorsiflexors on the right lower extremity due to a peripheral nerve injury. The PT notes foot drag and recommends a plastic ankle-foot orthosis (AFO). In general, an AFO uses what type of pressure system?

(A) One-point
(B) Two-point
(C) Three-point
(D) Four-point

185. Which practice schedule results in faster acquisition of a skill but poorer retention of the skill?

(A) Random practice
(B) Blocked practice
(C) Random and blocked practice both result in fast acquisition and poor retention.
(D) Neither random nor blocked practice results in fast acquisition and poor retention.

186. A physical therapist is treating a patient for shoulder pain and glenohumeral joint hypomobility. The patient also has secondary diagnoses of diabetes mellitus, heart disease, and osteoporosis. Which of the following would be the *MOST* appropriate intervention for this patient's impairments?

(A) Grade III glenohumeral joint mobilizations
(B) Thera-Band resistive strengthening exercise
(C) Active assistive range-of-motion exercises
(D) Isometric strengthening exercises

187. A physical therapist is reviewing the chart of a patient who is scheduled to go to court for damages that occurred in a motor vehicle accident. Following the rules of patient confidentiality, which one of the following people does *NOT* have the authority to review the physical therapy notes?

(A) The referring physician
(B) The defending lawyer
(C) The patient's spouse
(D) The patient's insurance carrier

188. A physical therapist is working on gait training with a patient who has a recent history of a stroke (six weeks ago). The patient demonstrates a steppage gait. The use of functional electrical stimulation may be beneficial at which of the following sites?

(A) Over the tibialis anterior
(B) Over the psoas major
(C) Over the gastrocnemius
(D) Over the biceps femoris

189. A physical therapist has been consulted for treatment of bilateral knee pain and difficulty walking in a patient with known RA. The patient complains of pain in her knees, wrists, and hands. She prefers to hold onto her husband or furniture when she walks. Which of the following assistive devices would be *MOST* appropriate for this patient?

(A) A wheelchair
(B) Crutches
(C) A cane
(D) A platform walker

190. A patient presents to physical therapy after being diagnosed with post-polio syndrome. The physical therapist takes a detailed medical history and asks about the course of the original poliomyelitis infection. The patient relates that he uses a right knee-ankle-foot orthosis for ambulation. He states that he has "no strength and a lot of pain" in the right leg. The therapist performs muscle testing. What muscles should the therapist test?

(A) Manual muscle testing of the entire body
(B) Gross manual muscle testing of only the large muscle groups
(C) Manual muscle testing of only the right lower extremity
(D) Manual muscle testing of everything except the right lower extremity, to avoid pain

191. A physical therapist has been asked to address a diabetic education class on the benefits of exercise. Which of the following is *NOT* a benefit of exercising for a patient with type 1 diabetes mellitus?

(A) Improved blood glucose control
(B) Improved weight reduction
(C) Decreased blood pressure
(D) Improved insulin binding and absorption

192. A patient is referred to physical therapy for wrist range of motion and progression to strengthening after six weeks of immobilization. She broke her wrist after a fall on the ice. Which of the following is *NOT* a result of prolonged immobilization (i.e., for longer than six weeks)?

(A) Atrophy of muscle
(B) Weakening of ligament
(C) Weakening of the joint capsule
(D) Weakening of the tendon

193. What health behavior change model theorizes that a person's motivations for health change are related to the behavior of influential people, called referents?

(A) Health belief model
(B) Transtheoretical model
(C) Theory of reasoned action
(D) Social cognitive theory

194. During an initial evaluation of a patient who has been discharged from an acute rehabilitation center to home, the physical therapist notes that the patient has difficulty expressing her thoughts verbally. The patient has difficulty with word-finding, and her speech often is nonsensical. She has difficulty communicating her answers to the therapist when she is asked a question. However, the patient is able to understand the therapist and is able to understand written material. With what dysfunction does this patient present?

(A) Wernicke's aphasia
(B) Broca's aphasia
(C) Global aphasia
(D) Dysarthria

195. A physical therapist is preparing to enter the hospital room of a patient who has active tuberculosis. What kind of personal protective equipment should the physical therapist be wearing?

(A) Gloves
(B) Gloves, gown, and mask
(C) Gown and mask
(D) None needed

196. A physical therapist has been providing exercise treatment to a patient who is concurrently undergoing chemotherapy treatments. Just before her physical therapy treatment session, the patient's labs come back showing her hemoglobin levels at 8 g/mL. The patient says she feels good today. Which exercise treatment plan would be *MOST* appropriate for this patient on this day?

(A) Moderate-intensity aerobic exercise for 10 minutes
(B) Low-intensity aerobic exercise for 20 minutes
(C) Low-weight resistive strengthening for 15 minutes
(D) No exercise is recommended.

197. An infant is seen extending his right arm, flexing his right arm, and holding his head to the right. What reflex is the infant demonstrating?

(A) Rooting reflex
(B) Asymmetric tonic neck reflex
(C) Symmetric tonic neck reflex
(D) Tonic labyrinthine reflex

198. What is the *MOST* likely description of a cough in a patient who has severe, advanced chronic bronchitis?

(A) Unproductive cough
(B) Productive cough intermittently
(C) Nocturnal cough only
(D) Near constant productive cough

199. A physical therapist is examining a patient with right lower quadrant pain. He remembers playing tennis yesterday and wonders if he strained a muscle but does not recall any point at which the pain began. The pain is worse with walking and bending over. On evaluation, the physical therapist notes tenderness over McBurney's point. What differential diagnosis does this finding support?

(A) Inguinal hernia
(B) Gallstones
(C) Abdominal muscle strain
(D) Appendicitis

200. A patient presents to physical therapy with Parkinson's disease. What symptoms should the physical therapist anticipate that this patient may demonstrate?

(A) Rigidity and intention tremor
(B) Rigidity and resting tremor
(C) Flaccidity and intention tremor
(D) Flaccidity and resting tremor

End of Section 4

IF YOU FINISH BEFORE TIME IS CALLED, YOU MAY CHECK YOUR WORK ON THIS SECTION ONLY. DO NOT TURN TO ANY OTHER SECTION IN THE TEST. **STOP**

Section 5

201. A physical therapist is identifying at-risk patients within his clinical caseload. Which one of the following patients is at greatest risk of decreasing bone mass progressing to osteoporosis?

(A) A 35-year-old female with a T score of –0.5
(B) A 16-year-old female cross-country runner who is amenorrheic
(C) A 75-year-old male whose primary mobility is in a wheelchair
(D) A 40-year-old male with bilateral OA of the knees

202. A patient is referred to physical therapy for Achilles tendon pain. He rates the pain as 6/10 with running or jumping and 3/10 at rest. He was initially given stretches and activity-modification instructions for home. He returns to report 4/10 pain with activity and 2/10 pain at rest. Which of the following exercise progressions is *MOST* appropriate?

(A) Standing heel raises
(B) Seated heel raises
(C) Ankle plantar flexion/dorsiflexion with Thera-Band
(D) Active ankle range of motion in the pain-free range

203. A physical therapist examines the workstation of a computer analyst whom he is also treating for neck pain. Which of the following is the proper position of the monitor in relation to eye level?

(A) Monitor at eye level
(B) Monitor just above eye level
(C) Monitor just below eye level
(D) Monitor slightly to the right

204. A patient is being treated by a physical therapist for pain and decreased ROM resulting from wrist sprain. Which of the following sequences of treatment interventions would achieve the *BEST* results to decrease pain and increase motion?

(A) Continuous ultrasound, manual stretching, exercise, ice
(B) Manual stretching, continuous ultrasound, exercise, ice
(C) Exercise, manual stretching, continuous ultrasound, ice
(D) Continuous ultrasound, manual stretching, ice, exercise

205. There are many ways for a researcher to collect data. In one research study, the lead researcher collects data by looking at patients' presence of lower extremity edema, but does not interact with the patients. What data collection technique is this person using?

(A) Survey
(B) Direct observation
(C) Indirect observation
(D) Participant observation

206. A patient in a nursing home needs physical therapy for abnormal gait and for falls. Which of the following exercises would have the greatest specificity of training for the weight-acceptance part of the gait sequence?

(A) Seated ankle dorsiflexion
(B) Standing ankle dorsiflexion
(C) Lunges
(D) Squats

207. A patient presents to physical therapy with a diagnosis of Brown-Séquard syndrome of a spinal cord injury. What symptoms does the physical therapist expect for this patient?

(A) Upper extremities more affected than the lower extremities bilaterally
(B) Motor, pain, and temperature loss bilaterally
(C) Loss of proprioception and vibration bilaterally
(D) Loss of motor, proprioception, and vibration ipsilaterally

208. A patient with dyspnea receives an order for physical therapy due to deconditioning. The physical therapist notes impaired mechanics of breathing and also notes abnormal diaphragm excursion with respiration. The therapist decides to teach the patient some diaphragmatic breathing exercises to improve the mechanics and ease of breathing. What is one of the goals of diaphragmatic breathing exercises?

(A) Increased respiratory rate

(B) Increased use of secondary muscles

(C) Decreased dyspnea

(D) Decreased exercise tolerance

209. Explicit knowledge means the same thing as what other term?

(A) Procedural knowledge

(B) Declarative knowledge

(C) Generalization of learning

(D) Transfer of learning

210. A physical therapist is evaluating a high-school pitcher who has left shoulder pain and stiffness. What position should the patient be in for the therapist to assess passive range of motion of the internal and external rotators of the shoulder?

(A) Supine with the shoulder abducted to 90°

(B) Seated with the shoulder abducted to 90°

(C) Supine with the shoulder in neutral

(D) Supine with the shoulder abducted to 45°

211. A physical therapist has chosen to use TENS as a method of pain management for a patient with chronic low-back pain. Which one of the following pain theories explains the mechanism of pain control with this type of electrotherapy?

(A) Endogenous opiate theory

(B) Gate control theory

(C) Hunting response theory

(D) Dorsal horn theory

212. A patient presents to physical therapy with low back pain of insidious onset. He complains of general muscular pain and sacral pain. When asked, he also describes pain with urination. Which differential diagnosis *BEST* describes his symptoms?

(A) Prostatitis

(B) Urinary tract infection

(C) Cauda equina syndrome

(D) Herniated lumbar disc

213. A patient who is exercising in cold ambient temperature can expect what adaptations of the skin?

(A) Dilation of skin blood vessels and increase in skin temperature

(B) Constriction of skin blood vessels and increase in skin temperature

(C) Dilation of skin blood vessels and decrease in skin temperature

(D) Constriction of skin blood vessels and decrease in skin temperature

214. A physical therapist chooses to use ice baths to decrease abnormal tone of an ankle. The therapist knows that ice immersion can decrease spasticity in the short term. After the ice immersion, the therapist plans to immediately stretch the ankle to reap the benefits of the ice. What is a contraindication to using ice immersion for tone reduction?

(A) Cerebrovascular accident

(B) Contracture

(C) Impaired sensation

(D) Muscular weakness

215. A 72-year-old patient who is exercising in the physical therapy clinic after repair of a rotator cuff tear starts to complain of severe pain and heaviness in his chest. He is diaphoretic and dyspneic. He also complains of lightheadedness and weakness. The physical therapist helps the patient lie down and immediately calls 911. With what condition are these signs and symptoms *MOST* critically associated?

(A) Cerebrovascular accident

(B) Chronic obstructive pulmonary disease

(C) Myocardial infarction

(D) Rib fracture

216. An 82-year-old patient presents to physical therapy with left-sided paralysis due to a CVA. The patient has good trunk control and good family support. The patient's family plans to take him out in the car frequently. The patient's goal is independence with wheelchair mobility. What wheelchair feature would be the *MOST* important for this patient to achieve his goals?

(A) Reclining back
(B) Rigid frame
(C) Power mobility
(D) One-arm drive

217. A patient enters the clinic with low back pain. She states the pain is worst with walking, moving from sit to stand, and bed mobility. Based on her subjective complaints of positional aggravators, which differential diagnosis would be *MOST* appropriate?

(A) Lumbar disc herniation
(B) SI joint dysfunction
(C) Hip osteoarthritis
(D) Spinal stenosis

218. A physical therapist is involved in ordering and arranging equipment in a brand-new physical therapy clinic. What special consideration must be taken for locating a highboy tank for hot or cold whirlpool treatments?

(A) Must plug into a GFI
(B) Must be on a tile floor only
(C) Must be on a carpeted floor only
(D) Can plug into any outlet

219. A physical therapist is using iontophoresis for a patient he is treating for greater trochanteric bursitis. He has chosen dexamethasone as the medication to be delivered for its anti-inflammatory benefits. Which of the following lead wires should be attached to the active, or medication-filled, electrode?

(A) White
(B) Black
(C) Red
(D) Yellow

220. A 28-year-old man is referred to physical therapy for bilateral hip, low back, and bilateral knee pain. He describes the pain as cyclic and better with low-level activity. On bad days, it prevents him from his regular exercise routine. He also gets some lower abdominal pain not long after the joint pain presents. What differential diagnosis may explain these presentations?

(A) Inflammatory bowel disease
(B) Hernia
(C) Appendicitis
(D) Irritable bowel syndrome

221. A physical therapist has been asked to provide a nursing-home restorative aide with recommendations for a senior exercise class. The nursing home wants to teach its residents why exercise is important. Which of the following is worsened by a lack of exercise?

(A) Depression
(B) Osteoporosis
(C) Cognitive function
(D) Balance

222. A patient is receiving physical therapy for gait training with a left transfemoral prosthesis. The patient ambulates independently without an assistive device. However, the patient vaults on the right lower extremity. The patient's physical therapist knows that a potential cause of this gait deviation is which of the following?

(A) The prosthetic foot is positioned in too much dorsiflexion.
(B) The prosthesis is too long.
(C) The prosthetic knee has insufficient friction.
(D) The prosthetic socket is too large.

223. A physician orders sharp debridement of a wound by physical therapy. The physical therapist uses tweezers to remove necrotic tissue. What color tissue should the therapist *NOT* remove?

(A) Black
(B) Brown
(C) Pink
(D) Yellow

224. A patient with a traumatic brain injury demonstrates decorticate rigidity posturing. What is this patient's position?

(A) Upper- and lower-extremity extension
(B) Upper- and lower-extremity flexion
(C) Upper-extremity flexion and lower-extremity extension
(D) Upper-extremity extension and lower-extremity flexion

225. A patient with pneumonia is receiving physical therapy for strengthening in a skilled nursing facility. During the first week of the patient's stay, she begins to cough. On evaluation, crackles and wheezes are auscultated. Her temperature is 102.1°F. She demonstrates impaired movement of the left side of the chest. On radiological evaluation, the patient is diagnosed with atelectasis. How is atelectasis defined?

(A) Increased amount of pleural fluid
(B) Free air leakage into the pleural space
(C) Collapse of lung tissue
(D) Bacterial infection

226. A physical therapist is evaluating a patient who has a chief complaint of left leg pain. The therapist has cleared the lower-extremity joints and is evaluating the patient in a seated position. He asks the patient to slouch down, extend his knee, and forward flex his neck. Which tissue could have increased tension in this position?

(A) Muscular
(B) Connective
(C) Vascular
(D) Neural

227. A physical therapist determines that a patient would benefit from electrical stimulation for pain management. The therapist's goal is to decrease pain transmission by inhibiting C-fiber action potentials. Which frequency of electrical stimulation would be *BEST* for this goal?

(A) 75 pps
(B) 150 pps
(C) 5 pps
(D) 50 pps

228. A physical therapist is treating a patient for patellofemoral pain resulting from muscle imbalance in the leg. The patient also takes insulin injections for diabetes mellitus. When advising the patient on the coordination of insulin with exercise in therapy, what recommendation should the therapist give regarding the injection site?

(A) "Inject in the quad since exercising it will increase absorption."
(B) "Inject in the stomach to avoid increased absorption by the quad."
(C) "Inject in the quad since exercising it will decrease absorption."
(D) "Inject in the stomach to avoid decreased absorption by the quad."

229. A physical therapist is dictating the initial evaluation of a patient he just assessed. Which of the following pieces of information would be put under the "O" part of the note?

(A) "Patient complains of pain in his left knee with walking."
(B) "ROM is 130° of flexion."
(C) "Treatment to be done 2 times/week."
(D) "Appears to be left knee medial collateral ligament sprain."

230. A patient is referred for physical therapy to evaluate and treat her low back pain. She is also 24 weeks pregnant. Which of the following exercises would be *MOST* appropriate for core stabilization for this patient?

(A) Supine bicycle with abdominal isometrics
(B) Quadripedal "fire hydrants" with abdominal isometrics
(C) Supine bridges with abdominal isometrics
(D) Side-lying mini–leg lifts with abdominal isometrics

231. A physical therapist is performing PROM on a patient's knee to assess the quality and quantity of motion. At the end of the available range of knee flexion, there is a soft end feel. What is the *MOST* probable explanation for this description?

(A) Approximation of the gastrocnemius and hamstring
(B) Tension from the patellar tendon
(C) Obstruction from the meniscus
(D) Contact between the tibia and femur

232. A sedentary 35-year-old man is thinking about starting an exercise program. He has not decided to change his behavior because he really does not like exercise, but he knows he is getting older and wants to remain healthy. This man is in what stage of change on the Transtheoretical Model?

(A) Precontemplation
(B) Contemplation
(C) Action
(D) Maintenance

233. A patient sustains a fall and fractures her right hip and right thumb. The orthopedic surgeon orders touch weight-bearing on the right lower extremity, weight-bearing through the right forearm, and non-weight-bearing on the right hand. What is the *MOST* appropriate assistive device for this patient?

(A) Axillary crutches
(B) Four-wheeled walker
(C) Cane
(D) Walker with platform attachment

234. A patient with a spinal cord injury at level C5 demonstrates signs and symptoms of autonomic dysreflexia. What should be the physical therapist's immediate response?

(A) Notify the patient's physician
(B) Stand the patient up
(C) Check for the source of the noxious stimulus
(D) Apply a nitroglycerin patch

235. A physical therapist analyzes the chest-wall motion of a patient who is hospitalized secondary to pneumonia. What type of chest-wall motion is expected in a normal, healthy person without lung disease?

(A) Upward and outward motion of the upper chest wall and compression of the abdominal viscera
(B) Downward motion of the rib cage without compression of abdominal viscera
(C) Compression of the abdominal viscera without movement of the rib cage
(D) Inward motion of the rib cage

236. A physical therapist is evaluating a patient who has knee pain. During the patient interview, the therapist notices the patient having dystonia, involuntary muscle jerks, and restlessness. These presentations are typical side effects of what type of drug therapy?

(A) NSAIDs
(B) Antipsychotics
(C) DMARDs
(D) Tricyclic antidepressants

237. A patient is referred for buttock pain that is present when she runs any distance. On evaluation, the physical therapist finds weakness of the patient's hamstrings in the prone position. When direct pressure is put on the sacroiliac joint, the hamstrings are strong and pain-free. What type of intervention would be *MOST* appropriate for this patient?

(A) Sacral joint mobilization
(B) Sacral stabilization
(C) Soft-tissue stretching
(D) Soft-tissue mobilization

238. A physical therapist reads a journal research article about the use of the timed "up and go" test. The article concludes that the test-retest reliability was high. What does this mean?

(A) High agreement of scores between two or more testers
(B) High agreement of scores when tested by the same tester on repeated administrations of the test
(C) High probability that the test measures balance and mobility
(D) High probability that this test is related to other tests

239. A physical therapist treating a child who has myelomeningocele notices that the child is able to roll supine to prone independently but is unable to roll prone to supine without minimum assistance. Specifically, what is the physical therapist examining?

(A) Sensation
(B) Autonomic function
(C) Tone
(D) Developmental sequence

240. A physical therapist is initiating treatment on a patient with a hamstring strain one week out. He is planning to start treatment with 20 minutes of moist heat applied to the painful area. Which treatment intervention would *NOT* be best suited to immediately follow heat application?

(A) Soft-tissue mobilization
(B) Passive stretching
(C) Active range of motion
(D) Resistive strengthening

241. A patient with a known history of schizophrenia has been treated for low back pain by a physical therapist for three weeks. The patient has shown good progress thus far, but today he presents as more withdrawn. He has a flat affect and answers all questions with "I don't know" What possible explanation could there be for this presentation?

(A) The patient is having delusions.
(B) The patient has stopped taking his medication.
(C) The patient has taken twice the dosage of his medication.
(D) The patient is showing signs of tardive dyskinesia.

242. A patient presents to physical therapy with pain in his upper arm resulting from lifting too much weight during off-season training. Which of the following muscles is *MOST* likely to be injured with improper upper-extremity weight training?

(A) Biceps brachii
(B) Deltoid
(C) Pectoralis major
(D) Brachialis

243. A patient with Parkinson's disease is prescribed relaxation techniques by her physical therapist. The physical therapy goal of relaxation is to decrease rigidity. What treatment technique can be used for relaxation?

(A) Slow rocking
(B) Quick stretch
(C) Electrical stimulation
(D) High-weight resistance exercise

244. A physical therapist notices a small sore on the plantar surface of the foot of a patient who has diabetes. The therapist spends one treatment on patient education and inspection and care of the foot, since the patient had not noticed the sore on his foot. The physical therapist knows that an ultimate result of an untreated neuropathic wound is what?

(A) Healing without treatment
(B) Low risk of infection
(C) Pain
(D) Amputation

245. Following a traumatic brain injury suffered in a motor vehicle accident, a patient scores a 5 out of a possible 15 on the Glasgow Coma Scale. What is the prognosis for this patient?

(A) Mild impairment, excellent rehab potential

(B) Severe impairment, excellent rehab potential

(C) Mild impairment, poor rehab potential

(D) Severe impairment, poor rehab potential

246. A patient has a diagnosis of epilepsy. What drug is *MOST* likely to be used to decrease the frequency of seizures?

(A) Dilantin (phenytoin)

(B) Paxil (paroxetine)

(C) Protonix (pantoprazole)

(D) Florinef (fludrocortisone)

247. If a patient's lung volumes are as follows, what is the patient's vital capacity? Tidal volume = 0.5 L, inspiratory reserve volume = 3.5 L, expiratory reserve volume = 1.0 L.

(A) 5.0 L

(B) 4.5 L

(C) 4.0 L

(D) 1.5 L

248. A physical therapist has chosen to use cryotherapy as a pain-reduction intervention for a patient with shoulder pain. Which rationale *BEST* explains how cryotherapy can decrease pain?

(A) Decreases muscle spindle activity

(B) A-beta and C-fiber stimulation

(C) A-delta and C-fiber stimulation

(D) Decreases the pain threshold

249. A physical therapy researcher is surveying 200 females with arthritis to find out how many have had hip fractures. What is the population being researched?

(A) 200 females

(B) All females with arthritis

(C) All people with arthritis

(D) All people

250. The internal carotid artery splits into what arteries to supply the majority of the cerebral hemispheres?

(A) Anterior cerebral and middle cerebral arteries

(B) Right and left vertebral arteries

(C) Posterior cerebral and middle cerebral arteries

(D) Anterior and posterior cerebral arteries

End of Section 5

IF YOU FINISH BEFORE TIME IS CALLED, YOU MAY CHECK YOUR WORK ON THIS SECTION ONLY. DO NOT TURN TO ANY OTHER SECTION IN THE TEST. **STOP**

Answers and Explanations For Practice Test 1

Section 1

1. **D.**

A patient must always provide informed consent for physical therapy evaluation and treatment. Even when educated as to the risks and benefits, the patient has the right to refuse treatment. Continued treatment without consent is unethical.
(Gabard, page 58)
Safety, Protection & Professional Roles

2. **D.**

It takes 25 lb of force to adequately elongate the cervical spine.
(Behrens, page 102)
Therapeutic Modalities

3. **A.**

When the output of the right side of the heart is greater than that of the left side, blood and fluid accumulate in the pulmonary veins, alveoli, and tissue spaces. This condition often accompanies congestive heart failure.
(Irwin, page 20)
Cardiac, Vascular, & Pulmonary Systems: Differential Diagnosis & Pathology

4. **C.**

Bone marrow suppression is a common side effect with chemotherapy and can put the patient at increased risk for osteoporosis and fractures. Aerobic and resistance exercise may be beneficial at decreasing other symptoms associated with chemo. Local superficial modalities are allowed as needed.
(Goodman/Pathology, page 253)
Multi-system: Differential Diagnosis & Pathology

5. **B.**

To maintain good posture with bending and lifting, the primary motion should occur in the lower extremities (i.e., bend at the knees). From the waist up, a neutral spine should be maintained. To prevent loss of balance, a wide base of support is necessary.
(Saunders, page 154)
Safety, Protection & Professional Roles

6. **C.**

Venous insufficiency typically presents with hemosiderin deposits that cause discoloration of the affected lower extremity. Pain typically worsens throughout the day. Skin may weep or remain dry. A risk factor for venous ulcer is previous or current deep vein thrombosis.
(Baranoski, page 280)
Integumentary System: Differential Diagnosis & Pathology

7. **D.**

An open-ended question does not have a limited choice of responses (i.e., yes or no) but allows for respondents to be expansive in their answers.
(Hicks, page 20)
Research & Evidence Based Practice

8. **C.**

In pregnancy, weight-bearing does shift to the heels in an attempt to compensate for the forward and upward shift of the center of gravity that occurs with anterior weight changes.
(Stephenson, page 125)
Multi-system: Differential Diagnosis & Pathology

9. **A.**

Subtalar neutral is the preferred position for ankle-foot orthosis.
(Nawoczenski, page 124)
Equipment & Devices

10. D.

Muscles attaching to the pelvis can become tight and have trigger points that can cause urgency for urination. Soft-tissue mobilization, trigger-point release, and stretching can improve this.
(Goodman/Pathology, page 707)
Genitourinary: Treatment Interventions

11. D.

Informed consent must be given prior to initiation of treatment. For this informed consent to be legal, the patient must not be a minor (under age of 18), the patient must be able to communicate, and the patient must be able to understand how the informed consent is presented (language). Informed consent is not dependent on insurance.
(Gabard, page 57)
Safety, Protection & Professional Roles

12. D.

Hydrocortisone is synthetically made cortisol and is primarily used for its anti-inflammatory effects. However, the ability to suppress inflammatory response also delays healing and bone formation. It does not affect the ability of skeletal muscle to contract.
(Goodman/Pathology, page 321)
Metabolic & Endocrine: Foundational Sciences & Background

13. D.

Clinical signs and symptoms of a deep vein thrombosis can include tenderness, swelling, redness, and tightness in the calf. Sometimes the patient is asymptomatic. Regardless, if symptoms occur soon after surgery it is crucial that the physician be notified.
(Goodman/Pathology, page 458)
Musculoskeletal System: Differential Diagnosis & Pathology

14. A.

The use of a TENS unit for pain management provides analgesia while the unit is on and for up to 30 minutes after treatment.
(Prentice, page 103)
Therapeutic Modalities

15. B.

Upper-extremity D1 begins in elbow extension, shoulder extension, and shoulder abduction. The shoulder is also internally rotated and the wrist is pronated and ulnarly deviated. It ends with shoulder flexed, adduced and externally rotated; the elbow extended and supinated; wrist radially deviated; and hand fisted. D1 extension is the reverse of D1 flexion.
(Voss, page 15)
Nervous System: Treatment Interventions

16. A.

In the early stage of controlled motion and beginning exercise, activities to strengthen the quad and hip flexors are appropriate. Exercise that stresses the ACL, such as short-arc quads (SAQs) or deep squats, should be avoided.
(Kisner, page 375)
Musculoskeletal System: Treatment Interventions

17. A.

Declarative knowledge is knowledge about objects or things. Procedural knowledge is knowledge about how to perform a task.
(Christiansen, page 429)
Teaching & Learning

18. C.

There has been no evidence that an MRI would have any adverse affects on a patient if needed for diagnostics.
(Magee/Scientific Differential Diagnosis & Pathology, page 574)
Multi-system: Differential Diagnosis & Pathology

19. A.

The rotator cuff assists with stabilization of the glenohumeral joint by providing an inferior pull to counteract the superior pull or compression of the joint by the deltoid.
(Norkin/Levangie, page 225)
Musculoskeletal System: Foundational Sciences & Background

20. B.

IFC is used primarily for pain management and should be sensory, not motor (as in choice D). The sensation should be strong and comfortable and may appear to lessen as the patient assimilates to the stimulation.
(Prentice, page 103)
Therapeutic Modalities

21. A.

To test for myotomal weakness, the isometric contraction must be maintained for at least five seconds to see if weakness develops.
(Magee, page 16)
Musculoskeletal System: Evaluation

22. C.

Sublingual nitroglycerin is the most common drug used to treat acute angina.
(Irwin, page 226)
Cardiac, Vascular, & Pulmonary Systems: Foundational Sciences & Background

23. B.

An inferior subluxation is the most common subluxation. Subluxation occurs due to severe weakness as the humeral head slips out of the glenoid fossa. The glenoid fossa is displaced due to muscular weakness, causing decreased shoulder stability.
(Umphred, page 771)
Nervous System: Evaluation

24. C.

A-delta fibers relay sharp, pricking pain sensations that are well localized. C fibers relay dull, burning sensation that is more poorly localized. Both are afferent neurons that are peripheral fibers.
(Behrens, page 10)
Therapeutic Modalities

25. C.

The myocardium is the cardiac muscular layer.
(Irwin, page 14)
Cardiac, Vascular, & Pulmonary Systems: Foundational Sciences & Background

26. D.

A hydrocolloid is used for autolytic debridement, promotion of moist wound environment, and protection of the wound from contamination.
(Brown, page 65)
Integumentary System: Treatment Interventions

27. A.

Electrocardiography measures the electrical activity of the heart.
(Irwin, page 178)
Cardiac, Vascular, & Pulmonary Systems: Differential Diagnosis & Pathology

28. C.

Adhesive capsulitis is a common musculoskeletal pathology in patients with diabetes mellitus (DM). Type II DM is typically adult-onset and most common in the obese population. Blurred vision and foot neuropathies are common symptoms associated with type II DM.
(Goodman/Pathology, page 345)
Metabolic & Endocrine: Differential Diagnosis & Background

29. B.

Borg's Rating of Perceived Exertion is used for its strong correlation of maximal oxygen uptake.
(Irwin, page 301)
Cardiac, Vascular, & Pulmonary Systems: Treatment Interventions

30. A.

The Oxford technique uses ten reps at full 10-RM, ten at 75 percent 10-RM, and ten at 50 percent 10-RM.
(Kisner, page 89)
Musculoskeletal: Treatment Interventions

31. D.

Exercises can be modified to accommodate patients' individual balance or endurance deficits. Since this patient needs this support, the physical therapist should assess his safety and independence with the stepping task and assess his need for an assistive device.
(Frownfelter, page 284)
Cardiac, Vascular, & Pulmonary Systems: Treatment Interventions

32. B.

Cranial nerve VII is the facial nerve, which supplies muscles of facial expression and eye closure. It also innervates tears, salivation, and taste.
(Martin, page 20)
Nervous System: Foundational Sciences & Background

33. B.

Manual muscle testing that finds weak, painless muscle action can indicate either a full muscle tear or injury to the nerve.
(Dutton, page 180)
Musculoskeletal System: Differential Diagnosis & Pathology

34. A.

Babinski sign is elicited by stroking the lateral part of the sole of the foot from the heel to the ball and then across the ball. Normally, in a patient older than six months the normal response is toe flexion. In infants less than six months and in patients with corticospinal tract dysfunction, the big toe extends and the other toes spread.
(Martin, page 18)
Nervous System: Evaluation

35. B.

Fever, pain, erythema, and edema are signs of infection. Osteomyelitis is infection in the bone and most commonly occurs in the long bones where bone formation occurs. Infections elsewhere in the body, as may occur with a dental procedure, can spread to the bone itself.
(Goodman/Clinical Medicine, page 576)
Musculoskeletal System: Differential Diagnosis & Pathology

36. B.

Myelomeningocele is the term used to describe spina bifida cystica in which the cyst contains spinal cord. Meningocele is the term used to describe spina bifida cystica in which the cyst contains only cerebrospinal fluid and meninges. Anencephaly is the condition where the brain does not developage Encephalocele is the condition where the brain projects from the skull.
(Martin, page 155)
Nervous System: Differential Diagnosis & Pathology

37. C.

These rotator cuff muscles are responsible for decelerating the arm as the ball is released during a throw.
(Donatelli, page 242)
Musculoskeletal System: Treatment Interventions

38. D.

Ataxia is uncoordinated movement. Lack of movement is akinesia. Weakness of one side of the body is hemiplegia. Slow movement is bradykinesia.
(Martin, page 285)
Nervous System: Differential Diagnosis & Pathology

39. B.

Slough and eschar are necrotic tissue that should be debrided. Pink or red tissue is granulation tissue that signals wound healing. Macerated tissue is peri-wound tissue that is wet and delicate.
(Brown, page 12)
Integumentary System: Treatment Interventions

40. C.

The motions to maximally open the facet joints are flexion, contralateral side-bending, and ipsilateral rotation.
(Behrens, page 106)
Musculoskeletal System: Foundational Sciences & Background

41. D.

Class 3 complete neurotmesis is a classification that indicates complete severance of a peripheral nerve. Regeneration is not possible without surgical repair. However, a patient should be able to gain function through physical therapy treatment using orthotics, stretching, and compensatory techniques.
(Rothstein, page 295)
Nervous System: Differential Diagnosis & Pathology

42. C.

Econcentric exercise is specific to two-joint muscles. In this case, the biceps is the two-joint muscle and flexes the elbow. By moving the shoulder into an extended position, it lengthens the biceps to allow safe elbow flexion strengthening in a position that could potentially be one of injury. If the shoulder were flexed, the biceps would be shortened and not in the appropriate functional position.
(Magee/Scientific Differential Diagnosis & Pathology, page 447)
Musculoskeletal System: Foundational Sciences & Background

43. C.

In high environmental temperatures, the body dilates skin blood vessels and increases sweat production.
(Serup, page 34)
Integumentary System: Foundational Sciences & Background

44. A.

Functional training involves repeated practice of functional activities to improve these activities.
(Umphred, page 73)
Nervous System: Treatment Interventions

45. B.

Knee flexion contracture causes excessive knee flexion in the affected knee.
(Lusardi, page 737)
Equipment & Devices

46. D.

The transverse humeral ligament of the shoulder holds the biceps tendon in the bicipital groove. The rupture of this ligament allows the biceps tendon to slip into and out of the groove, sometimes causing irritation of the tendon.
(Donatelli, page 56)
Musculoskeletal Systems: Foundational Sciences & Background

47. A.

The transtheoretical model describes these six stages that persons progress and digress through when making a health behavior change.
(Bastable, page 176)
Teaching & Learning

48. D.

Prostaglandin is a vasodilator, which allows an increase of blood flow to the area in need.
(Magee/Scientific Differential Diagnosis & Pathology, page 10)
Multi-system: Foundational Sciences & Background

49. A.

The Berg Balance Scale is one standardized measure that is used as an outcomes measure. Proprioceptive neuromuscular facilitation, neurodevelopmental treatment, and craniosacral therapy are all treatment techniques.
(Cole, page 36)
Research & Evidence Based Practice

50. B.

An incident report should be filled out and added to the patient's chart. In some facilities the clinic supervisor or medical director also signs the incident report.
(Gabard, page 217)
Safety, Protection & Professional Roles

Section 2

51. A.

During forward flexion, both facet joints open. In extension, both facet joints close. In side-bending right, the right facet closes and the left facet opens; in side-bending left, the left facet closes and the right facet opens.
(Saunders, page 268)
Musculoskeletal System: Differential Diagnosis & Pathology

52. D.

Duchenne muscular dystrophy is an x-linked recessive gene; only males exhibit symptoms. Symptoms include profound and progressive weakness, especially of the shoulder and pelvis girdles; cardiac and respiratory muscle weakness; scoliosis; and contractures.
(Umphred, page 399)
Nervous System: Differential Diagnosis & Pathology

53. A.

Volumetric water displacement is a general way to measure edema of a hand or foot. If the water displaced was more, the volume of the foot was greater, thus indicating increased edema.
(Behrens, page 31)
Therapeutic Modalities

54. A.

Rheumatoid arthritis (RA) is a systemic disease. Nodules and inflammation associated with RA can occur in locations other than just synovial joints. Osteoarthritis affects primarily weight-bearing joints, COPD affects primarily the pulmonary system, and fibromyalgia is a musculoskeletal system connective-tissue disorder.
(Goodman/Pathology, page 102)
Multi-system: Differential Diagnosis & Pathology

55. C.

The temporal lobe contains the primary auditory cortex and Wernicke's area.
(Martin, page 11)
Nervous System: Foundational Sciences & Background

56. C.

Regular exercise is beneficial for this patient during times of symptoms and when no symptoms of pain are present. Benefits are twofold in that regular exercise can help with the movement of bowels through the GI tract and relieve stress (a trigger for IBS).
(Goodman/Pathology, page 652)
Gastrointestinal: Foundational Sciences & Background

57. A.

Motor learning is needed to teach the patient which muscles need to contract to stop or slow the flow of urine. Once the patient is better able to isolate these muscles, strengthening can occur. Strengthening of the pelvic floor muscles can decrease the frequency of incontinence.
(Goodman/Pathology, page 725)
Genitourinary: Foundational Sciences & Background

58. B.

Hyperthyroidism is characterized by unexplained weight loss, intolerance to heat, tremor, poor balance and coordination, and changing moods. An overactive thyroid may be enlarged (a goiter). Musculoskeletal presentation may include calcific tendonitis or inflammation of structures around a joint.
(Goodman/Pathology, page 329)
Metabolic & Endocrine: Differential Diagnosis & Pathology

59. C.

Injury to the common peroneal nerve presents with inability to dorsiflex and evert the foot. Patients with this peripheral nerve injury present with foot drop during gait. Pain is usually not present.
(Rothstein, page 357)
Nervous System: Differential Diagnosis & Pathology

60. C.

The peroneal nerve is supplied by the S1 nerve root and when injured, such as in a freeze mechanism, can cause weakness of the ankle everters and numbness on the lateral side of the foot.
(Hoppenfeld/Orthopaedic, page 59)
Musculoskeletal System: Differential Diagnosis & Pathology

61. A.

Tenodesis is the passive shortening of the finger flexors as the wrist extends. This passive motion can replace active grippage. Care should be taken to avoid finger flexor stretching while the wrist is extended to maintain some tension to achieve tenodesis graspage.
(Umphred, page 498)
Nervous System: Treatment Interventions

62. A.

To increase the intervertebral foraminal space, 25° of flexion is optimal. Too much flexion or even small amounts of extension can decrease interforaminal space.
(Behrens, page 105)
Therapeutic Modalities

63. D.

Duchenne muscular dystrophy is an x-linked recessive gene. Only males exhibit symptoms. Symptoms include profound and progressive weakness (especially of the shoulder and pelvis girdles), cardiac and respiratory muscle weakness, scoliosis, and contractures.
(Umphred, page 399)
Nervous System: Differential Diagnosis & Pathology

64. D.

Glucocorticoids are used to decrease inflammation but can hinder healing and the body's ability to fight infection by decreasing the inflammatory response. In all cases, care must be taken with passive mobilizations and stretches so as not to injure the area while the inflammatory response is suppressed.
(Goodman/Pathology, page 95)
Multi-system: Foundational Sciences & Background

65. B.

Pain resulting from an injury causes the muscles to react by tightening or guarding to prevent further injury. This muscle guarding can then cause dysfunction of the muscle and joint, thus causing more pain. It can be a circle of one thing causing another.
(Behrens, page 4)
Therapeutic Modalities

66. D.

Buttock, posterior leg, and foot pain can be referred from anything innervated by the L5 nerve root. This includes the L4 facet as it articulates with the L5 facet. The L4 nerve root, however, supplies a dermatomal area over the front of the thigh.
(Behrens, page 8)
Musculoskeletal System: Differential Diagnosis & Pathology

67. A.

Nominal level simply puts data in groups. Ordinal level allows data to be ranked. Interval level allows data to be ranked and assumes equal intervals between the rankings. Ratio level has an absolute zero.
(Hicks, page 34)
Research & Evidence Based Practice

68. C.

The glenohumeral (GH) joint itself contributes 120° of elevation motion for flexion and abduction. The remaining 60° motion for full range comes from rotation of the scapulothoracic (ST) joint. This makes the ratio 2° of GH motion for every 1° of ST motion.
(Norkin/Levangie, page 229)
Musculoskeletal System: Foundational Sciences & Background

69. D.

The greatest risk factor for developing COPD is cigarette smoking.
(Irwin, page 147)
Cardiac, Vascular, & Pulmonary Systems: Differential Diagnosis & Pathology

70. D.

Gastrocnemius is considered primarily a movement muscle. It crosses over two joints and is made up of primarily type IIa muscle fibers. The remaining choices are all postural stabilizers and are considered endurance muscles.
(Dutton, page 16)
Musculoskeletal System: Foundational Sciences & Background

71. C.

Since the pain appears to be coming from an L4 nerve supply, it would be most appropriate to ultrasound the area over the L4 nerve root. For the best thermal effects, an area no larger than twice the size of the sound head should be used.
(Behrens, page 74)
Therapeutic Modalities

72. A.

Following anterior shoulder dislocation, the motions of abduction and external rotation away from neutral should be avoided. Internal rotation coupled with adduction also moves the humeral head anterior to an uncomfortable position. Cane-assisted shoulder flexion is the appropriate exercise for this patient at this time.
(Kisner, page 256)
Musculoskeletal System: Treatment Interventions

73. A.

All goals should be specific, objective, and measurable. Short-term goals are usually achieved in two to four weeks and are purposeful in moving toward a long-term goal. Long-term goals are also specific, objective, and measurable and should also be functional. Choices B and D are not specific and objectively measurable. Choice C is an example of a long-term goal.
(Shamus, page 129)
Safety, Protection & Professional Roles

74. D.

Normally, the diastolic blood pressure increases less than 10 mm Hg, remains the same, or decreases less than 10 mm Hg.
(Irwin, page 87)
Cardiac, Vascular, & Pulmonary Systems: Foundational Sciences & Background

75. D.

Long, complicated surveys are less likely to be returned. Follow-up for unreturned surveys is helpful. Spring and fall are better times of year to improve return of surveys. A well-written and informative cover letter can increase the rate of return.
(Bork, page 200)
Research & Evidence Based Practice

76. C.

A respiratory rate above 20 breaths per minute is considered to be tachypneic. A respiratory rate below ten breaths per minute is described as bradypneic. Apnea is the absence of breath. Eupnea is normal rate of breathing.
(Irwin, page 288)
Cardiac, Vascular, & Pulmonary Systems: Evaluation

77. B.

Side-lying is more comfortable than prone in cases of severe low back pain. Gentle rotational mobilization can increase movement of the vertebral joints, thus decreasing pain and muscle spasm.
(Saunders, page 258)
Musculoskeletal System: Treatment Interventions

78. A.

Chest radiography is the most commonly used imaging technique in the assessment of patients' lung disease.
(Irwin, page 211)
Cardiac, Vascular, & Pulmonary Systems: Differential Diagnosis & Pathology

79. D.

The hypoglossal nerve functions to move the tongue.
(Martin, page 20)
Nervous System: Foundational Sciences & Background

80. A.

It is difficult to establish treatment goals that involve independent decision-making or action by the patient when dementia is involved. The patient tends to forget the recommendations or may be unable to follow through with home programs.
(Lewis, page 83)
Multi-system: Differential Diagnosis & Pathology

81. A.

If a patient is unable to perform standardized tests and measurements, a therapist can use nonstandardized methods to record a baseline measurement. For example, if the patient has difficulty donning a shirt and cannot lift his left shoulder high enough to place the left arm in the shirt after the right arm, the therapist can document this in the notes and document change with physical therapy treatment interventions.
(Glickstein, page 164)
Nervous System: Evaluation

82. D.

With pursed-lip breathing, the patient inhales through the nose and then slowly exhales through pursed lips.
(Irwin, page 311)
Cardiac, Vascular, & Pulmonary Systems: Treatment Interventions

83. C.

Definitive diagnosis of diabetes mellitus includes having the classic signs and symptoms of diabetes and a nonfasting blood plasma glucose concentration >200 mg/dL. Fasting blood glucose levels are diabetic if they are >126 mg/dL.
(Goodman/Pathology, page 351)
Metabolic & Endocrine: Evaluation

84. A.

Upper extremity flexion is described as scapular retraction; elevation; shoulder external rotation and abduction; elbow, wrist, and finger flexion; and forearm supination. Lower extremity flexion is described as hip flexion, abduction, and external rotation; knee flexion; ankle dorsiflexion and inversion; and toe extension.
(Martin, page 287)
Nervous System: Differential Diagnosis & Pathology

85. B.

Sudoriferous glands are sweat glands. The evaporation of sweat assists in thermoregulation.
(Hanumadass, page 18)
Integumentary System: Foundational Sciences & Background

86. C.

The brachioradialis reflex is specific for C6 disc herniation with nerve root involvement. The biceps reflex tests C5 and triceps tests C7.
(Hoppenfeld/Orthopedic, page 33)
Musculoskeletal System: Evaluation

87. D.

The ankle-brachial index is used to compare the blood pressure of the ankle with the blood pressure of the arm and measures arterial perfusion of the leg.
(Baranoski, page 291)
Integumentary System: Differential Diagnosis & Pathology

88. A.

Hold-relax is a specific PNF technique that can target range of motion. The antagonist is isometrically contracted in a shortened range, followed by a relaxation and movement into a lengthened position of the agonist.
(Voss, page 304)
Nervous System: Treatment Interventions

89. A.

Mechanical debridement may be painful for the patient. Wetting the dry dressing before removing it defeats the purpose of debridement. Wet-to-dry dressings are often used in conjunction with other treatments and other debridement techniques. Wet-to-dry dressings are nonselective and can remove both necrotic and viable tissue.
(Baranoski, page 119)
Integumentary System: Treatment Interventions

90. C.

A reclining-back wheelchair to achieve the 60° hip flexion restriction is needed.
(Sussman, page 373)
Equipment & Devices

91. C.

Upper limb tension testing can identify neural involvement in the arm or neck. It can be further specified by ulnar, median, or radial bias.
(Magee/Orthopedic, page 165)
Musculoskeletal System: Evaluation

92. C.

For a very large and/or dependent transfer, a hydraulic lift is the safest mode of transfer.
(Pierson, page 88)
Equipment & Devices

93. B.

This is classic Pavlovian, or respondent, conditioning. A neutral stimulus is added to a behavior (music playing with sit-to-stand) and the music becomes a conditioned stimulus to the conditioned response (sit-to-stand).
(Bastable, page 45)
Teaching & Learning

94. A.

The physical therapy assistant is the only one licensed to instruct and perform exercises as part of physical therapy treatment. If any of the other choices were to supervise the exercise, it would not be considered a physical therapy service.
(Pagliarulo, page 55)
Safety, Protection & Professional Roles

95. A.

Solid ankle-foot orthoses resist hyperextension of the knee.
(Edelstein, page 42)
Equipment & Devices

96. A.

To stretch the hamstrings, the hip must be flexed with the knee extended as in a straight leg raise. To stabilize the pelvis, the other leg can be stabilized in the extended position. Some may prefer the method of 90/90 to avoid back strain, but it is not truly meant to stretch the hamstrings.
(Kisner, page 137)
Musculoskeletal System: Evaluation

97. D.

Droplet nuclei only travel approximately three feet through the air before dissipating. If the patient covers his mouth while coughing, contamination should not be a problem.
(Duesterhaus, page 14)
Safety, Protection & Professional Roles

98. A.

Explicit learning includes not only procedural knowledge but also knowledge only known to the learner, such as coordination and force generation.
(Christiansen, page 430)
Teaching & Learning

99. D.

Heart rate is the dependent variable. The dependent variable is the observed variable that is changed due to manipulation of the independent variable.
(Hicks, page 70)
Research & Evidence Based Practice

100. B.

As part of the patient interview, the therapist may ask, "Are you in a safe relationship?" If the patient indicates that he or she is not, the physical therapist should have information readily available for treatment interventions. If the patient denies any domestic abuse, the observation of unexplained contusions should be documented.
(Gabard, page 77)
Safety, Protection & Professional Roles

Section 3

101. D.

In the cervical spine, side-bending and rotation occur in opposite directions. Therefore, to increase right rotation, left side-bending can also be improved with side glides toward the left.
(Dutton, page 1087)
Musculoskeletal System: Treatment Interventions

102. C.

Segmental breathing exercises work by providing pressure to an area of lung on the chest wall and instructing the patient to improve the expansion of that area. This treatment can be used in patients with atelectasis.
(Irwin, page 311)
Cardiac, Vascular, & Pulmonary Systems: Treatment Interventions

103. D.

The cardinal signs of inflammation are erythema, increased tissue temperature, edema, loss of function, and pain. Low-grade fever is a systemic response and can indicate other pathology, including infection.
(Behrens, page 6)
Therapeutic Modalities

104. A.

The Dix-Hallpike test indicates there is pathology of the left posterior canal. The appropriate treatment would be an Epley maneuver that starts with the head to the left.
(Umphred, page 650)
Nervous System: Treatment Interventions

105. A.

The best approach to take when educating an obese patient on the benefits and need for exercise is the overall improved health viewpoint. Many patients who are obese do not have the motivation to exercise just for weight loss or to become athletic. It is also possible that some obese patients do not enjoy walking or athletics. A broad list of health benefits is best.
(Goodman/Pathology, page 33)
Multi-system: Differential Diagnosis & Pathology

106. A.

An inguinal hernia occurs when abdominal tissue or organs push through a weakened area of the abdominal muscle wall. There is pain with exertion that causes the abdominals to pinch on the herniated tissue. In this case, the weakened abdomen could be a result of the tackle, and the herniation may have occurred during his lifting.
(Goodman/Pathology, page 658)
Gastrointestinal: Differential Diagnosis & Pathology

107. B.

Neglect is inattention to one side of the body.
(Umphred, page 831)
Nervous System: Differential Diagnosis & Pathology

108. A.

Endometriosis can produce implants on the iliopsoas and pelvic floor muscles, causing pain with muscle testing of each of those. The presence of cyclic pain clues you in to the endometriosis.
(Goodman/Clinical Med, page 561)
Genitourinary: Differential Diagnosis & Pathology

109. A.

An assistive orthosis can pre-position the thumb to assist with grip and prehension.
(Edelstein, page 125)
Equipment & Devices

110. A.

Lung cancer is most likely to metastasize to one of the long bones or lumbar spine.
(Goodman/Clinical Med, page 575)
Multi-system: Differential Diagnosis & Pathology

111. A.

Alternating isometrics, slow reversals, and agonistic reversals are all specific techniques used in proprioceptive neuromuscular facilitation. Also included are contract-relax, hold-relax, hold-relax active movement, rhythmic initiation, rhythmic rotation, rhythmic stabilization, slow reversal hold, and slow reversals.
(Martin, page 255)
Nervous System: Treatment Interventions

112. A.

Lidocaine is different from the other choices due to its local analgesic and anti-inflammatory effects.
(Michlovitz, page 117)
Therapeutic Modalities

113. D.

Random practice schedules involve scheduling tasks in a random order.
(Christiansen, page 433)
Teaching & Learning

114. C.

Interval level allows data to be ranked and assumes equal intervals between the rankings. Ratio level has an absolute zero. Nominal level simply puts data in groups. Ordinal level only allows data to be ranked.
(Hicks, page 37)
Research & Evidence Based Practice

115. C.

Secondary osteoporosis can present after prolonged use of certain medications. Heparin, Coumadin, steroids, and aspirin are a few of these. Secondary osteoporosis occurs as a result of some other modifiable risk factors.
(Goodman/Pathology, page 872)
Metabolic & Endocrine: Treatment Interventions

116. B.

The left facet joint is stuck in an open position or cannot close. In extension, the right transverse process closes as it should while the left facet remains open. The right transverse process will be more posterior.
(Saunders, page 268)
Musculoskeletal System: Evaluation

117. A.

Equal and upward motion of the lower ribs is the normal motion with inspiration. The flattening of the diaphragm that is commonly seen with chronic obstructive pulmonary disease results in equal and inward motion of the lower margin of the ribs.
(Irwin, page 297)
Cardiac, Vascular, & Pulmonary Systems: Evaluation

118. A.

The loss of fluid associated with the flu can cause an imbalance in the electrolytes within the body. Muscle weakness, cramping, and paresthesia are all resultant signs and symptoms of inadequate electrolyte availability.
(Goodman/Pathology, page 111)
Multi-system: Differential Diagnosis & Pathology

119. D.

Lying supine puts the least amount of pressure on the disc; walking and standing both provide second-least; and sitting puts the greatest pressure on the disc.
(Saunders, page 125)
Musculoskeletal System: Treatment Interventions

120. C.

To elicit a motor response, the most appropriate electrode setup would be a smaller electrode over the motor point of the muscle and a larger electrode over the muscle belly.
(Behrens, page 170)
Therapeutic Modalities

121. A.

The APTA Guide for Professional Conduct guidelines say gifts and favors should not be accepted that affect professional judgment. In this case, the patient is on her last treatment session and is offering a small token of appreciation. It is correct to accept the gift so it will not appear unappreciated.
(Gabard, page 152)
Safety, Protection & Professional Roles

122. B.

Pressure from immobilization on the radial nerve can elicit symptoms similar to those of C7 nerve root immobilization. However, in this case, the aggravating factor is the cast, not anything in the lumbar spine.
(Hoppenfeld/Orthopedic, page 14)
Musculoskeletal System: Differential Diagnosis & Pathology

123. A.

Kehr sign is pain in the left shoulder referred from a lacerated or ruptured spleen. The symptoms of bloatedness and weakness (most likely due to a bleed) support the organ involvement. Immediate referral is indicated.
(Goodman/Pathology, page 631)
Gastrointestinal System: Differential Diagnosis & Pathology

124. D.

Tidal volume is the volume of air inspired or expired during a normal breathing cycle. The volume of air that can be inspired after normal inspiration is the inspiratory reserve volume. The volume of air that can be expired after normal expiration is the expiratory reserve volume. The volume of air that remains in the lungs after maximal expiration is residual volume.
(Irwin, page 44)
Cardiac, Vascular, & Pulmonary Systems: Foundational Sciences & Background

125. D.

A Trendelenburg gait indicates a gluteus medius weakness during stance. Hip abduction itself strengthens the hip in an abducted position, which does not carry over as well to the function of the gluteus medius in an adducted position during gait. Single-leg stance more closely simulates that function.
(Magee/Pathology, page 455)
Musculoskeletal System: Treatment Interventions

126. B.

Pulmonary emphysema results from destruction of bronchioles, alveolar ducts, and septa that creates large airspaces that are unavailable for gas exchange. Cystic fibrosis is a genetic disorder that affects lung secretions. Asthma is a hyperreactivity of smooth muscle of the bronchioles.
(Irwin, page 148)
Cardiac, Vascular, & Pulmonary Systems: Differential Diagnosis & Pathology

127. D.

Exercise is known to decrease blood pressure, decrease resting heart rate, decrease the progression or onset of osteoporosis, and increase walking endurance and walking speed.
(Goodman/Clinical Med, page 443)
Musculoskeletal System: Foundational Sciences & Background

128. D.

Orthostatic hypotension is often seen after prolonged bed rest, and patients should be monitored for changes in vital signs and tolerance for activity when allowed to progress to more upright positions after bed rest.
(Irwin, page 272)
Cardiac, Vascular, & Pulmonary Systems: Treatment Interventions

129. B.

The parietal lobe is the primary sensory cortex and also plays a role in short-term memory.
(Martin, page 11)
Nervous System: Foundational Sciences & Background

130. D.

The convex-concave rule states that if one joint surface is concave related to another, the slide is in the same direction as the motion of the bone. If the joint surface is convex, the slide is in the opposite direction to the motion of the bone.
(Dutton, page 81)
Musculoskeletal System: Foundational Sciences & Background

131. B.

Homonymous hemianopia is the loss of vision of half the visual field. Diplopia is double vision. Nystagmus presents as eyes moving rapidly horizontally or vertically. Visual agnosia is the inability to recognize familiar objects.
(Martin, page 285)
Nervous System: Evaluation

132. C.

Cohorting is when patients with similar diagnoses are grouped together to avoid infection to others when space or transport is needed. Patients with airborne precautions should remain isolated in single rooms.
(Duesterhaus, page 96)
Safety, Protection & Professional Roles

133. C.

Physical therapists cannot diagnose medical conditions but can diagnose nonmedical conditions such as developmental delay, sensory integrative dysfunction, and postural dysfunction.
(Farber, page 108)
Nervous System: Evaluation

134. B.

According to the Rule of Nines, the posterior trunk accounts for 18 percent and an entire arm accounts for 9 percent. The total surface area is 27 percent.
(Hanumadass, page 8)
Integumentary System: Evaluation

135. B.

Plethysmography records volume changes in the limb and is used to assess the severity of venous insufficiency.
(Baranoski, page 293)
Integumentary System: Differential Diagnosis & Pathology

136. C.

With vertebral compression fractures it is essential to avoid flexion activities that will further compress the vertebral body, causing pain. The further into extension the motion is, the more uncomfortable it can be due to distraction stresses. The best position is neutral spine.
(Saunders, page 135)
Musculoskeletal System: Treatment Interventions

137. B.

The posterior columns convey information on proprioception, vibration, two-point discrimination, and deep touch. The spinothalamic tract conveys pain and temperature information. The corticospinal tract is the primary motor pathway. The tectospinal tract carries information on orientation of the head toward a sound or object.
(Martin, page 16)
Nervous System: Foundational Sciences & Background

138. B.

In this position the ulnar nerve is at its greatest tension.
(Magee/Orthopedic, page 165)
Musculoskeletal System: Differential Diagnosis & Pathology

139. D.

Leg exercises are important for patients with venous insufficiency to improve the muscle pump mechanism.
(Baranoski, page 305)
Integumentary System: Treatment Interventions

140. B.

Neurodevelopmental treatment is based on facilitation of normal postural control while inhibiting abnormal posture and muscle tone. The therapist directs movements so that the patient can experience normal movement. Once tone is normalized, functional activities and movements are added.
(Stokes, page 320)
Nervous System: Treatment Interventions

141. A.

Phantom pain is pain in the amputated limb.
(Carroll, page 37)
Equipment & Devices

142. D.

When reading research articles, the physical therapist should consider how the study will affect the management and care of her own patients.
(Helewa, page 81)
Research & Evidence Based Practice

143. D.

Increased intracranial pressure can be due to swelling of the brain itself, thereby pressing the brain against the skull and possibly resulting in herniation through openings of the cranial cavity. Increased blood or fluid in the ventricles may also place increased pressure on the brain tissue. Increased intracranial pressure results in a poor prognosis.
(Umphred, page 417)
Nervous System: Differential Diagnosis & Pathology

144. D.

The benefits of exercise while undergoing chemotherapy are many. However, bone marrow suppression is a side effect of the chemotherapy drugs and is not listed as a benefit of exercise during treatment.
(Goodman/Pathology, page 259)
Multi-system: Foundational Sciences & Background

145. B.

Although all of these features may be desirable, the foot exit feature is the most important for the patient's mobility.
(Wilson, page 22)
Equipment & Devices

146. A.

Cognitive learning theorists do not rely on rewards. Cognitive learning theory emphasizes an individual's perception, thought, memory, motivation, and past experience and how this relates to learning.
(Bestable, page 50)
Teaching & Learning

147. B.

Scapular depression is the movement used to perform a wheelchair push-up for pressure relief. Other techniques for pressure relief include a side lean or forward lean. For patients who cannot perform pressure relief independently, wheelchair positioning and special equipment may be needed to avoid skin breakdown.
(Umphred, page 510)
Nervous System: Treatment Interventions

148. D.

The first step should be to perform a detailed literature review, before completing a proposal, creating a hypothesis, or establishing control groups.
(Currier, page 36)
Research & Evidence Based Practice

149. B.

The Occupational Safety and Health Administration (OSHA) establishes health and safety standards for the workplace. Workers are given the right to register a complaint or refuse to work in unsafe conditions without risking consequences or retaliation from the employer.
(Gabard, page 215)
Safety, Protection & Professional Roles

150. B.

All equipment used in the clinic should be checked regularly for proper function and calibration. For this type of maintenance, the biomedical department and the equipment manufacturer are the best options.
(Behrens, page 69)
Safety, Protection & Professional Roles

Section 4

151. A.

Ice is considered a conduction mechanism of energy exchange because heat is conducted from the body to the ice in an attempt to warm the cold ice.
(Behrens, page 38)
Therapeutic Modalities

152. B.

Toe raises are meant to strengthen the gastrocnemius-soleus complex. The calf is a major stabilizer of the ankle from mid to late stance, and calf weakness can contribute to instability.
(Braddom, page 105)
Musculoskeletal Systems: Treatment Interventions

153. A.

Brandt-Daroff exercises are designed to habituate an abnormally functioning vestibular system.
(Umphred, page 650)
Nervous System: Treatment Interventions

154. A.

Localized erythema, edema, pain, and decreased ROM are all normal responses to tissue injury from the arthroplasty. Purulent or yellow discharge from the wound would be more indicative of fever.
(Goodman/Pathology, page 130)
Musculoskeletal System: Treatment Interventions

155. C.

A pulmonary embolus most commonly forms following the development of a deep vein thrombosis.
(Irwin, page 166)
Cardiac, Vascular, & Pulmonary Systems: Differential Diagnosis & Pathology

156. C.

Of the four options given, walking on the treadmill offers the greatest chance of aggravating joint pain with the repetitive trauma from pounding on the joints. Aquatic therapy and cycling offer non-weight-bearing or partial weight-bearing aerobic exercise to save the joints. Resistive strength training can strengthen as well as offer "stress" to the bones to prevent progression toward osteopenia.
(Goodman/Pathology, page 33)
Multi-system: Differential Diagnosis & Pathology

157. B.

Some gastric pathologies may refer to the lower thoracic spine. If the patient is not responding properly to physical therapy treatment interventions, or if there are other systemic complaints, a non-musculoskeletal pathology may be the culprit.
(Dutton, page 211)
Gastrointestinal: Differential Diagnosis & Pathology

158. C.

Pia mater is the innermost layer of the meninges; it adheres to the brain.
(Martin, page 10)
Nervous System: Foundational Sciences & Background

159. D.

Endometriosis can occur only in women who are in the childbearing years. It is more prevalent in women who have not had children or are pregnant later in life.
(Goodman/Clinical Med, page 559)
Genitourinary: Differential Diagnosis & Pathology

160. D.

Resistance training that is specific to the site of bone loss can help to improve bone density. Cycling and aquatic therapy are non-weight-bearing and do not stimulate bone growth.
(Goodman/Pathology, page 881)
Metabolic & Endocrine: Treatment Interventions

161. C.

Volar glides of the radius on the humerus will increase elbow flexion.
(Kisner, page 177)
Musculoskeletal System: Treatment Interventions

162. C.

Trial and error allows the patient to experience normal and abnormal movement patterns and to be involved in evaluation, modification, and repetition of the movement pattern. The learner/patient is allowed to experience mistakes and then is an active participant in solving problems.
(Umphred, page 438)
Teaching & Learning

163. D.

The recommendation is to work at 60 to 70 percent of the safe maximal heart rate. To determine the safe maximal heart rate, subtract the patient's age from 220. In this case, 220 – 32 = 188, so the safe maximal heart rate is 188 bpm; 60 percent of 188 = 113; and 70 percent of 188 = 131. Thus, 125 bpm falls into the target range.
(Stephenson, page 129)
Multi-system: Differential Diagnosis & Pathology

164. B.

Concentric contractions require more motor units than the other choices to move against the same resistance.
(Magee/Scientific Differential Diagnosis & Pathology, page 445)
Musculoskeletal System: Foundational Sciences & Background

165. B.

Heat application can increase local blood flow to the treatment area. If the treated area is also an insulin injection site, it can accelerate the absorption of insulin and cause hypoglycemia. Symptoms of hypoglycemia can include headache, decreased coordination, and lethargy.
(Goodman/Pathology, page 359)
Metabolic & Endocrine: Treatment Interventions

166. B.

During active flexion of the knee, the tibia moves posteriorly on a fixed femur in an open chain position, following the convex-concave rule.
(Kisner, page 194)
Musculoskeletal System: Treatment Interventions

167. C.

Mottling is a sign of overheating of the tissues, so more towels should be added to prevent a burn injury. Mottling does not mean heat can no longer be used.
(Behrens, page 25)
Therapeutic Modalities

168. A.

Type 1 diabetes is characterized by the fact that it is insulin-dependent. It is essentially not improved with exercise and requires medication for control of blood sugar. It is most often juvenile-onset.
(Goodman/Pathology, page 344)
Metabolic & Endocrine: Differential Diagnosis & Pathology

169. C.

The ulnar nerve has sensory distribution to the pinky and ulnar half of the ring finger. The median nerve distributes to the middle finger. The radial nerve distributes to the thumb and index fingers and the radial half of the middle finger.
(Dutton, page 40)
Musculoskeletal System: Evaluation

170. B.

Graves' disease is a form of hyperthyroidism. Musculoskeletal manifestations can include periarthritis with joint pain and stiffness. Calcific tendonitis can also occur, further limiting function.
(Goodman/Pathology, page 329)
Metabolic & Endocrine: Differential Diagnosis & Pathology

171. B.

Cardiac output equals the product of heart rate and stroke volume: CO = HR × SV. So:
$CO = 60 \text{ bpm} \times 0.1 \text{ L}$
$CO = 6 \text{ L/min}$
(Irwin, page 30)
Cardiac, Vascular, & Pulmonary Systems: Foundational Sciences & Background

172. B.

The close-packed position of the shoulder is abduction and external rotation. In a close-packed position, the ligaments of a joint are most tightened and are therefore at greatest risk of injury.
(Dutton, page 83)
Musculoskeletal System: Foundational Sciences & Background

173. C.

Tricyclic antidepressants significantly increase heart rate during exercise. This may mean that although such patients do not perceive the exercise as exerting, their heart rate must be monitored to avoid activity that pushes them over the desired increase.
(Goodman/Pathology, page 57)
Multi-system: Foundational Sciences & Background

174. B.

The ADA has assembled a list of necessary adjustments to allow for the use of a wheelchair in the home and community setting. Doorways should be more than 32 inches wide and toilets should be 17–19 inches tall. In this case, a handrail is not as good a choice as a ramp, and the 16-inch-high recliner is too low for him to rise from.
(Deusterhaus, page 483)
Safety, Protection & Professional Roles

175. A.

Elbow flexion is innervated by the C5 nerve root.
(Martin, page 381)
Nervous System: Foundational Sciences & Background

176. B.

Pulse oximetry measures arterial oxygen saturation.
(Irwin, page 206)
Cardiac, Vascular, & Pulmonary Systems: Evaluation

177. A.

The function of L2 myotome is hip flexion, with the dermatome affecting the anteromedial thigh above the knee.
(Magee/Orthopedic, page 552)
Musculoskeletal System: Foundational Sciences & Background

178. B.

This patient is at risk of developing heart disease and would benefit from physical therapy for prevention and risk reduction. The other patients presented here are beyond prevention; they have active cardiac or pulmonary disease.
(Irwin, page 262)
Cardiac, Vascular, & Pulmonary Systems: Treatment Interventions

179. B.

Since the patient is spending less time on the painful leg, he is working to get the unaffected leg down for added support. The shortened stance time on the injured side will cause a shortened step length on the opposite side.
(Magee/Orthopedic, page 963)
Musculoskeletal System: Evaluation

180. D.

The Modified Ashworth Scale is used to grade spasticity. A grade of 3 indicates considerable increase in muscle tone, and passive range of motion is difficult.
(Umphred, page 430)
Nervous System: Evaluation

181. A.

Increased or increasing intracranial pressure is a contraindication to chest percussion. Presence of secretions, cystic fibrosis, and mechanical ventilation are all indications for postural drainage and manual percussion.
(Frownfelter, page 333)
Cardiac, Vascular, & Pulmonary Systems: Treatment Interventions

182. A.

Vital signs such as blood pressure, heart rate, and respiratory rate can be used to assess the autonomic nervous system.
(Farber, page 109)
Nervous System: Evaluation

183. **B.**

This position allows the heels of the feet and the elbows to be "on air" so as not to cause pressure areas that can become sore.
(Deusterhaus, page 118)
Safety, Protection & Professional Roles

184. **B.**

To address muscle guarding and spasticity, the goal is to fatigue the muscle to facilitate muscle relaxation. Less rest time is necessary, since strength is not a goal.
(Behrens, page 183)
Therapeutic Modalities

185. **A.**

The patient needs to anteriorly shift the weight of the body to stand up. The pelvis should be in neutral, rotated neither posteriorly nor anteriorly. The therapist may need to facilitate upward displacement of the pelvis.
(Bly, page 69)
Nervous System: Treatment Interventions

186. **A.**

Increasing the amount of time that a patient spends in bed may cause impairment of respiratory function and status, putting him at risk of respiratory infections and complications.
(Irwin, page 274)
Integumentary System: Treatment Interventions

187. **D.**

Autonomic dysreflexia happens in spinal cord–injured patients whose injury is above the level of T6. A noxious stimulus results in a dramatic rise in blood pressure due to sympathetic nervous system overflow.
(Martin, page 386)
Nervous System: Treatment Interventions

188. **B.**

Ankle-foot orthosis offers the support this patient needs without the extra support and bulkiness that he does not require.
(Seymour, page 381)
Equipment & Devices

189. **C.**

The subject is entitled to withdraw from the study at any time. The subject should give informed consent and should be made aware of any risks of the study. A control group that receives a placebo is appropriate for this study.
(Currier, page 73)
Research & Evidence Based Practice

190. **D.**

Myelin increases the speed of nerve impulses. A patient with multiple sclerosis has multiple lesions or plaques of the central nervous system.
(Umphred, page 595)
Nervous System: Differential Diagnosis & Pathology

191. **B.**

A forearm cuff is used to treat lateral epicondylitis and to decrease stress on the forearm flexors.
(Edelstein, page 134)
Equipment & Devices

192. **C.**

Learning is specific. By the therapist's creating the same conditions that the patient will encounter at home, the patient is able to learn specific techniques that apply to her home situation.
(Christiansen, page 429)
Teaching & Learning

193. **D.**

Passive range of motion is indicated for this patient. Quick movements during change of position, Trendelenburg position, and chest percussions are all contraindicated.
(Umphred, page 708)
Nervous System: Treatment Interventions

194. **A.**

Constant feedback is feedback that is given after every trial.
(Christiansen, page 434)
Teaching & Learning

195. **D.**

Standard deviation measures the average amount that a set of scores deviates from the mean.
(Hicks, page 55)
Research & Evidence Based Practice

196. C.

A keloid scar is raised and extends beyond the original wound boundaries.
(Sussman, page 95)
Integumentary System: Evaluation

197. B.

Countercoup lesions are on the opposite side of the brain, not the impacted side, and are a result of deceleration. Coup lesions are damage to the same side of the brain as the impact to the head.
(Martin, page 31)
Nervous System: Differential Diagnosis & Pathology

198. C.

Sharp debridement via tweezers is an example of selective debridement. Wet-to-dry dressings, whirlpool, and wound irrigation are examples of nonselective debridement and may result in removing viable tissue as well as the necrotic tissue.
(Baranoski, page 120)
Integumentary System: Treatment Interventions

199. B.

A positive correlation means that two variables increase or decrease together. A negative correlation means that as one variable increases, the other variable decreases. Correlation, however, does not necessarily indicate that one variable causes the other.
(Hicks, page 80)
Research & Evidence Based Practice

200. A.

If the knees and hips cannot be at 90° angles, this is the best position to maintain a neutral spine and avoid postural injury.
(Saunders, page 372)
Safety, Protection & Professional Roles

Section 5

201. D.

Spondylolisthesis is the forward slippage of one vertebra on another. Spondylosis is when the two vertebrae are showing degenerative changes that appear anvil-like on X-ray. Spondylolysis is a defect in the pars.
(Dutton, page 1217)
Musculoskeletal System: Foundational Sciences & Background

202. D.

Presence of a pacemaker is a contraindication to electrical stimulation in this area. Electrical stimulation is used to increase blood flow, decrease edema, and encourage wound contraction.
(Sussman, page 491)
Integumentary System: Treatment Interventions

203. A.

High-level exercise is contraindicated for patients diagnosed with pericarditis.
(Irwin, page 10)
Cardiac, Vascular, & Pulmonary Systems: Treatment Interventions

204. D.

Application of moist heat may actually inhibit muscle strength for the first 30 minutes after its use. It also decreases muscle endurance. It does aid in increasing tissue extensibility, decreasing pain, and decreasing muscle spasm.
(Behrens, page 42)
Therapeutic Modalities

205. B.

Habituation exercises overstimulate the vestibular system to "reset" the system and decrease symptoms of dizziness.
(Umphred, page 650)
Nervous System: Foundational Sciences & Background

206. A.

Metastatic cancer often shows up in the long bones or lumbar vertebrae. Signs and symptoms that do not add up and night pain should be red flags for referral to the physician.
(Magee/Scientific Differential Diagnosis & Pathology, page 244)
Multi-system: Differential Diagnosis & Pathology

207. B.

Uncontrolled inflammation that remains in an injured joint can have detrimental effects on otherwise healthy tissue surrounding the injured area. It is the injury itself that causes laxity and immobilization that causes capsular tightness, and vasodilation is a primary effect of the inflammatory response.
(Magee/Scientific Differential Diagnosis & Pathology, page 41)
Musculoskeletal System: Treatment Interventions

208. B.

A healthy individual should be able to maintain non-weight-bearing to go from sit to stand and then pivot to the chair. No assistance should be necessary.
(Deusterhaus, page 246)
Safety, Protection & Professional Roles

209. A.

Maceration is the softening of tissue by soaking. Macerated tissue appears white and is thin and fragile.
(Sussman, page 96)
Integumentary System: Evaluation

210. A.

The supine position allows the stomach to slide up in the abdominal cavity and push into the diaphragm, irritating the symptoms. A wedge behind the patient can allow recumbent exercise without worsening symptoms.
(Goodman/Pathology, page 633)
Gastrointestinal: Treatment Interventions

211. C.

Endocrine pathologies affect the glands of the body that secrete hormones. Depending on the type of pathology, either too much or too little hormone may be excreted, causing a multitude of signs and symptoms.
(Goodman/Pathology, page 324)
Metabolic & Endocrine: Foundational Sciences & Background

212. A.

Resistive exercise can be done every other day for a basic strengthening with aerobic exercise on the off days to improve cardiovascular health.
(Hall, page 80)
Musculoskeletal Systems: Treatment Interventions

213. A.

Since the pulling motion is less strenuous on the back than a push, most of the help should be pulling so that the one who assists with a push does not have much load to move.
(Duesterhaus, page 226)
Safety, Protection & Professional Roles

214. A.

Brunnstrom has described synergy patterns seen in the upper and lower extremities, flexion, and extension. This patient demonstrates a classic upper-extremity flexion synergy.
(Rothstein, page 466)
Nervous System: Evaluation

215. A.

A lower frequency will elicit a stronger contraction in this denervated muscle. The lower frequency may be more uncomfortable.
(Robinson, page 178)
Therapeutic Modalities

216. D.

When tightened, the transverse abdominis, multifidus, and pelvic floor provide stability to the lumbar spine. The rectus abdominis does not attach to the spine and does not provide the stabilization that the transverse abdominis does.
(Magee/Scientific Differential Diagnosis & Pathology, page 395)
Musculoskeletal System: Treatment Interventions

217. C.

The PTA has the knowledge and background to follow through with an exercise regimen as instructed and supervised by a physical therapist and is familiar with what to look for as adverse reactions to the exercise.
(Gabard, page 250)
Safety, Protection & Professional Roles

218. C.

If a patient who was previously independent with mobility presents with limitations, functional training is one technique to address this. Strength and endurance training can also help.
(Irwin, page 359)
Cardiac, Vascular, & Pulmonary Systems: Treatment Interventions

219. B.

Myelin increases the speed of nerve impulses and insulates the axons.
(Martin, page 10)
Nervous System: Foundational Sciences & Background

220. C.

Based on the desired depth of penetration (superficial), the 3 MHz frequency is most suitable. Based on the fact that the injury is still in the acute inflammatory stage, nonthermal pulsed effects are most desirable.
(Behrens, page 70)
Therapeutic Modalities

221. A.

As pregnancy progresses, the center of gravity moves anterior and superior.
(Kisner, page 554)
Multi-system: Differential Diagnosis & Pathology

222. C.

It is the responsibility of the physical therapist to respect the patient's wishes regarding a male or female therapist. There may be religious, ethnic, or other reasons for the patient's preference.
(Gabard, page 92)
Safety, Protection & Professional Roles

223. B.

The right lung has three lobes: upper, middle, and lower. The left lung has two lobes: upper and lower.
(Irwin, page 41)
Cardiac, Vascular, & Pulmonary Systems: Foundational Sciences & Background

224. D.

Whirlpool is used for wounds with thick exudate, slough, and necrotic tissue. It should be discontinued when the necrotic tissue is cleared.
(Brown, page 29)
Integumentary System: Treatment Interventions

225. D.

Dysphagia is difficulty with swallowing.
(Martin, page 285)
Nervous System: Differential Diagnosis & Pathology

226. B.

Motivation is key in this situation. Patient A has a husband who is eager to help her. Patient B needs to do this movement by herself in order to go home independently. Motivation is necessary.
(Umphred, page 17)
Teaching & Learning

227. C.

The slump test assesses neural tension of the lower extremity.
(Magee/Orthopedic, page 497)
Musculoskeletal System: Evaluation

228. A.

Pleural effusion is the condition of an increased amount of fluid occupying the pleural space. Pneumothorax is a condition of free air leaked into the pleural space. Atelectasis is the collapse of lung tissue.
(Irwin, page 172)
Cardiac, Vascular, & Pulmonary Systems: Differential Diagnosis & Pathology

229. C.

Rancho Los Amigos Cognitive Functioning Scale is used to describe a patient's cognitive function. The Modified Ashworth Scale is used to measure spasticity. The Glasgow Coma Scale is used to rate a patient's level of arousal and cortical function. Brunnstrom's stages of recovery identify the levels of a patient's recovery from hemiplegia.
(Martin, page 358)
Nervous System: Evaluation

230. A.

A pancoast tumor is in the apex of the lung; when large enough, it can put pressure on surrounding structures, giving the described signs and symptoms.
(Goodman/Pathology, page 610)
Multi-systems: Differential Diagnosis & Pathology

231. B.

Inter-rater reliability is the degree to which there is agreement in measurement between raters.
(Currier, page 167)
Research & Evidence Based Practice

232. C.

Dysdiadochokinesia is defined as impaired ability to produce rapid alternating movements. Ataxia is defined as impaired muscular coordination. Bradykinesia is defined as a slowness of movement. Dysphagia is defined as impaired swallowing.
(Umphred, page 724)
Nervous System: Differential Diagnosis & Pathology

233. B.

To predict maximal heart rate, subtract the patient's age from 220; in this case, 220 – 72 = 148. Certain medications such as beta-blockers and sympathomimetics blunt or exaggerate the heart rate response and this formula cannot be used. Following a heart transplant, the heart is denervated and will have an abnormal heart-rate response.
(Irwin, page 84)
Cardiac, Vascular, & Pulmonary Systems: Evaluation

234. D.

Multidirectional weight-shifting with and without arm support can address dynamic sitting balance goals. Patients should be challenged to progress into higher levels of maintaining balance.
(Umphred, page 732)
Nervous System: Treatment Interventions

235. A.

The epidermis is the outer layer of the skin.
(Moffat, page 1)
Integumentary System: Foundational Sciences & Background

236. D.

A patient with Alzheimer's disease has memory and cognitive deficits. A caregiver should be educated on the exercise program in order to help the patient to correctly complete the exercises.
(Glickstein, page 66)
Nervous System: Treatment Interventions

237. B.

A hand serves a more cosmetic function. An active terminal device is able to open and close without the use of the sound hand.
(Carroll, page 143)
Equipment & Devices

238. D.

Any indication of systemic signs such as fatigue or proximal muscle weakness (inability to sit up at her desk, and a heavy feeling while lifting her legs) should caution the physical therapist to look beyond the musculoskeletal diagnosis. Lack of appropriate response to therapy treatment interventions should also indicate something more global.
(Goodman/Pathology, page 324)
Metabolic & Endocrine: Differential Diagnosis & Pathology

239. B.

In this case, either the right facet will not close or the left facet is stuck open. It will be the left transverse process that can be palpated in extension.
(Saunders, page 269)
Musculoskeletal System: Evaluation

240. C.

A four-point pattern uses alternate and reciprocal movement of the crutches and the opposite lower extremity.
(Pierson, page 110)
Equipment & Devices

241. C.

Generalization refers to learning one skill and being able to complete a closely related skill.
(Christiansen, page 429)
Teaching & Learning

242. B.

Qualitative research avoids numbers and can help look at other people's views or opinions.
(Hicks, page 7)
Research & Evidence Based Practice

243. B.

The capsular pattern of the shoulder is external rotation > abduction > internal rotation.
(Magee/Orthopedic, page 232)
Musculoskeletal System: Foundational Sciences & Background

244. C.

If the results are statistically significant, it is unlikely that the difference is due to chance. Also, the treatment may be clinically important if the change is large enough for therapists to change the way they treat patients.
(Helewa, page 87)
Research & Evidence Based Practice

245. C.

The deep peroneal nerve can become compressed by fluid accumulation in the anterior compartment, causing numbness, pain, and foot drop.
(Magee/Orthopedic, page 900)
Musculoskeletal System: Differential Diagnosis & Pathology

246. A.

Decreased potassium levels inhibit normal muscle function by limiting the effectiveness of the sodium-potassium pump needed for muscle contraction. Electrolyte loss is common, with flulike symptoms of diarrhea and vomiting.
(Goodman/Pathology, page 631)
Multi-system: Foundational Sciences & Background

247. D.

Proprioception is the ability to identify the position of the body or a body part without looking.
(Umphred, page 430)
Nervous System: Evaluation

248. C.

Asking another therapist to measure the range of motion without the second therapist knowing why creates a blind procedure. In a blind test, the examiner is not aware of the hypothesis. This can eliminate any possible bias on the part of the examiner.
(Hicks, page 100)
Research & Evidence Based Practice

249. D.

A person's locus of control can be external or internal. A person with an external locus of control believes that events are caused by fate and powerful others. They tend to respond to directions from an expert.
(Davis, page 192)
Teaching & Learning

250. B.

The capsular pattern of the hip is restriction of flexion, abduction and medial rotation. These motion restrictions indicate capsular involvement. The order of restriction may vary.
(Magee/Orthopedic, page 33)
Musculoskeletal System: Differential Diagnosis & Pathology

Answers and Explanations For Practice Test 2

Section 1

1. **D.**

   The therapist should be positioned at a 45° angle behind the patient, able to guard and catch the patient if necessary but not in the patient's way during mobility. Most loss of balance is to the posterior or side, making this a good guarding position.
   (Duesterhaus, page 14)
   Safety, Protection & Professional Roles

2. **C.**

   The two terminal lymphatic vessels are the right lymphatic duct and the thoracic duct.
   (Thibodeau, page 339)
   Cardiac, Vascular, & Pulmonary Systems: Foundational Sciences & Background

3. **C.**

   Aspirin, acetaminophen, and NSAIDs are all non-narcotic drugs that can be used for pain relief. Medications such as codeine, morphine, and hydrocodone are narcotic analgesics and can produce tolerance and addiction.
   (Behrens, page 7)
   Musculoskeletal System: Foundational Sciences & Background

4. **A.**

   Stress incontinence occurs when there is stress on the pelvic floor musculature, such as in sneezing, coughing, lifting, or exercise.
   (Goodman/Pathology, page 722)
   Genitourinary System: Differential Diagnosis & Pathology

5. **B.**

   A cohort study identifies subjects who have a risk factor for development of a particular condition and follows them to establish which subjects develop that condition.
   (Helewa, page 20)
   Research & Evidence Based Practice

6. **A.**

   The patient has reddening of the skin and does not need surgery. A patient should not toilet herself if her hygiene techniques are inadequate. Bathing regularly (more often than biweekly) is a must for good skin care. This patient should follow a toileting schedule, and nursing staff should apply protective ointment to the impaired skin.
   (Brown, page 133)
   Integumentary System: Foundational Sciences & Background

7. **A.**

   This particular PNF pattern is called rhythmic stabilization and uses isometric contractions of antagonist to facilitate movement.
   (Voss, page 302)
   Nervous System: Treatment Interventions

8. **C.**

   Compression wraps are an appropriate treatment intervention for patients with lymphedema.
   (Irwin, page 445)
   Cardiac, Vascular, & Pulmonary Systems: Treatment Interventions

9. **B.**

   A seat that is too wide can cause difficulty with propulsion, difficulty with transfers, difficulty due to increased overall width, and postural problems.
   (Pierson, page 154)
   Equipment & Devices

10. D.

Questions should be easy for the respondent to understand and should avoid medical jargon. Questions should not be leading. Questions should be clear. Choice C may be unclear, as it does not delineate inpatient versus outpatient physical therapy.
(Hicks, page 20)
Research & Evidence Based Practice

11. D.

CPT codes indicate what services the physical therapist has provided. ICD-9 codes are the diagnostic codes. In this case, rotator cuff tear is the medical diagnosis and shoulder pain is the physical therapy diagnosis.
(Shamus, page 44)
Safety, Protection & Professional Roles

12. A.

The patellar tendon reflex is specific to L4 nerve root involvement. The Achilles tendon reflex is S1, and there is no reflex specific to L5.
(Hoppenfeld/Orthopedic, page 68)
Musculoskeletal System: Evaluation

13. B.

The quick isometric contractions work to strengthen the fast-twitch fibers of the pelvic floor musculature that must contract when a stress event such as coughing occurs. Increasing the length of hold can help with urge incontinence and can decrease the amount of urinary loss.
(Goodman/Pathology, page 726)
Genitourinary System: Intervention

14. B.

The health of connective tissues is directly affected by hormone production and metabolism, which are controlled by the endocrine system.
(Goodman/Pathology, page 322)
Metabolic & Endocrine System: Treatment Interventions

15. B.

Pneumothorax is the condition that results when free air is allowed to leak into the space between the visceral and parietal pleura.
(Irwin, page 172)
Cardiac, Vascular, & Pulmonary Systems: Differential Diagnosis & Pathology

16. D.

The obturator nerve is part of the lumbosacral plexus, not the brachial plexus.
(Martin, page 21)
Nervous System: Foundational Sciences & Background

17. C.

Procedural knowledge is knowledge of how to do something.
(Christiansen, page 429)
Teaching & Learning

18. D.

Although it appears the patient can be transferred from the bed, pulsatile lavage may be the most appropriate. The patient's wound is small so this method will allow the most direct method of wound care without introducing bacteria from other body parts, which may occur in a whirlpool.
(Behrens, page 93)
Therapeutic Modalities

19. A.

The capsular pattern of the hip is flexion > abduction > internal rotation. Backward walking and bridging assess hip extension, and side-stepping assesses hip abduction and adduction. Squatting to the floor best assesses the hip flexion range of motion. This does not rule out a capsular pattern.
(Magee/Orthopedic, page 659)
Musculoskeletal System: Evaluation

20. A.

The presence of malaise, fever, and fatigue indicates some systemic pathology, usually infection or an abnormal response within the body.
(Goodman/Clinical Medicine, page 534)
Genitourinary System: Differential Diagnosis & Pathology

21. B.

Energy conservation is the best way to decrease muscular work and enable the patient to perform necessary functional tasks. Physical therapists should educate the patient on combining trips to get maximum benefit from any exertion, decreasing the difficulty of activities by changing positions, and getting help from a caregiver.
(Umphred, page 584)
Nervous System: Treatment Interventions

22. **D.**

Potassium, magnesium, sodium, and calcium are the primary electrolytes whose excessive presence or complete absence in the body can cause multisystem dysfunction. Selenium is not an electrolyte.
(Goodman/Pathology, page 107)
Multi-System: Foundational Sciences & Background

23. **C.**

Traction can irritate hypermobile joints and their supporting structures.
(Behrens, page 113)
Therapeutic Modalities

24. **C.**

The APTA Guide for Professional Conduct gives guidelines stating that gifts and favors that affect (or attempt to affect) professional judgment should not be accepted. In this case, it appears the patient is bringing a gift in order to influence the physical therapist's decision to continue care; accepting such a gift would be unethical.
(Gabard, page 152)
Safety, Protection & Professional Roles

25. **B.**

Macrotrauma is a quick, one-time force that is great enough to cause injury, in this case to the ACL. Microtrauma is caused by repetitive stress causing injury; this stress in a one-time occurrence is not enough to cause injury. Transection is a laceration, and compression is a contusion.
(Magee/Scientific Differential Diagnosis & Pathology, page 5)
Musculoskeletal System: Foundational Sciences & Background

26. **B.**

Necrotic tissue is dead and may inhibit wound healing. As it becomes dry, it becomes brown or black, thick, and hard.
(Baranoski, page 89)
Integumentary System: Differential Diagnosis & Pathology

27. **D.**

A corrective orthosis is used to increase or correct contractures.
(Edelstein, page 128)
Equipment & Devices

28. **A.**

T12 discogenic pathology can refer pain to the L5-S1 area. Nerve root involvement would refer pain into the lower extremities, and facet pain is very localized to that level.
(Grant, page 78)
Musculoskeletal System: Differential Diagnosis & Pathology

29. **A.**

Exercise or activity that increases intra-abdominal pressure may exacerbate the pain associated with diverticulosis. One of the first exercises from which this patient would benefit is instruction in diaphragmatic breathing to avoid increased pressures.
(Goodman/Pathology, page 653)
Gastrointestinal System: Treatment Interventions

30. **D.**

An electroencephalogram is used to measure brainwave activity and to diagnose seizure activity and type of seizure.
(Rothstein, page 418)
Nervous System: Differential Diagnosis & Pathology

31. **D.**

Homan's test is used to detect the presence of deep vein thrombosis in the lower leg.
(Rothstein, page 186)
Cardiac, Vascular, & Pulmonary Systems: Evaluation

32. **A.**

The ACL is considered a static stabilizer of the knee because it provides passive support. The muscles surrounding the knee are considered dynamic stabilizers.
(Norkin/Levangie, page 364)
Musculoskeletal System: Foundational Sciences & Background

33. **D.**

MODS is an end-stage syndrome where organs essentially shut down. If physical therapy intervention is sought, it will be for skin precautions to avoid breakdown. Mobility and strengthening are not appropriate goals.
(Goodman/Pathology, page 104)
Multi-system: Differential Diagnosis & Pathology

34. **A.**

The 3 MHz frequency reaches superficial soft tissues only. For maximal thermal benefits to decrease spasm and increase tissue mobility, continuous ultrasound is recommended.
(Behrens, page 60)
Therapeutic Modalities

35. **A.**

Exercise done in the position of necessary muscle action has the best carryover into functional activity. In this case, ankle dorsiflexors, ankle plantar flexors, and hip abductors play a key role in balance. Strengthening them in a standing position works them in a functional position.
(Magee/Scientific Differential Diagnosis & Pathology, page 73)
Musculoskeletal System: Treatment Interventions

36. **A.**

This population could be at risk for falls, and it is not recommended to have them practice their balance without something nearby to hold onto for safety. Single-leg stance may help improve balance but is most safely practiced holding onto something.
(Bottomly, page 445)
Safety, Protection & Professional Roles

37. **C.**

An IPOP is predominantly used for young patients who have suffered a trauma and have no skin or balance impairments.
(Seymour, page 127)
Equipment & Devices

38. **A.**

The functional reach test is used to test balance. In this test the therapist measures the distance a standing person can reach with an outstretched arm. The nine-hole peg test and Frenchay arm test examine upper limb function. The Mini-Mental State Exam tests cognition.
(Umphred, page 629)
Nervous System: Evaluation

39. **B.**

Tendons contain 3–5 percent elastin, which is more than any of the other choices.
(Magee/Scientific Differential Diagnosis & Pathology, page 15)
Musculoskeletal System: Differential Diagnosis & Pathology

40. **A.**

A randomized clinical trial is the most powerful research design to determine efficacy of treatment. A case study has a sample size of one. A descriptive study has no scientific power but can describe a new condition. A cohort study groups subjects by a common characteristic and therefore is not randomized.
(Helewa, page 20)
Research & Evidence Based Practice

41. **D.**

If a wound has moisture, the drainage should be absorbed. If necrotic tissue is present, it should be debrided. If the wound is dry, moisture should be added.
(Baranoski, page 132)
Integumentary System: Treatment Interventions

42. **C.**

If the left hip abductors are weak, the contralateral hip may drop with left stance phase. This is referred to as Trendelenburg gait.
(O'Sullivan, page 330)
Nervous System: Evaluation

43. **D.**

The use of positive high-volt pulsed current stimulation over an edematous area is thought to push the positively charged edema away from the injured site.
(Michlovitz, page 114)
Therapeutic Modalities

44. **A.**

This patient is exercising at roughly 60 percent of her maximum heart rate, which follows guidelines for exercise during pregnancy.
(Stephenson, page 120)
Multi-system: Differential Diagnosis & Pathology

45. **B.**

When designing an exercise program, the exercises should simulate the desired end-range function or activity. Muscle strengthening occurs specific to the action it is performing.
(Magee/Scientific Differential Diagnosis & Pathology, page 73)
Musculoskeletal System: Foundational Sciences & Background

46. A.

A patient with Parkinson's disease has the main manifestations of bradykinesia, rigidity, tremor, and postural instability.
(Martin, page 444)
Nervous System: Differential Diagnosis & Pathology

47. A.

With use of outcome measures, a physical therapist can document progress (or lack of progress) and goal achievement. The use of outcome measures can increase the therapist's efficiency by directing treatment and thus decreasing the number of therapy visits.
(Cole, page 167)
Research & Evidence Based Practice

48. B.

Factors that influence self-efficacy are a person's own experiences; observations of others' experiences; and support from friends, family members, and others.
(Davis, page 193)
Teaching & Learning

49. C.

Guillain-Barré syndrome is a demyelinating neurological disorder that results in flaccid weakness and hyporeflexia. Weakness begins distally and progresses proximally. Autonomic dysfunction is also often seen.
(Umphred, page 387)
Nervous System: Differential Diagnosis & Pathology

50. C.

Forward flexion of the trunk with arms supported in front is a position known to decrease the work of breathing.
(Irwin, page 308)
Cardiac, Vascular, & Pulmonary Systems: Treatment Interventions

Section 2

51. D.

It is normal for a patient to experience dizziness and sometimes nausea during treatment. As long as the patient is able to continue, the repositioning should not be stopped—but the dizziness should lessen before the patient moves to the next position.
(Umphred, page 650)
Nervous System: Treatment Interventions

52. D.

There are more differences than similarities between OA and RA. RA always involves inflammation, whereas OA usually does not. RA is bilateral and symmetrical in presentation; OA is not. OA is primarily in weight-bearing joints; RA is not. Both conditions, however, can be genetically linked.
(Goodman/Pathology, page 947)
Multi-system: Differential Diagnosis & Pathology

53. A.

Posture muscles are made up primarily of slow-twitch, oxidative fibers (type I). These muscles are considered endurance muscles because they are called upon to remain active for longer periods of time. They are prone to weakness and can fatigue if they are too weak to maintain a posture.
(Dutton, page 16)
Musculoskeletal System: Foundational Sciences & Background

54. C.

The pulse rate or frequency determines the rate of motor nerve stimulation. Higher pulse rates lead to stronger contraction and rapid fatigue. A strong contraction is needed to increase resultant muscle strength, but the muscle needs rest to avoid fatigue. The duty cycle determines how much time the muscle is active versus its rest time and should be decreased to allow more rest time.
(Behrens, page 178)
Therapeutic Modalities

55. B.

The ICD-9 code is the PT diagnosis that is prompting the patient to seek physical therapy. This should not be confused with the physician's medical diagnosis. The choices of PT evaluation, therapeutic exercise, and manual therapy are CPT codes.
(Shamus, page 44)
Safety, Protection & Professional Roles

56. D.

Correlation coefficient denotes strength of correlation. Negative numbers indicate negative correlation. Positive numbers indicate positive correlation. Zero indicates no relation. The closer the number is to 1.0, the stronger the correlation.
(Hicks, page 77)
Research & Evidence Based Practice

57. **A.**

Fast-twitch oxidative-glycolytic muscle fibers are recruited after one hour of moderate-intensity activity or interval training involving bouts of high-intensity exercise.
(Magee, Zachazewski, page 365)
Musculoskeletal System: Treatment Interventions

58. **B.**

The cerebellum is located inferior to the occipital lobe and in the posterior portion of the cranium.
(Martin, page 14)
Nervous System: Foundational Sciences & Background

59. **D.**

Postural drainage in the Trendelenburg position, chest percussion, and vibration are contraindicated due to the patient's rib and vertebral fractures.
(Frownfelter, page 333)
Cardiac, Vascular, & Pulmonary Systems: Treatment Interventions

60. **D.**

The armrest should be removable to allow positioning of the sliding board for patient transfer.
(Pierson, page 158)
Equipment & Devices

61. **D.**

Alginates function to pack a wound and absorb exudate. Adequate exudate must be present to convert the alginate into a gel. This helps to maintain a moist wound environment. A shallow wound does not need to be packed, but a deep wound does require both packing and absorption.
(Brown, page 61)
Integumentary System: Treatment Interventions

62. **B.**

Grade III mobilizations are large-amplitude movements into tissue stretch or resistance end range.
(Saunders, page 239)
Musculoskeletal System: Treatment Interventions

63. **C.**

Physical therapists should evaluate whether the research results are applicable to their own patient population. Isometric strength of 20-year-old males is applicable to this therapist's practice.
(Helewa, page 89)
Research & Evidence Based Practice

64. **C.**

Faded feedback is provided extensively as the new skill is taught, and then feedback is decreased as the skill is being learned and practiced.
(Christiansen, page 434)
Teaching & Learning

65. **A.**

Older patients who are taking tricyclic antidepressants may be at greater risk of heat stroke in warmer temperatures. Exercise in a heated pool may put additional stress on the system and may have adverse effects. A phone call to the physician, making him aware of this risk and recommending modified treatment in the clinic or in a nonheated pool, may be appropriate.
(Goodman/Pathology, page 57)
Multi-system: Foundational Sciences & Background

66. **B.**

Nonmodifiable risk factors for osteoporosis are female gender, age >50, and Caucasian. General inactivity and caffeine intake are modifiable risk factors for osteoporosis. The fact that this woman has a compression fracture in the thoracic spine should trigger the suspicion of bone pathology.
(Goodman/Pathology, page 872)
Metabolic & Endocrine System: Differential Diagnosis & Pathology

67. **B.**

Progressive resistance exercise is shown to increase strength and slow the progression of osteoporosis in a frail elderly person.
(Magee/Scientific Differential Diagnosis & Pathology, page 342)
Musculoskeletal System: Treatment Interventions

68. C.

A clinical stimulator is necessary to generate the power needed to facilitate contraction. With pulse widths and frequencies essentially the same, it is the on/off time that is crucial. For muscle reeducation, there must be a 1:3 work-to-rest ratio to avoid fatigue.
(Behrens, pages 177 and 180)
Therapeutic Modalities

69. B.

This runner has symptoms of dehydration.
(Moffat, page 22)
Integumentary System: Foundational Sciences & Background

70. C.

PNF emphasizes diagonal movement patterns.
(Voss, page 1)
Nervous System: Treatment Interventions

71. C.

Cystic fibrosis is a genetic disorder of endocrine gland function that results in abnormally thick secretions of bronchial mucous glands, sweat glands, and the pancreas.
(Irwin, page 156)
Cardiac, Vascular, & Pulmonary Systems: Differential Diagnosis & Pathology

72. B.

A standing frame is appropriate for a patient with C7 paraplegia.
(Edelstein, page 78)
Equipment & Devices

73. C.

The sternocleidomastoid can be injured with forced hyperextension, such as in a car accident. When it is in spasm it causes the head to rotate and extend to the affected side.
(Hoppenfeld, page 111)
Musculoskeletal System: Evaluation

74. C.

Validity is the degree to which an instrument measures what it is intended to measure. Probability is the likelihood for random error in a set of results. Inter-rater reliability is the degree to which there is agreement between different examiners. Intra-rater reliability is the degree of agreement when the same examiner obtains the same measurement on different attempts.
(Currier, page 171)
Research & Evidence Based Practice

75. B.

By educating the patient on the severity of the risk of disobeying the precautions and the costs that could be incurred if injury does occur, the therapist can change the patient's perceptions of the health threat.
(Davis, page 192)
Teaching & Learning

76. C.

The measurements should be taken on both the affected and unaffected legs at several sites. Taking a picture without taking measurements is inadequate for comparison at a later date.
(Sussman, page 97)
Integumentary System: Evaluation

77. B.

The lateral femoral cutaneous nerve is the more superficial portion of the femoral nerve and when compressed, can cause sensory change to the lateral thigh. Nerve compression would not respond to treatment unless whatever was causing the compression was addressed, as nerves need space to function.
(Magee/Orthopedic, page 702)
Musculoskeletal System: Differential Diagnosis & Pathology

78. D.

Intra-abdominal pressures are increased with activities that cause strain and with Valsalva maneuver. Of the choices listed, walking causes the least amount of increased pressures. The other activities can be done successfully with education on breathing techniques and body mechanics.
(Goodman/Pathology, page 633)
Gastrointestinal System: Foundational Sciences & Background

79. A.

Microtrauma injuries are caused by repetitive stress to the injured area. One repetition of these stresses would not necessarily injure the tissues, but cumulative trauma causes tissue injury.
(Magee/Scientific Differential Diagnosis & Pathology, page 5)
Musculoskeletal System: Differential Diagnosis & Pathology

80. C.

In this case, the pelvic floor is responding well to treatment, but the bladder continues to feel the need to empty too often. The use of a progressive voiding schedule can retrain the bladder that it does not need to empty as often. Water consumption needs to be maintained at a high level so that the bladder can stretch and fill without the urge to empty.
(Goodman/Pathology, page 726)
Genitourinary System: Foundational Sciences & Background

81. C.

It is unethical to fail to provide treatment because of an individual's religious beliefs. Accommodations must be made, if possible, to adhere to a patient's values. If evaluation or treatment cannot be done without compromising these viewpoints, the patient must be informed and given the choice to continue.
(Gabard, page 93)
Safety, Protection & Professional Roles

82. C.

There is no known benefit of using TENS on the proximal end of the residual limb. Use of TENS on the distal end of the limb or over the nerve root will stimulate the hypersensitive nerve. Stimulation of the non-amputated limb may see some crossover to relieve the phantom limb pain on the amputated leg.
(Prentice, page 94)
Therapeutic Modalities

83. D.

Obesity, diabetes, and arteriosclerosis are all systemic conditions that delay healing because of inability to adequately deliver blood and nutrients to the tissues. Pregnancy has no such effect on healing.
(Magee/Scientific Differential Diagnosis & Pathology, page 15)
Multi-system: Differential Diagnosis & Pathology

84. D.

All of the choices involve pain and dysfunction of the affected tendon. Tendinosis is the only one that is non-inflammatory.
(Magee/Scientific Differential Diagnosis & Pathology, page 64)
Musculoskeletal System: Differential Diagnosis & Pathology

85. B.

There should be approximately 1.5 to 2 inches, or three to four finger-widths, from the seat to the popliteal fossa.
(Pierson, page 153)
Equipment & Devices

86. B.

Amyotrophic lateral sclerosis is a progressive neuromuscular disorder with both upper motor neuron and lower motor neuron signs. Classic presentation is symptoms of fatigue and weakness. Exercise can be used to prevent disuse atrophy, although weakness will still progress. Care should be used to avoid overexertion.
(Umphred, page 373)
Nervous System: Treatment Interventions

87. C.

Cardiac output equals stroke volume multiplied by heart rate: $CO = SV \times HR$.
(Irwin, page 30)
Cardiac, Vascular, & Pulmonary Systems: Foundational Sciences & Background

88. D.

The screw home mechanism "locks" the knee into place in full extension. To truly test knee extension strength, the knee must be "unlocked"; i.e., in 5° flexion.
(Norkin/Levangie, page 357)
Musculoskeletal System: Evaluation

89. D.

The rooting reflex is a response to a stimulus to an infant's cheek. A normal response is for the infant to turn the head toward the side of the stimulus and open the mouth. This response is normally present from 28 weeks of gestation to three months of age.
(Farber, page 163)
Nervous System: Evaluation

90. B.

Pulling puts less strain on the low back than pushing. There is still a load to move even though the load is on the cart, due to the coefficient of friction.
(Duesterhaus, page 14)
Safety, Protection & Professional Roles

91. B.

A heart rate of less than 60 bpm is considered to be bradycardia. Normal resting heart rate is between 60 and 100 bpm.
(Irwin, page 30)
Cardiac, Vascular, & Pulmonary Systems: Evaluation

92. D.

The Achilles reflex tests neurologic level S1-S2.
(Magee/Orthopedic, page 52)
Nervous System: Evaluation

93. A.

The patient is demonstrating foot drop, and the muscles that dorsiflex the foot should be tested.
(Stokes, page 37)
Nervous System: Evaluation

94. B.

Transfer of training refers to being able to learn a new skill in one environment and perform the same skill in a different environment. Practicing in many different environments helps maximize transfer of training.
(Christiansen, page 429)
Teaching & Learning

95. B.

Heterotopic ossification is associated with brain injury and is defined as abnormal bony growth at a joint. It presents as decreased range of motion and increased pain. The joint may also be warm to the touch. The physical therapist should begin aggressive range of motion exercises and therapy to avoid contracture development.
(Montgomery, page 93)
Nervous System: Differential Diagnosis & Pathology

96. B.

Diuretics are used to decrease fluid buildup within the body. The downside of their use is that they can actually cause too much loss of fluid and a depletion of electrolytes needed for muscle function.
(Goodman/Pathology, page 110)
Multi-system: Foundational Sciences & Background

97. C.

Injured ligaments respond best to low-load exercise for strengthening. Immobilization actually weakens ligaments, and non-weight-bearing exercise does not provide the necessary loading.
(Magee/Scientific Differential Diagnosis & Pathology, page 41)
Musculoskeletal System: Treatment Interventions

98. D.

Athetosis is defined as impaired timing, coordination, and force production of both the limbs and the trunk. Postural impairments are commonly seen.
(Umphred, page 264)
Nervous System: Differential Diagnosis & Pathology

99. D.

Upper-extremity exercise increases blood pressure more than lower-extremity exercises. Position of the body can also cause changes in blood pressure.
(Irwin, page 34)
Cardiac, Vascular, & Pulmonary Systems: Treatment Interventions

100. B.

Informed consent is not legal if the patient cannot understand what is written or spoken.
(Gabard, page 56)
Safety, Protection & Professional Roles

Section 3

101. B.

Levodopa is typically used to treat Parkinson's disease.
(Mosby, page 607)
Nervous System: Foundational Sciences & Background

102. A.

A four-wheeled walker can only add support for this patient, and the basket gives her a place to put a small portable oxygen tank for transport. She probably wouldn't need to haul more than one at a time.
(Irwin, page 314)
Cardiac, Vascular, & Pulmonary Systems: Treatment Interventions

103. B.

In the right side-lying position, the contents of the stomach cannot easily move into the esophagus and cause reflux.
(Goodman/Pathology, page 635)
Gastrointestinal System: Treatment Interventions

104. B.

With the bed rails lowered, the patient has the chance of falling out of bed or may be tempted to get out of bed without assistance. Either of these could cause injury to the patient.
(Goodman/Pathology, page 338)
Safety, Protection & Professional Roles

105. C.

During isotonic contractions, the sarcomeres shorten as a result of the actin sliding over the myosin filaments in a ratchet-like motion, using cross-bridges to pull the actin along the myosin.
(Dutton, page 14)
Musculoskeletal System: Foundational Sciences & Background

106. C.

Conversion is the transformation of high-frequency electrical or mechanical energy into heat. Ultrasound uses mechanical energy to increase tissue temperatures.
(Behrens, page 39)
Therapeutic Modalities

107. C.

If a patient is unable to move through full range of motion against gravity, the next position should be gravity-eliminated. In this case, that position would be side-lying.
(Hislop, page 209)
Musculoskeletal System: Evaluation

108. A.

An untreated UTI can spread infection to any other area of the body that is susceptible. Osteoporosis does not occur as the result of an infection.
(Goodman/Clinical Med, page 534)
Genitourinary System: Differential Diagnosis & Pathology

109. B.

Low levels of TSH in combination with other physical findings that include balance and coordination problems and heat intolerance indicate a hyperfunctioning thyroid. High TSH levels are indicative of hypothyroidism.
(Goodman/Pathology, page 330)
Metabolic & Endocrine System: Evaluation

110. B.

Iontophoresis is an example of direct current where there is unidirectional flow of current. One electrode is always positive and one is always negative.
(Behrens, page 142)
Therapeutic Modalities

111. D.

Walking the stairs would put too much stress on the patient's weight-bearing joints, possibly aggravating joint pain or causing joint injury.
(Goodman/Pathology, page 33)
Multi-system: Differential Diagnosis & Pathology

112. D.

This sequence prevents the transfer of infectious material to the physical therapist or to the outside of the room.
(Duesterhaus, page 103)
Safety, Protection & Professional Roles

113. C.

In the case of tendinopathies, the primary concern is to change whatever is causing the irritation. Choices A, B, and D actually make changes to the function of the patellar tendon. The use of modalities may be adjunct but does not change the negative factors.
(Magee/Scientific Differential Diagnosis & Pathology, page 68)
Musculoskeletal System: Treatment Interventions

114. A.

The therapist's funny story is anecdotal and should not be considered scientific.
(Hicks, page 136)
Research & Evidence Based Practice

115. A.

Pressure on the medial pubic ramus can cause an abducted gait pattern.
(Seymour, page 230)
Equipment & Devices

116. A.

Increase a patient's mobility to improve function and blood flow. Use of upper-body machines may pose risk of skin tears. Use of assistive devices will protect patients from falls and skin tears. Throw rugs do not offer padding and can cause falls from tripping.
(Brown, page 202)
Integumentary System: Treatment Interventions

117. A.

In standing, the facets are in maximal contact and, if degeneration is present, the most painful. Vascular compromise would elicit greater pain with walking, and herniation would be painful in sitting.
(Saunders, page 107)
Musculoskeletal System: Differential Diagnosis & Pathology

118. C.

After this period of immobilization and bed rest, the patient may demonstrate signs and symptoms of orthostatic hypotension. The use of a tilt table or a tilt-in-space wheelchair can help to acclimatize the patient to the upright position.
(Palmer, page 19)
Nervous System: Treatment Interventions

119. A.

Operant conditioning focuses on behavior and employs reinforcement of desired behaviors and non-reinforcement of unwanted behaviors.
(Bastable, page 47)
Teaching & Learning

120. A.

Signs and symptoms of congestive heart failure are orthopnea, unproductive cough, sudden weight gain of 6 to 10 lb, dyspnea, presence of a third heart sound, exertional dyspnea upon minimal exercise, and crackles in the lungs.
(Irwin, page 142)
Cardiac, Vascular, & Pulmonary Systems: Differential Diagnosis & Pathology

121. C.

A posterolateral disc herniation typically causes the patient to shift away from the affected side. It is more common than a posteromedial disc herniation. A direct posterior herniation is even less common and can cause the patient to shift or flex forward.
(Magee/Orthopedic, page 538)
Musculoskeletal System: Differential Diagnosis & Pathology

122. B.

In following the ethical considerations for patient confidentiality, information about a patient's health or any evaluation or treatment they are having cannot be discussed with any other person without that patient's permission. Exceptions to this include other members of the patient's health-care team or the patient's insurance carriers.
(Gabard, page 63)
Safety, Protection & Professional Roles

123. C.

Acetone, or fruity, breath is a classic sign of hyperglycemia; if ignored, it could progress to ketoacidosis or diabetic coma. During exercise, poor hormone control of glucose circulating in the blood can cause hyperglycemia.
(Goodman/Pathology, page 355)
Metabolic & Endocrine System: Foundational Sciences & Background

124. C.

A stage III wound is a full-thickness wound that extends to the underlying fascia.
(Brown, page 97)
Integumentary System: Evaluation

125. B.

Mobility is the lowest stage of motor control, followed by stability, controlled mobility, and finally skill.
(Martin, page 255)
Nervous System: Treatment Interventions

126. D.

Econcentric muscle contraction combines a concentric contraction at one joint and an eccentric contraction at an adjacent joint of a two-joint muscle. Two-joint muscles such as the gastroc are the most commonly injured.
(Magee/Scientific Differential Diagnosis & Pathology, page 446)
Musculoskeletal System: Treatment Interventions

127. C.

The age of the patients with knee replacements is the independent or manipulated variable. Knee range of motion after knee replacement is the dependent variable.
(Hicks, page 66)
Research & Evidence Based Practice

128. C.

To best isolate the pelvic floor for strengthening, contractions should be done without co-contraction of the surrounding musculature. It is difficult to tell whether contraction is adequate when other, nearby muscles are working at the same time.
(Goodman/Pathology, page 726)
Genitourinary System: Treatment Interventions

129. B.

During expiration, lung tissue and the chest wall recoil elastically after inspiration to return to the resting position.
(Irwin, page 50)
Cardiac, Vascular, & Pulmonary Systems: Foundational Sciences & Background

130. A.

Quadriplegia affects the entire body; typically, the upper extremities are more affected than the lower extremities. Diplegia typically affects only the lower extremities and trunk. Hemiplegia is seen when only one side of the body is affected.
(Martin, page 126)
Nervous System: Differential Diagnosis & Pathology

131. A.

This patient is showing signs and symptoms consistent with peroneal nerve palsy. Crossing her legs puts pressure directly on the fibular head where the peroneal nerve becomes superficial.
(Magee/Orthopedic, page 806)
Musculoskeletal System: Differential Diagnosis & Pathology

132. B.

The median is the mid-score of a set of data, when placed in order of magnitude. So for the sequence of 10, 25, 36, 82, and 100, the median is 36.
(Hicks, page 50)
Research & Evidence Based Practice

133. B.

A ventricular shunt drains cerebrospinal fluid from the ventricles to either the heart or the peritoneum to prevent increased intracranial pressure.
(Umphred, page 455)
Nervous System: Differential Diagnosis & Pathology

134. C.

Classic signs and symptoms of rheumatoid arthritis include bilateral joint pain with associated inflammation, morning stiffness with or without activity, and nonpainful nodules (rheumatoid nodules), typically on the extensor tendons of the joint.
(Goodman/Pathology, page 947)
Multi-system: Differential Diagnosis & Pathology

135. C.

Even though the results of the MRI are written for the physical therapist to view, it is not in the physical therapist's scope of practice to release the results of radiologic reports.
(Gabard, page 62)
Safety, Protection & Professional Roles

136. A.

The opiate pain control theory postulates that electrical stimulation releases enkephalins and beta-endorphins to the area of pain.
(Prentice, page 103)
Therapeutic Modalities

137. A.

Instability can occur at the atlantoaxial joint, causing decreased range of motion and the symptoms described here. Care must be taken in this case, as the joint is unstable and any excessive movement could compress on the brain stem and/or spinal cord.
(Goodman/Pathology, page 953)
Multi-system: Differential Diagnosis & Pathology

138. D.

An air cell cushion provides the greatest pressure relief.
(Baranoski, page 198)
Equipment & Devices

139. A.

Burns can limit a joint's range of motion. Staging is not performed on a burn.
(Moffat, page 63)
Integumentary System: Differential Diagnosis & Pathology

140. C.

The most cephalic structure is the midbrain and the most caudal is the medulla.
(Martin, page 15)
Nervous System: Foundational Sciences & Background

141. B.

VO_2 max decreases due to multiple factors; decreased blood volume and decreased peripheral nervous system input are two of these factors. Generally, patients can also have decreased functional activities; however, this is not a physiologic change.
(Irwin, page 274)
Cardiac, Vascular, & Pulmonary Systems: Differential Diagnosis & Pathology

142. B.

Forward-shoulders posture places the humeral head in an anterior position in the glenoid fossa, putting pressure on the anterior joint capsule. Rotator cuff weakness inhibits the inferior movement of the humeral head during elevation. Scapular weakness or immobility requires greater superior movement of the humeral head to reach overhead. Deltoid weakness does not cause impingement but just causes difficulty maintaining overhead position.
(Magee/Scientific Differential Diagnosis & Pathology, page 59)
Musculoskeletal System: Differential Diagnosis & Pathology

143. C.

This is an example of blocked practice, where tasks are blocked together when practiced.
(Christiansen, page 433)
Teaching & Learning

144. D.

The Peabody Development Motor Scales are a standardized tool used to assess gross and fine motor abilities of children from birth through age 83 months.
(Umphred, page 461)
Nervous System: Evaluation

145. C.

A three-point gait pattern is used when the assistive device is advanced first, followed by the affected lower extremity, and then the unaffected lower extremity.
(Pierson, page 112)
Equipment & Devices

146. D.

Barrel-chested presentation suggests obstructive lung disease and is caused by hyperinflation of the lungs. The sternocleidomastoid and trapezius are secondary muscles of inspiration and can increase in size with prolonged dyspnea. Digital clubbing can indicate cardiopulmonary disease.
(Irwin, page 288)
Cardiac, Vascular, & Pulmonary Systems: Evaluation

147. A.

The stimulus for clonus is rapid dorsiflexion of the ankle. A positive response is prolonged alternating dorsiflexion and plantar flexion of the ankle.
(Rothstein, page 379)
Nervous System: Evaluation

148. C.

In most cases of tuberculosis, the patient can prevent the spread by covering the mouth when coughing. In cases of the patient being unable to do so, a mask can serve as a barrier.
(Deusterhaus, page 105)
Safety, Protection & Professional Roles

149. B.

NSAIDs, when used in combination with antihypertensive medications, may decrease the ability of the antihypertensive to control hypertension. This should alert the physical therapist that the blood pressure may not be as controlled as it should be and that aerobic exercise or high-intensity exercise may need to be monitored or avoided.
(Goodman/Pathology, page 91)
Multi-system: Foundational Sciences & Background

150. A.

As the patient reaches toward the left side, the right lateral trunk musculature must act eccentrically.
(Umphred, page 764)
Nervous System: Treatment Interventions

Section 4

151. C.

There are eight cervical nerves and seven cervical vertebrae, and each nerve exits just below the corresponding vertebra.
(Hoppenfeld/Orthopaedic, page 28)
Musculoskeletal System: Foundational Sciences & Background

152. B.

Objective findings during evaluation are listed in the objective portion of the note. These can include measures, palpation, special tests, observations, and comments on quality or abnormality of motions and functional mobility.
(Kettenbach, page 39)
Safety, Protection & Professional Roles

153. A.

Electrical safety in the clinic should involve yearly maintenance and equipment checks by biomedical staff. Extension cords should never be used in the clinic for patient equipment. Ground fault interrupter outlets are preferred for electrical equipment and are required for whirlpool equipment.
(Behrens, page 156)
Therapeutic Modalities

154. C.

A peptic ulcer can refer pain specifically to the lateral border of the right scapula. The heart and pancreas refer pain to the left shoulder, and the kidneys are associated with low back pain.
(Dutton, page 248)
Gastrointestinal System: Differential Diagnosis & Pathology

155. B.

Hypertonicity can cause muscle imbalances, and impaired motor control can result in joint contractures if not addressed. Pain may also occur.
(Umphred, page 766)
Nervous System: Treatment Interventions

156. D.

The lower lobes are best cleared with the patient in side-lying or prone position with the lower part of the bed raised 18 inches higher than the head of the bed.
(Irwin, page 321)
Cardiac, Vascular, & Pulmonary Systems: Treatment Interventions

157. A.

The anatomical snuffbox can be palpated with thumb abduction just distal to the radial styloid process.
(Hoppenfeld, page 66)
Musculoskeletal System: Evaluation

158. A.

Oral interview is an example of nonexperimental research that permits data collection without rigid control or manipulation of variables.
(Currier, page 117)
Research & Evidence Based Practice

159. C.

By adjusting the mat, you can allow some success for the patient in both sit-to-supine and sit-to-stand. This allows the patient to experience success while learning the movements.
(Umphred, page 17)
Teaching & Learning

160. B.

New scar tissue is bright pink. The physical therapist should be sure to educate the patient on the care of the scar.
(Sussman, page 95)
Integumentary System: Evaluation

161. B.

Crossing the ankles and raising the arms up toward the ceiling helps with independent rolling. The patient can use a rocking motion to initiate the rolling over.
(O'Sullivan, page 968)
Nervous System: Treatment Interventions

162. B.

Patients with spinal stenosis prefer flexion because extension further closes the interspinous foramina.
(Saunders, page 137)
Musculoskeletal System: Differential Diagnosis & Pathology

163. C.

Proper sequence in descending stairs is to place the assistive device on the step below, then the affected leg, then the unaffected leg. This allows the strongest leg to lower the body weight onto the step below.
(Deusterhaus, page 304)
Safety, Protection & Professional Roles

164. D.

Rhabdomyolysis is the destruction of skeletal muscle tissue. Other signs and symptoms include blood in the urine.
(Goodman/Pathology, page 334)
Metabolic & Endocrine System: Treatment Interventions

165. A.
The axillary vessels and nerves are at risk of injury if the patient places pressure in the axilla by using the crutches incorrectly.
(Pierson, page 104)
Equipment & Devices

166. C.
The face has a large representation on the sensory homunculus compared to its actual size.
(Martin, page 12)
Nervous System: Foundational Sciences & Background

167. C.
If a patient's oxygen saturation falls below 88 percent, the administration of supplemental oxygen and/or discontinuation of exercise is indicated.
(Irwin, page 100)
Cardiac, Vascular, & Pulmonary Systems: Treatment Interventions

168. C.
The intervertebral disc swells up to 20 percent at night (during sleep). This can cause increased pain when the patient first sits or stands beside the bed, due to increased intradiscal pressures.
(Braddom, page 892)
Musculoskeletal System: Differential Diagnosis & Pathology

169. A.
A normal distribution results in a bell-shaped curve. This is a graph of frequency distributions.
(Hicks, page 48)
Research & Evidence Based Practice

170. C.
Digital clubbing indicates cardiopulmonary disease or small-bowel disease.
(Irwin, page 288)
Cardiac, Vascular, & Pulmonary Systems: Evaluation

171. D.
A DXA score of –2.0 is indicative of osteopenia, and the patient received this score five years ago. Sharp pain in the thoracic area could indicate a fracture; this is a classic pathology related to osteoporosis.
(Goodman/Pathology, page 879)
Metabolic & Endocrine System: Differential Diagnosis & Pathology

172. D.
To maintain strength gains, the same intensity and duration must be maintained, but the frequency can decrease by one-third of what it was during active training. In this case, the patient went from eight workouts per week to five workouts per week.
(Magee/Scientific Differential Diagnosis & Pathology, page 367)
Musculoskeletal System: Treatment Interventions

173. B.
A 120 lb patient weighs approximately 60 lb below the waist. With the coefficient of friction at 50 percent, 30 lb of force is needed to move the pelvis and legs. To get 40 lb of traction force, the unit must be set at 70 lb. (Calculation: 70 lb traction force applied, minus the 30 lb needed to overcome the coefficient of friction, equals 40 lb of traction force).
(Behrens, page 102)
Therapeutic Modalities

174. C.
Since the spill is an unknown liquid, it should not be cleaned up without proper precautions. If the material is hazardous, it could be dangerous to the person cleaning it up or could cause damage with disposal. Notifying the unit supervisor, who will then notify the hazardous materials team, is the correct plan of action.
(Deusterhaus, page 92)
Safety, Protection & Professional Roles

175. A.
Dizziness getting into and out of bed is indicative of positional vertigo. The Dix-Hallpike test will assess the change in head/body position and its effect on dizziness.
(Umphred, page 634)
Nervous System: Evaluation

176. B.
Facial grimacing, tremors, and shuffling gait are signs associated with tardive dyskinesia. This is a side effect of the drug therapy that is necessary in treating psychotic disorders such as schizophrenia.
(Bonder, page 96)
Multi-system: Differential Diagnosis & Pathology

177. C.

The purpose of the orthoses to treat congenital hip dysplasia is to position the femoral head in the acetabulum. Avascular necrosis is a risk of these orthoses.
(Nawoczenski, page 248)
Equipment & Devices

178. A.

For wounds with large amounts of exudate, the physical therapist should use an absorbent dressing to absorb the exudate. Exudate tends to macerate the peri-wound area.
(Brown, page 37)
Integumentary System: Treatment Interventions

179. C.

Prevention of fractures is key for children with osteogenesis imperfecta.
(Umphred, page 293)
Nervous System: Treatment Interventions

180. C.

The ligamentum flavum is the only one of the lumbar ligaments that runs longitudinally between the vertebrae along the facet and transverse process. The other ligaments do not interfere with the spinal foramina.
(Magee/Orthopedic, page 517)
Musculoskeletal System: Foundational Sciences & Background

181. A.

To calculate the mean of a set of ROM measures, the numbers are added together and then divided by the total number of measures taken, so 85.2° is the mean for this set of measurements.
(Hicks, page 51)
Research & Evidence Based Practice

182. A.

The intrinsic impulse of the heart begins at the SA node, then spreads to the AV node, the bundle of His, and the bundle branches, and it terminates in the Purkinje fibers.
(Irwin, page 29)
Cardiac, Vascular, & Pulmonary Systems: Foundational Sciences & Background

183. A.

Anterior cord syndrome tends to happen with a flexion injury of the cervical vertebral spine. The result is loss of movement, pain, and temperature sensation bilaterally below the level of the injury. Choice B describes Brown-Séquard syndrome. Choice C describes posterior cord syndrome. Choice D describes cauda equina injury.
(Martin, page 385)
Nervous System: Differential Diagnosis & Pathology

184. C.

An AFO uses a three-point pressure system: anterior force at the calf shell; a posterior force on the dorsal surface of the foot, supplied by the shoe; and a superior force from the shoe/orthosis.
(Edelstein, page 39)
Equipment & Devices

185. B.

Blocked practice results in faster acquisition but poorer retention of a skill.
(Christiansen, page 433)
Teaching & Learning

186. C.

Joint mobilizations are contraindicated in patients with osteoporosis due to the risk of fracture. Hypomobility of a joint requires ROM exercise to increase tissue extensibility and muscle length. Isotonic or isometric strengthening exercises tighten down muscle tissue and could add to hypomobility of the joint.
(Kisner, page 156)
Musculoskeletal System: Treatment Interventions

187. C.

In the case of a lawsuit involving a motor vehicle accident, the lawyer and insurance carriers have access to the patient's medical records, as they are relevant to the case. Health-care professionals directly involved in the patient's care also have access. Without the patient's permission, the spouse cannot look at the medical records.
(Gabard, page 64)
Safety, Protection & Professional Roles

188. A.

The tibialis anterior is the primary ankle dorsiflexor that is generally inactive in a steppage gait. Functional electrical stimulation over the tibialis anterior motor point during gait can facilitate ankle dorsiflexion during heel strike and the swing phase.
(Robinson, page 178)
Therapeutic Modalities

189. D.

Due to the multi-joint, bilateral involvement of RA, an assistive device that takes pressure off the painful joints is most appropriate. Both a cane and crutches put pressure through the wrist and hand that may exacerbate symptoms. The wheelchair may decrease the patient's mobility too much and may precipitate deconditioning.
(Goodman/Pathology, page 953)
Multi-system: Differential Diagnosis & Pathology

190. A.

Manual muscle testing should be performed on the entire body. Since the patient has relied so heavily on other body parts to compensate for a weakened extremity, other movements and muscles may have become weak. Care should be taken in positioning the patient and performing the muscle testing to avoid causing the patient pain.
(Umphred, page 580)
Nervous System: Evaluation

191. A.

Exercise has not been shown to improve blood sugar control in type 1 diabetes mellitus. It does assist in weight control and insulin absorption. Blood pressure also decreases with regular exercise.
(Goodman/Pathology, page 354)
Metabolic & Endocrine System: Foundational Sciences & Background

192. C.

During prolonged periods of immobilization, there is an increase in the cross-linking of the fibers of the joint capsule, making it more stiff and tight.
(Magee/Scientific Differential Diagnosis & Pathology, page 35)
Musculoskeletal System: Foundational Sciences & Background

193. C.

The theory of reasoned action emphasizes that behavior is related to attitudes toward the behavior itself and the motivation to comply with influential people.
(Bestable, page 177)
Teaching & Learning

194. B.

Broca's aphasia is an expressive aphasia. Patients have difficulty expressing themselves even though they know what to say. A patient with Broca's aphasia is able to comprehend the written and spoken word.
(Rothstein, page 441)
Nervous System: Evaluation

195. D.

In most cases of tuberculosis, the patient can prevent the spread of the disease by covering the mouth when coughing. In cases of the patient being unable to do so, a mask can serve as a barrier.
(Deusterhaus, page 105)
Safety, Protection & Professional Roles

196. C.

Hemoglobin levels under 10 g/mL related to concurrent chemotherapy indicate caution should be used with aerobic exercise.
(Goodman/Pathology, page 259)
Multi-system: Foundational Sciences & Background

197. B.

Asymmetric tonic neck reflex occurs with rotation of the head and results in extension of the ipsilateral extremities and flexion of the contralateral extremities. This reflex is normally present from birth to approximately age four to six months.
(Martin, page 133)
Nervous System: Evaluation

198. D.

Chronic bronchitis is defined as a productive cough on most days for three consecutive months of a year for at least two consecutive years. The cough starts gradually but progresses to nearly constant productive coughing.
(Irwin, page 150)
Cardiac, Vascular, & Pulmonary Systems: Differential Diagnosis & Pathology

199. D.

Tenderness over McBurney's point is indicative of appendicitis. McBurney's point is halfway between the ASIS and the umbilicus on the right side of the lower abdomen.
(Goodman/Pathology, page 662)
Gastrointestinal System: Differential Diagnosis & Pathology

200. A.

Patients with Parkinson's disease typically demonstrate cogwheel rigidity, intention tremor, bradykinesia or akinesia, and impaired posture.
(Umphred, page 671)
Nervous System: Differential Diagnosis & Pathology

Section 5

201. B.

Weight-bearing activity by a young female athlete without menstruation puts her at greater risk for osteoporotic changes and increased risk for fracture.
(Goodman/Pathology, page 882)
Metabolic & Endocrine System: Differential Diagnosis & Pathology

202. D.

In treating tendinopathies, active loading should be avoided until there is no pain at rest.
(Magee/Scientific Differential Diagnosis & Pathology, page 69)
Musculoskeletal System: Treatment Interventions

203. A.

If the monitor is too high or low it causes increased neck flexion or extension to see the monitor, which can then cause neck pain and further poor posture positions.
(Saunders, page 372)
Safety, Protection & Professional Roles

204. A.

Continuous ultrasound is used for its thermal effects. These include increased tissue temperature and increased tissue extensibility. The most appropriate time to use ultrasound is right before tissue stretching. It is also thought that ultrasound and ice actually have opposite effects, so should not be used immediately after one another.
(Behrens, page 67)
Therapeutic Modalities

205. B.

Direct observation involves the researcher observing the subject but not interacting with the subject. Indirect observation is observation of subjects without the subjects' knowledge. Participant observation involves interaction between the researcher and subject.
(Bork, page 97)
Research & Evidence Based Practice

206. C.

Since walking is a closed-chain activity, a closed-chain exercise is most appropriate. Lunges incorporate the weight acceptance of a load onto the heel of one leg similar to walking.
(Magee/Scientific Differential Diagnosis & Pathology, page 456)
Musculoskeletal System: Treatment Interventions

207. D.

Brown-Séquard syndrome affects half of the spinal cord and results in loss of motor, proprioception, and vibration sensation ipsilaterally. Pain and temperature sensation are lost on the contralateral side a few segments below the lesion.
(Martin, page 384)
Nervous System: Differential Diagnosis & Pathology

208. C.

The goals of diaphragmatic breathing are to decrease dyspnea, decrease the work of respiration, decrease secondary muscle activity, and decrease the respiratory rate.
(Irwin, page 310)
Cardiac, Vascular, & Pulmonary Systems: Treatment Interventions

209. B.

Explicit knowledge is knowledge of information that can be named and recited (or declared). Explicit knowledge and declarative knowledge have the same meaning.
(Christiansen, page 430)
Teaching & Learning

210. A.

To best assess shoulder rotation range of motion without substitution, the supine position is preferred. In supine, the scapula is stabilized. Once in that position, internal and external rotation are best assessed at 90 degrees of abduction for the most "pure" rotation motion.
(Magee/Orthopedic, page 260)
Musculoskeletal System: Evaluation

211. B.

The gate control theory proposed by Melzack and Wall says that the patient's perception of pain is dependent on the excitatory and inhibitory effects on the transmission of the signal to the brain. The theory proposes that electrical stimulation can close the "gate" to prevent the relay of the pain sensation.
(Behrens, page 12)
Therapeutic Modalities

212. B.

Pain or difficulty with urination should always elicit the thought that a urinary tract infection (UTI) may be the culprit for any back or flank pain. Further musculoskeletal testing can rule out other pathology, and physician referral for labs can confirm a UTI.
(Goodman/Clin Med, page 548)
Genitourinary System: Differential Diagnosis & Pathology

213. D.

Peripheral blood vessels are constricted, which results in shunting heat to the body's core and a decrease in skin temperature.
(McArdle, page 549)
Integumentary System: Foundational Sciences & Background

214. C.

Impaired sensation is a contraindication to the use of ice immersion of a body part.
(Stokes, page 400)
Nervous System: Treatment Interventions

215. C.

Symptoms of an acute myocardial infarction include severe chest pain, pressure, or heaviness, which may extend to the jaw, neck, upper extremities, and upper back. Other signs and symptoms are nausea and vomiting, diaphoresis, dyspnea, lightheadedness, and weakness. Many myocardial infarctions, however, are asymptomatic.
(Irwin, page 136)
Cardiac, Vascular, & Pulmonary Systems: Differential Diagnosis & Pathology

216. D.

A one-arm-drive wheelchair allows for independence with manual propulsion by using one upper and one lower extremity. A reclining-back wheelchair is not needed for someone who is medically stable with good trunk control. A rigid frame and power mobility are not ideal for folding the wheelchair to place it in the car.
(Pierson, page 150)
Equipment & Devices

217. B.

Sacroiliac pathologies are most painful with transitional movements that cause shearing to the joint. Such movements as getting up from a chair, rolling over in bed, and walking are most irritating to the back.
(Saunders, page 162)
Musculoskeletal System: Differential Diagnosis & Pathology

218. A.

Any piece of electrical equipment that may purposefully come into contact with water should be plugged into a ground-fault interrupter (GFI) plate. This prevents injury or death from electric shock by shutting off the circuit.
(Behrens, page 156)
Safety, Protection & Professional Roles

219. B.

The black lead is the negative electrode and should be used to drive the negatively charged dexamethasone into the desired area.
(Michlovitz, page 117)
Therapeutic Modalities

220. A.

Inflammatory bowel disease (IBD) can be preceded by multi-joint arthritic pain. The arthralgia can present before the IBD or during exacerbations of IBD. Pain in the lower intestines can refer to the lower right quadrant or to the hip or knee. If the patient is not aware of IBD, some questions on family history and bowel function may indicate the need for physician referral.
(Goodman/Pathology, page 649)
Gastrointestinal System: Differential Diagnosis & Pathology

221. B.

Progressive resistance exercise using the joints of bones affected by osteoporosis can decrease the progression of the disease. Exercise does not stop the progression altogether but can hinder it.
(Magee/Scientific Differential Diagnosis & Pathology, page 347)
Musculoskeletal System: Foundational Sciences & Background

222. B.

The prosthesis is too long.
(Seymour, page 231)
Equipment & Devices

223. C.

A pink or red color indicates viable tissue.
(Sussman, page 199)
Integumentary System: Treatment Interventions

224. C.

Decorticate rigidity results in general upper-extremity flexion and lower-extremity extension. Decerebrate rigidity results in upper- and lower-extremity extension.
(Umphred, page 418)
Nervous System: Differential Diagnosis & Pathology

225. C.

Atelectasis is the condition that results in the collapse of alveoli and an abnormal volume of lung tissue for gas exchange.
(Irwin, page 173)
Cardiac, Vascular, & Pulmonary Systems: Differential Diagnosis & Pathology

226. D.

There is no muscle, vessel, or connective tissue that runs continuously from the neck to the foot. The only tissue that has origin in the neck and runs to the foot is neural tissue—the spinal cord and peripheral nerves.
(Magee/Orthopedic, page 497)
Musculoskeletal System: Evaluation

227. C.

Inhibiting C-fiber action potentials is accomplished through the endogenous opioid theory of pain management. A frequency of 1–5 pps is most appropriate for reaching this goal.
(Behrens, page 216)
Therapeutic Modalities

228. B.

Insulin injection sites should be away from the muscle that is exercising.
(Goodman/Pathology, page 356)
Metabolic & Endocrine System: Differential Diagnosis & Pathology

229. B.

The objective portion of the initial assessment lists things that can be measured, observed, or palpated by the physical therapist. The other choices are all subjective in nature or are future plans.
(Shamus, page 35)
Safety, Protection & Professional Roles

230. D.

During pregnancy, exercise in the supine position for longer than three minutes should be avoided. Also, any exercise in which the pelvis is above the head such as in a "fire hydrant." can be potential for an air embolus. The safest position of the choices is in side-lying with controlled hip abduction.
(Stephenson, page 129)
Multi-system: Differential Diagnosis & Pathology

231. A.

A soft end feel at the end of knee flexion is soft-tissue approximation of muscle. Patellar tendon tension would give a tissue-stretch end feel, meniscus obstruction would give a springy end feel, and bony contact would give a hard end feel. The latter two would be abnormal end feels in the knee.
(Magee/Orthopedic, page 31)
Musculoskeletal System: Evaluation

232. B.

This man is contemplating a health behavior change. He has not yet made a decision or started the change.
(Davis, page 195)
Teaching & Learning

233. D.

A walker with a platform attachment allows for weight-bearing through the elbow and forearm without weight-bearing on the wrist.
(Pierson, page 105)
Equipment & Devices

234. C.

The first response should be to check for the source of the noxious stimulus. Autonomic dysreflexia is an emergency situation. If the painful stimulus cannot be identified, methods to decrease the patient's blood pressure—such as standing the patient up or applying a nitroglycerin patch—should be used. Finally, the patient's physician should be notified.
(Martin, page 386)
Nervous System: Treatment Interventions

235. A.

The chest wall normally moves upward and outward in the upper portion (like a pump-handle) and the downward motion of the diaphragm compresses the abdominal viscera.
(Irwin, page 297)
Cardiac, Vascular, & Pulmonary Systems: Evaluation

236. B.

Antipsychotic medications can cause pyramidal effects and movement disorders during use.
(Goodman/Pathology, page 57)
Multi-system: Foundational Sciences & Background

237. B.

Compression of the sacroiliac joint, causing improvement in muscle strength and decreased pain, indicates that the patient is in need of stabilization. Strengthening of the muscles that compress the sacroiliac joint will provide added stability.
(Hall, page 360)
Musculoskeletal: Treatment Interventions

238. B.

Test-retest reliability is the degree to which scores agree after repeated administration of the test under stable conditions.
(Cole, pages 28 and 39)
Research & Evidence Based Practice

239. D.

The therapist is assessing gross motor milestones of the developmental sequence.
(Farber, page 110)
Nervous System: Evaluation

240. D.

The use of heat on muscles actually reduces muscular strength and endurance. Heat is useful in increasing tissue extensibility prior to stretching or range of motion exercise.
(Behrens, page 42)
Therapeutic Modalities

241. B.

When a patient stops taking his medication for a psychotic disorder, he may become more passive and withdrawn and may easily become agitated.
(Goodman/Pathology, page 57)
Multi-system: Differential Diagnosis & Pathology

242. A.

Two joint muscles are at greater risk of injury because of movement at both ends of the muscle. Combined joint motions of the two-joint muscle can put excessive strain on these muscles. Of these, the biceps is the only two-joint muscle listed here.
(Magee/Scientific Differential Diagnosis & Pathology, page 446)
Musculoskeletal System: Treatment Interventions

243. A.

Slow rocking is one technique that can be used to encourage relaxation and decrease rigidity. After rigidity is decreased, mobility can be addressed.
(Umphred, page 675)
Nervous System: Treatment Interventions

244. D.

Over 50 percent of lower-extremity amputations are performed on diabetic patients and are preceded by a foot ulcer.
(Brown, page 179)
Integumentary System: Differential Diagnosis & Pathology

245. D.

The Glasgow Coma Scale is used to rate the severity of coma. A score of less than 8 indicates that the person is in a coma and has had a severe brain injury.
(Umphred, page 422)
Nervous System: Evaluation

246. A.

Dilantin is an antiseizure medication.
(Mosby, page 816)
Nervous System: Foundational Sciences & Background

247. A.

Vital Capacity = Tidal Volume + Inspiratory Reserve Volume + Expiratory Reserve Volume, or VC = TV + IRV + ERV. So:
VC = 0.5 + 3.5 + 1.0
VC = 5.0 L
(Irwin, page 45)
Cardiac, Vascular, & Pulmonary Systems: Foundational Sciences & Background

248. B.

Cryotherapy actually elevates the pain threshold by stimulating A-beta and C fiber. Decreasing muscle spindle activity helps to reduce muscle spasm.
(Behrens, page 49)
Therapeutic Modalities

249. B.

The population is the entire group of individuals who possess the researched characteristic. In this case, the researcher is looking at females with arthritis.
(Hicks, page 25)
Research & Evidence Based Practice

250. A.

The internal carotid artery splits into the anterior cerebral and middle cerebral arteries. These supply the blood to the majority of the cerebrum.
(Martin, page 25)
Nervous System: Foundational Sciences & Background

References

1. American Academy of Orthopedic Surgeons. *Joint Motion: Method of Measuring and Recording.* AAOS, Chicago. 1965.
2. American Physical Therapy Association. *Guide to Physical Therapist Practice, revised 2nd Edition.* Phys Therap. 2003.
3. Bailey Dina M. *Research for the Health Professional: A Practical Guide.* F.A. Davis Company, Philadelphia. 1991.
4. Baranoski S and Ayello E. *Wound Care Essentials: Practice Principles.* Lippincott Williams & Wilkins, Philadelphia. 2004.
5. Bastable, Susan. *Nurse as Educator: Principles of Teaching and Learning for Nursing Practice.* Jones & Bartlett Publishers, Inc., Sudbury, MA. 2003.
6. Behrens BJ and Michlovitz SL. Physical Agents Theory and Practice 2nd Ed. FA Davis Company, Philadelphia. 2006.
7. Bly L and Whiteside A. *Facilitation Techniques based on NDT Principles.* Therapy Skill Builders, San Antonio, TX. 1999.
8. Boissonnault WG. *Examination in Physical Therapy Practice, 2nd Edition.* Churchill Livingstone, New York, 1995.
9. Bork Christopher (Ed.). *Research in Physical Therapy.* J.B. Lippincott Company, Philadelphia, PA. 1993.
10. Brown DE and Neumann, RD. *Orthopedic Secrets, 2nd Ed.* Hanley & Belfus, Philadephia. 1999.
11. Brown P and Maloy J. *Quick Reference to Wound Care, Second Edition.* Jones and Bartlett Publishers, Sudbury, MA. 2005.
12. Burr HS, Taffel M, Harvey WC. An Electrometric Study of Wound Healing in Man. *Yale Journal of Biologic Medicine.* 1940; 12;483.
13. Campbell Suzann. *Decision Making in Pediatric Neurologic Physical Therapy.* Churchill Livingston, Philadelphia, PA. 1999.
14. Chastain P. The effect of deep heat on isometric strength. *Physical Therapy.* 1978; 58: 543.
15. Christiansen C, Baum C, and Bass-Haugen J (Eds.). *Occupational Therapy: Performance, Participation, and Well-being, Third Edition.* Slack Incorporated, Thorofare, NJ. 2005.
16. Ciccone CD. *Pharmacology in Rehabilitation, 3rd Edition.* Perspectives in Rehabilitation, 2002.
17. Cole B, Finch E, Gowland C, and Mayo N. *Physical Rehabilitation Outcome Measures.* Canadian Physiotherapy Association, Canada. 1994.
18. Currier Dean. *Elements of Research in Physical Therapy.* Williams & Wilkins, Baltimore, MD. 1990.
19. Curtis Kathleen. *Physical Therapy Professional Foundations: Keys to Success in School and Career.* Slack Incorporated, Thorofare, NJ. 2002.
20. Davis Carol. *Patient Practitioner Interaction: An Experiential Manual for Developing the Art of Healthcare Fourth Edition.* Slack Incorporated, Thorofare, NJ. 2006.
21. DeTurk W and Cahalin L. *Cardiovascular and Pulmonary Physical Therapy, AN Evidenced-based Approach.* McGraw-Hill Companies, Incorporated, New York. 2004.
22. Dirckx John. *Stedman's Concise Medical Dictionary for the Health Professions, Third Edition.* Williams & Wilkins, Baltimore, MD. 1997.
23. Domholdt Elizabeth. *Rehabilitation Research: Principles and Applications.* Elsevier Saunders, St. Louis. 2005.
24. Duesterhaus Minor MA and Duesterhaus Minor S. *Patient Care Skills, 2nd Ed.* Appleton & Lange, East Norwalk, CT. 1990.
25. Edelstein J and Bruckner J. *Orthotics: A Comprehensive Clinical Approach.* SLACK Incorporated, Thorofare, NJ. 2002.
26. Edwards H, et al. Effect of temperature on muscle energy metabolism and endurance during successive isomtric contractions, sustained to fatigue, of the quadriceps muscle in man. *Journal of Physiology.* 1972; 220:335.
27. Frownfelter D and Dean E. *Cardiovascular and Pulmonary Physical Therapy: Evidence and Practice, Fourth Edition.* Mosby Elsevier, St. Louis. 2006.

28. Glickstein J. *Therapeutic Interventions in Alzheimer's Disease, Second Edition.* Aspen Publishers, Inc, Gaithersburg, MD. 1997.
29. Goldberg Stephen. *Clinical Neuroanatomy made ridiculously simple.* MedMaster, Miami. 1995.
30. Goodman CC and Snyder TEK. *Differential Diagnosis for Physical Therapists: Screening for Referral.* Saunders, St.Louis, 2007.
31. Goodman CC, Fuller KS and Boissonnault WG. *Pathology: Implications for the Physical Therapist.* Saunders, Philadephia, 2007.
32. Hanumadass M and Ramakrishnan K. *The Art and Science of Burn Wound Management.* Anshan Ltd., Kent, UK. 2005.
33. Hecox B, Mehreteab TA, Weisberg J, Sanko J. Integrating Physical Agents in Rehabilitation, 2nd Ed. Pearson Prentice Hall, Upper Saddle River NJ. 2006.
34. Helewa A and Walker J. *Critical Evaluation of Research in Physical Rehabilitation Towards Evidence-Based Practice.* W.B. Saunders Company, Philadelphia. 2000.
35. Henderson JM. Ruling out danger: Differential diagnosis of thoracic spine. *Phys. Sportsmed.* 20:124-132, 1992.
36. Hicks Carolyn. *Research Methods for Clinical Therapists: Applied Project Design and Analysis.* Churchill Livingstone, Edinburgh 2004.
37. Hillegass EA and Sadowsky HS. *Essentials of Cardiopulmonary Physical Therapy Second Edition.* W.B. Saunders Company, Philadelphia. 2001.
38. Hislop HJ and Montgomer J. *Daniels and Worthingham's Muscle Testing, 6th Ed.* WB Saunders Company, Philadelphia. 1995.
39. Hoppenfeld S. *Physical Examination of the Spine & Extremities.* Appleton-Century-Crofts, Norwalk, CT. 1976.
40. Horve-Willoughby Christine. *Aquatic Therapy: Effective Strategies for Patient Care.* Cross Country University. 2003.
41. Irwin S and Tecklin J. *Cardiopulmonary Physical Therapy: A Guide to Practice, Fourth Edition.* Mosby, St. Louis. 2004.
42. Kandel ER, Schwartz JH, and Jessell TM (Eds.). *Principles of Neural Science, Third Edition.* Elsevier, New York. 1991.
43. Karacoloff L, Hammersley C, and Schneider F. (Eds.). *Lower Extremity Amputation: A Guide to Functional Outcomes in Physical Therapy Management, Second Edition.* Aspen Publishers, Inc., Gaithersburg, MD. 1992.
44. Kettenbach Ginge. *Writing SOAP Notes, Second Edition.* F.A. Davis Company, Philadelphia. 1995.
45. Kisner C and Colby LA. *Therapeutic Exercise: Foundations and Techniques, 2nd Ed.* FA Davis Company, Philadelphia. 1985.
46. Kloth LC, McCulloch JM, Feedar JA. *Wound Healing: Alternatives in Management.* F.A. Davis Company, Philadelphia. 1990.
47. Lewis C and Bottomley J. *Geriatric Rehabilitation: A Clinical Approach, Third Edition.* Appleton & Lange, Norwalk, CT. 2008.
48. Lusardi M, and Nielsen C. *Orthotics and Prosthetics in Rehabilitation, Second Edition.* Saunders Elsevier Inc., St. Louis. 2007.
49. Luttgens K, Deutsch H, and Hamilton N. *Kinesiology: Scientific Basis of Human Motion, 8th Ed.* Brown & Benchmark Publishers, Madison, WI. 1992.
50. Magee David. *Orthopedic Physical Assessment Third Edition.* W.B. Saunders Company, Philadelphia. 1997.
51. Magee DJ, Zachazewski JE, and Quillen WS. *Scientific Foundations and Principles of Practice in Musculoskeletal Rehabilitation.* Saunders-Elsevier, St. Louis. 2007.
52. Magec DJ. *Orthopedic Physical Assessment, 4th Edition.* Elsevier, Philadelphia. 2002.
53. Maitland GD. *Peripheral manipulation, 2nd Edition.* Butterworth, Boston. 1977.
54. Maitland GD. *Vertebral Manipulation.* Butterworths, London. 1973.
55. Martin S, and Kessler M. *Neurologic Interventions for Physical Therapy, Second Edition.* Saunders Elsevier Inc., St. Louis. 2007.
56. McArdle W, Katch F, and Katch V. *Exercise Physiology: Energy, Nutrition, and Human Performance, Third Edition.* Lea & Febiger, Philadelphia. 1991.
57. Melzack R and Wall PD. Pain Mechanisms: A New Theory. *Science.* 150:971, 1965.
58. Michlovitz SL and Nolan TP. Modalities for Therapeutic Intervention, 4th ED. FA Davis Company, Philadelphia. 2005.
59. Moffat Marilyn (Ed). *Integumentary Essentials, Applying the Preferred Physical Therapist Practice Patterns.* SLACK Incorporated, Thorofare, NJ. 2006.
60. Montgomery Jacqueline (Ed.). *Physical Therapy for Traumatic Brain Injury.* Churchill Livingstone Inc., New York. 1995.

61. Nawoczenski D, & Epler M. *Orthotics in Functional Rehabilitation of the Lower Limb.* W.B. Saunders Company, Philadelphia. 1997.
62. Norkin CC and Levangie PK. *Joint Structure & Function, 2nd Ed.* FA Davis Company, Philadelphia. 1992.
63. Norkin CC and White DJ. *Measurement of Joint Motion: A Guide to Goniometry, 2nd Ed.* FA Davis, Philadelphia. 1995.
64. O'Sullivan S and Schmitz T. *Physical Rehabilitation, Fifth Edition.* F.A. Davis Company, Philadelphia. 2007.
65. Palmer S, Kriegsman K, and Palmer J. *Spinal Cord Injury: A Guide for Living,* Johns Hopkins Press Health Book. Johns Hopkins University Press, Baltimore. 2000.
66. Pierson F. *Principles and Techniques of Patient Care.* W.B. Saunders Company, Philadelphia. 1994.
67. Prentice WE. Therapeutic Modalities for Physical Therapists, 2nd Ed. McGraw-Hill, New York, NY. 2002.
68. Pryor J and Prasad SA (Eds). *Physiotherapy for Respiratory & Cardiac Problems: Adults and Paediatrics, Third Edition.* Churchill Livingstone, Edinburgh. 2002.
69. Robinson AJ and Snyder-Mackler L. Clinical Electrophysiology: Electrotherapy & Electrophysiologic testing, 2nd Ed. Williams & Wilkins, Baltimore. 1995.
70. Rothstein JM, Roy SH, and Wolf SL. *The Rehabilitation Specialist's Handbook, Second Edition.* F.A. Davis Company, Philadelphia. 1998.
71. Saunders HD and Saunders R. *Evaluation, Treatment and Prevention of Musculoskeletal Disorders.* The Saunders Group, Chaska, MN. 1993.
72. Serup J, Jemec G and Grove G (Eds.). *Handbook of Non-Invasive Methods and the Skin, Second Edition.* CRC Press, Taylor & Francis Group, Boca Raton, FL. 2006.
73. Stokes M Editor. *Physical Management in Neurological Rehabilitation, Second Edition.* Elsevier Mosby, Edinburgh. 2004.
74. Sussman C and Bates-Jensen B (Eds.). *Wound Care, A Collaborative Practice Manual for Physical Therapists and Nurses, Second Edition.* Aspen Publishers, Inc., Gaithersburg, MD. 2001.
75. Thibodeau GA and Patton KT. *Structure & Function of the Body, Thirteenth Edition.* Mosby Elsevier, St. Louis, MO. 2008.
76. Thibodeau GA and Patton KT. *Structure & Function of the Body, 13th Edition.* Mosby Elsevier, St. Louis, 2008.
77. Tierney LM, McPhee SJ, and Papadakis MA. *Current Medical Diagnosis & Treatment 37th Edition.* Appleton & Lange, Stamford, CT. 1998.
78. Voss D, Ionta M, and Myers B. *Proprioceptive neuromuscular Facilitation Patterns and Techniques, Third edition.* Harper & Row, Publishers, Inc., Philadelphia. 1985.
79. Wilson Angela. *Strategies & Interventions for Skin & Wound Management.* PESI, LLC, Eau Claire, WI. 2006.
80. Yanagisawa O, Miyanaga Y, Shiraki H, et al. The effects of various therapeutic measures on shoulder range of motion and cross-sectional areas of rotator cuff muscles after baseball pitching. *Journal of Sports Medicine and Physical Fitness.* 2003;43: 356-366.
81. www.acsm.org
82. www.cancer.org
83. www.cdc.gov

About the Authors

Bethany Chapman received a bachelor's degree in Biology and Athletic Training from the University of Northern Iowa, and a master's degree in Physical Therapy from the University of Iowa. She practiced as a physical therapist for 8 years before taking on her current position at an outpatient physical therapy clinic. She also teaches Anatomy & Physiology for Kaplan University online.

Mary Fratianni received a bachelor's degree in Exercise Science and master's of Physical Therapy from the University of Iowa. She currently is the rehabilitation director of Mill-Pond Retirement Community in Ankeny, Iowa and teaches physical therapy courses for Kaplan University online. She resides in West Des Moines with her husband and two young sons.

NOTES